## DEATH AND COMPASSION

Is compassion an appropriate motive for ending life?
Can euthanasia ever be justified as an act of benevolence?
Can euthanasia allow a person to die with dignity?

*Death and Compassion* offers a systematic exploration of the role of the virtues within medical ethics and practice – presenting a critique of principle-based ethical systems within the context of modern medicine. Focusing specifically on terminal care and the ethical problems surrounding euthanasia, and drawing on Aristotle's teleological account of the virtues, the author develops an argument in favour of a systematic incorporation of the virtues of compassion, benevolence and respectfulness in medical practice – transcending the shortcomings of principles of beneficence, non-maleficence and respect for patient autonomy.

By presenting new ways of conceptualising and reasoning about ethical issues such as the termination of life-support, physician-assisted suicide and euthanasia, *Death and Compassion* offers new insights for a radical rethink of the dominant mode of thinking in contemporary bioethics and the practice of modern medicine.

Liezl van Zyl is a lecturer in the Department of Philosophy at the University of Waikato, New Zealand.

# ASHGATE STUDIES IN APPLIED ETHICS

Scandals in medical research and practice; physicians unsure how to manage new powers to postpone death and reshape life; business people operating in a world with few borders; unprofessional conduct in scientific research; damage to the environment; concern regarding the welfare of animals - all have prompted an international demand for ethical standards which go beyond matters of personal taste and opinion.

The *Ashgate Studies in Applied Ethics* series presents leading international research on the most topical areas of applied and professional ethics, recognizing that the revival of interest in applied ethics is a return to an important role for philosophers: a concern with justice and good conduct in all spheres of life. Focusing particularly on professional, business, environmental, medical and bio-ethics, the series draws from many diverse interdisciplinary perspectives including: philosophical, historical, legal, medical, environmental and sociological. Exploring the intersection of theory and practice, books in this series will prove of particular value to researchers, students, and practitioners worldwide.

# Death and Compassion

## A virtue-based approach to euthanasia

LIEZL VAN ZYL
*University of Waikato, New Zealand*

**Ashgate**
Aldershot • Burlington USA • Singapore • Sydney

Published by
Ashgate Publishing Ltd
Gower House
Croft Road
Aldershot
Hants GU11 3HR
England

Ashgate Publishing Company
131 Main Street
Burlington, VT 05401-5600 USA

Ashgate website: http://www.ashgate.com

**British Library Cataloguing in Publication Data**
Van Zyl, Liezl
Death and compassion : a virtue-based approach to euthanasia. - (Ashgate studies in applied ethics)
1. Euthanasia - Moral and ethical aspects
I. Title
179.7

**Library of Congress Cataloging-in-Publication Data**
Van Zyl, Liezl L.
Death and compassion : a virtue-based approach to euthanasia / Liezl van Zyl.
p.cm.
Includes bibliographical references and index.
ISBN 0-7546-1231-7
1. Euthanasia--Moral and ethical aspects. 2. Assisted suicide--Moral and ethical aspects. 3. Terminal care--Moral and ethical aspects. I. Title.

R726.V36 2000
179.7--dc21

00-044142

ISBN 0 7546 1231 7

Printed in Great Britain by
Antony Rowe Ltd, Chippenham, Wiltshire

*To Paul*

# Contents

# Summary


The aim of this book is to provide a critique of principle-based ethical systems within the context of modern medicine, focusing specifically on end-of-life decisions. In an attempt to transcend the shortcomings of principles as they operate within both utilitarian and deontological ethical theories, I argue for an incorporation of the virtues in medical practice, drawing from and developing Aristotle's teleological account of the virtues.

Since Greek antiquity to the present, scientific knowledge and technological skills have undergone significant advances, completely transforming the role of medicine. Medical practice shifted from being an art or craft to an endeavour requiring vast and sophisticated technical competence and scientific knowledge. These changes are paralleled by a shift in the framework within which ethical issues are raised and addressed. Ethical thinking, once grounded in the virtues and centred in the character and dispositions of the moral agent, came to be anchored in rules and principles of right action.

The shortcomings of a principle-based ethic are identified and discussed, using the problems surrounding euthanasia as a vehicle for radically rethinking the dominant mode of thinking in contemporary bioethics. Three pertinent questions concerning the morality of euthanasia are raised, each invoking a typical feature of human suffering, which leads to an analysis of a moral virtue that addresses each of these features of suffering.

The first question is whether euthanasia or 'mercy-killing' can ever be seen as an expression of compassion or love. As an alternative to the impersonality of a principle-based ethic and its rejection of compassion as an appropriate moral motivation, I develop an Aristotelian account of compassion as a response to suffering as solitude.

The second question concerns the ends or goals of medicine, namely whether the prolongation of life is always beneficial, and whether the termination of life can ever be seen as an act of benevolence, that is, as allowing someone to die a 'good death'. In light of a critique of the notions of harm and benefit in Western medicine and of universal principles and rules of beneficence and non-maleficence as they operate within deontological and utilitarian theories, I develop an account of 'responsible benevolence' that is sensitive to particular circumstances, and a response to suffering as helplessness and dependence.

Third, the question arises whether euthanasia can ever be seen as showing respect for a person, allowing that person to 'die with dignity'. In the light of the shortcomings of the principle of respect for patient autonomy and the notion of informed consent, I develop a teleological account of the virtue of respectfulness that allows a more satisfactory response to suffering as loss of self-respect.

Finally, suffering as despair introduces the re-examination of the problems of euthanasia in terms of the virtues of compassion, benevolence and respectfulness, demonstrating how an Aristotelian theory of the virtues constitutes a more satisfactory approach to these problems through judging by criteria responsive to an individual, existential situation, rather than criteria that consider individual cases as instances for the application of universal and impersonal principles and duties.

# Acknowledgements

I am grateful to Janine Neustroski and Jay Corwin for their help in proofreading the manuscript; Anton van Niekerk, Willie Esterhuyse and Willem Landman for their comments on a previous version of this text; and the University of Waikato, the Centre for Science Development and the University of Stellenbosch for financial assistance. In particular, I would like to thank Paul Flood for his invaluable help in proofreading and formatting the manuscript, for his critical comments and suggestions, and for his general love and support throughout this project.

Hamilton, New Zealand
March 2000

# Introduction

## Medicine and Euthanasia

W.H.S. Jones begins his introduction to one of the most well-known Hippocratic treatises as follows: 'The little treatise called *The Art* has as its object to prove that there is such a thing as an art of medicine' (1923, vol. II:186). All but the most sceptical of modern readers would find this a very strange pursuit – medicine has long proved itself to be a respectable discipline. Yet the writer of *The Art* seems to take the charges brought against the art of medicine very seriously, developing his defence in a rigorous and systematic fashion, reminiscent of the style of the pre-Socratic philosophers. One of the charges brought against the Hippocratic physician was that cures were merely a matter of luck, since some patients recovered without medical help while others died despite being treated by a physician. The refusal by many physicians to treat terminally-ill patients was taken as further proof that physicians were aware of their own lack of power in the face of disease. The prevailing view amongst critics was that disease was caused by the gods, and could therefore only be cured by them. By contrast, Hippocratic physicians rejected metaphysical explanations of illness as divine punishment. Disease, they believed, was caused by an imbalance in the natural constituents of the human body, and was usually corrected by nature. Man could assist this process if he understood the workings of nature. The writer of *The Art* argues that what appears to be a spontaneous or miraculous cure is actually nature's way of correcting an imbalance, and added that this process would occur much faster with the help of a physician. Yet he does not make any attempt to deny the limitations of medicine. The physician's task is a modest one, namely to act as nature's assistant. The art of medicine consists not only of relieving suffering caused by disease, but also of refusing to treat incurable disorders. To undertake desperate cases is a sign of incompetence: It indicates a failure to realise that the illness is stronger than the means at the disposal of medicine. In the same way that Socrates's wisdom was based on an awareness of his own ignorance, a wise physician recognises the limits of his art:

> For if a man demand from an art a power over what does not belong to the art, or from nature a power over what does not belong to nature, his ignorance is more allied to madness than to lack of knowledge.... Whenever therefore a man suffers from an ill which is too strong for the means at the disposal of medicine, he surely must not even expect that it can be overcome by medicine (*The Art* VIII).

Today such prudent modesty is rare amongst physicians. Medical science and technology have undergone tremendous progress, allowing far greater accuracy in diagnosis and success in treatment. Since many conditions previously thought desperate can now be cured, a physician who fails to do so can be charged with incompetence or negligence. Increasingly, however, and in stark contrast to previous eras, it is the very ability and commitment of medical professionals to prolong human life that lies at the basis of sceptical attitudes towards medical progress. It is often pointed out that developments in medical technology have made it possible to sustain life almost indefinitely, but that methods of pain management have lagged behind. This has given rise to a number of moral questions not encountered before, or not encountered with such urgency: 'Should human life be maintained for as long as possible?', 'When, if ever, is withdrawal of life-sustaining treatment morally justifiable?', and 'Is it ever permissible to end human life as quickly and painlessly as possible?'

Over the last few decades the moral acceptability of euthanasia has become one of the most widely debated issues in medical ethics. The changes that have occurred in the meaning and use of the term 'euthanasia' suggest that its emergence as a central moral issue is relatively recent. The word 'euthanasia' was coined in the seventeenth century from the Greek *eu thanatos*, literally, 'a good death', and was commonly used to describe the nature of the *dying process* a person or institution undergoes. For example, euthanasia could refer to a gentle and easy death (as opposed to a violent, painful or torturous death) or a heroic death (as opposed to a cowardly death). It is only at the end of the nineteenth century, with the publication of an essay by Dr. S.D. Williams in 1872, that the term came to be used in the modern sense of the *act* of painlessly putting to death those suffering from terminal conditions. Williams argued that it would be the highest triumph of the physician to take care of the needs and desires of a dying human being by affecting euthanasia, but very few of his colleagues agreed. The vast majority of physicians saw euthanasia as a form of 'professional murder', often supporting their position with reference to the Hippocratic injunction against administering deadly drugs to patients. The issue was laid to rest, for the most part, until the 1960s, when advances in medical technology made it possible to prolong the lives of many patients who had no hope of recovery. It was at this time that the distinction was drawn between 'active' and 'passive' euthanasia, giving rise to the question of whether there is a morally significant difference between allowing a person to die by withholding or withdrawing treatment (passive euthanasia) and killing someone by administering a lethal injection (active euthanasia).

The changing connotation of the term 'euthanasia' suggests that its appearance as a central moral issue in medicine is linked to developments in biotechnology, together with the over-zealous efforts of physicians who refuse to admit defeat. Some critics cite the discrepancy between the development of life-prolonging technologies and methods of pain management as the main cause of appeals to legalise euthanasia. Others blame the dehumanising effects of modern technology. For instance, in an essay entitled 'Euthanasia and the tyranny of technology', Furlow (1975) argues that the progress made possible by the rational, scientific method of modern medicine has resulted in physicians losing sight of one of their foremost duties to mankind, which is 'to prepare the sick and dying to accept irreversible disease and the natural conclusion to life – death'. Another by-product of medical progress that distorts the perspective on dying, he argues, is 'the ever lengthening twilight that divides life from death'. Artificial life-support systems only create and sustain the semblance of life, 'man has increasingly become dehumanised, to the point that truly worthwhile aspects of late life are no more'.

The call for legalised euthanasia cannot, however, be wholly attributed to the development of life-prolonging technologies. Suffering, whether from physical pain, incapacity or loss of independence, has always been a central feature of human life, and it is implausible to suggest that humans suffer more, or more intensely, from disease, disability or their treatment than in previous centuries. History books are filled with examples of people who died prolonged and agonising deaths, yet few considered ending their lives. What have changed, then, are our attitudes and expectations in the face of death and suffering.

Over the centuries human beings have devised a variety of strategies in an attempt to cope with and find meaning in their experiences of death and suffering. The attempt to cure disease and prevent death through medication and surgery is only one such strategy. Given the choice, not all societies would have appreciated the power of modern medicine to prolong life and to manage pain. During the Middle Ages, for example, the dying man had a priest at his side, not a physician, since it was considered infinitely more important to secure one's place in heaven than to prolong one's earthly existence or to avoid earthly suffering. Hence the prominence of versions of a treatise entitled *Ars Moriendi* (*The Art of Dying*), which gave clear directions for dying a good death: One had to accept and endure suffering as God's rightful punishment for one's sins, obtain God's forgiveness, and resist surrender to diabolical temptations such as despair, vanity, infidelity and an attachment to material possessions.

The ancient Greeks would have had a greater appreciation for modern medicine, but only to the extent to which it allowed them to live a good or virtuous life. Human life was not considered valuable in itself, and did not need to be preserved at all costs. In general, the pre-Socratic philosophers lamented the brevity of life and the inevitability of death, yet at the same time they applauded those who died heroically. To die in battle was the ultimate show of courage; it was a way of attaining immortality, if only in the minds of future generations. For Socrates the challenge of living was not to escape death but to avoid wrongdoing, so that in the end he chose to die rather than sacrifice his integrity. In Plato's *Republic* Socrates criticises Herodicus, a physical-education instructor who, afflicted with a chronic illness, combined the arts of medicine and physical exercise to doctor himself. This venture allowed him no time to fulfil his responsibilities as a good citizen or to live a rewarding life. '[T]hanks to his cleverness', Socrates says, 'he reached old age, but had one foot constantly in the grave' (*Republic* 406b). Even Aristotle, who had a far greater appreciation of life, nevertheless believed that life was not preferable to death if it could be procured only at the cost of virtue.

Underlying modern medical practice is a set of cultural values, ideals and beliefs that provides the impetus for its growth, guides the direction of its development, and governs its use. Three significant and closely related shifts characterise the development of modern medical practice and have radically impacted on modern man's experience and expectations in the face of death and suffering. The first of these is the transformation of medicine from an *art* into a *science*. This shift can be attributed to the Enlightenment ideal of emancipating reason from the yoke of religious belief, superstition and emotion, to attain knowledge that is universal, objective and value-free. The Greek physician relied for the most part on his powers of intuition to ascertain the cause of a patient's suffering, to predict its outcome and to provide care and comfort. With the application of scientific methods to health and physiology it became possible to successfully alter the disease process in ways that can be predicted and duplicated. The demonstrated benefits of modern medicine inspired great confidence in its ability to improve our quality of life and to prevent death. Today we no longer hope and pray to live our lives free from considerable or chronic pain; we expect to live and die comfortably, and demand that the benefits of modern medicine reach all of those affected by ill health.

At the same time that the critical attitude underlying a secularised world view brought forth the growth of scientific medicine, the loss of religious faith also created a need for alternative ways of coping with pain and suffering. For most enlightened people, the Stoic belief in the power of the rational mind to liberate us from pain and fear of death through apathy, or the early Christian view that man through his sinfulness deserves to suffer and die (but might through the grace of God continue to live in a blissful state after death), are no longer appealing answers to the problem of pain, its meaning or significance. Suffering as a result of disease and injury is today most often viewed as utterly meaningless, as a tragedy which we attribute to accident, error or injustice. The greater degree of certainty made possible by modern prognostic equipment has also robbed many of the hope of recovery that often accompanies ignorance. Medicine has become the only means of responding to suffering and our only source of hope – '*there must be something they can do*'.

Therefore, one way of understanding the appeal to legalise euthanasia is as an acknowledgement of the failure of medicine to realise the Enlightenment ideal of completely eliminating pain and suffering through scientific methods. Ironically, it is this ideal which has also robbed us of the ability to find meaning in suffering. Having reached the limits of medicine, the question arises, 'What lies beyond?', 'When we cannot go back to the days of strength and vitality and can no longer find solace in the bliss that awaits us in the Hereafter, where do we go?', and 'When our medicine no longer puts an end to the horror, how do we respond?'

The second shift in medical practice occurred with the incorporation of Enlightenment ideals into the sphere of medical ethics. The Modern period saw a gradual development from *virtue-based ethical systems*, exemplified by the ancient Greek philosophers (most notably Plato and Aristotle), the ancient Stoics and some sections of the early Christian church, to *principle-based ethics*, most notably deontological and utilitarian approaches. For virtue-ethicists the central moral question is: 'What sort of person should I become?' The Hippocratic Corpus provides numerous guidelines on how to become an excellent physician, one who would serve as an example to inspire others and would be trusted and admired by patients. The good physician of Graeco-Roman antiquity was expected to be medically knowledgeable, benevolent, honourable and trustworthy, but could use his discretion to decide how (and even whether) to treat a specific patient. There were no penalties for malpractice in the Greek states, so the physician who transgressed risked only his good reputation. A good physician did not simply follow rules. Instead, he was sensitive to the detail of his patients' moral lives and disposed by character to behave appropriately in particular circumstances.

Enlightenment thinkers rejected this approach to morality as subjective, sentimental, and hence, irrational. Moral philosophers, if they were to be taken seriously, had to show that moral judgements can be true or false and that moral values exist independently of the feelings of particular individuals. Whereas virtue-based theories centre on the character of persons, most modern theories of morality – whether deontological, consequentialist or contractarian – have as their focus the formulation of rules of right action. Although deontologists and utilitarians usually do make room for an account of virtue in their theories, it is only by way of supplementing the main task of formulating the ultimate principles and rules of morality. Kant, for example, believed that virtue consists in the disposition to obey what duty requires, whereas utilitarians value virtues insofar as they tend to maximise utility.

Over the past few decades much effort has been put into specifying the responsibilities of health-care professionals in terms of principles and rules. The 'four-principles approach' developed by Tom Beauchamp and James Childress has become the dominant approach to ethical problems in health care. The fourth edition of their *Principles of Biomedical Ethics* appeared in 1994, and their approach has formed the subject matter of numerous journal articles and books, including an enormous volume edited by Ranaan Gillon, *Principles of Health Care Ethics* (1994). This approach shares with utilitarian and Kantian theories an emphasis on universally-valid principles of obligation, but does not identify one supreme, absolute principle which is to support all other action-guides in the system. Instead, the four principles are seen as non-absolute or *prima facie*, meaning that they are always binding unless they conflict with the obligations required by another of the four principles, in which case it is necessary to balance the demands of the two principles. The four principles included in the framework are beneficence (the obligation to provide benefits and balance benefits against risks), non-maleficence (the obligation to avoid the causation of harm), respect for patient autonomy (the obligation to respect the decision-making capacities of autonomous persons) and justice (obligations of fairness in the distribution of benefits and risks). Beauchamp and Childress claim that, whatever your personal philosophy, religion, moral theory or political stance, you will be able to commit yourself to the four principles. They devote the last chapter of their book to a discussion of the virtues, which they see as complimenting the four principles. The virtues are given a special place on the sideline.

The incorporation of the principle of respect for patient autonomy in this foursome is the outcome of a third major shift in medical practice: *Patients* have become clients or *agents* of decision-making. Respect for persons has traditionally been understood to require, first and foremost, respect for the sanctity of human life or respect for a person's right to life. Today the predominant conception of respect in Western medicine is that the wishes of patients as autonomous persons have to be adhered to. The independent, self-determining and rational individual emerged in England during the seventeenth century, when the scientific ideals of unfettered rationality, objective experimentation and autonomous observation were incorporated and translated into the political and moral spheres. It was only in the 1960s, however, that this liberal ideal of self-determination began to show a definite impact in the medical context. Increasingly, the physician's assumption of authority to make decisions on behalf of patients came to be rejected as paternalistic and disrespectful. Viewing patients as decision-making agents, it was argued, is necessitated by the pluralism of beliefs and values characteristic of contemporary societies and compounded by the relative anonymity of the physician-patient interchange. Since it is the patient's values and goals that determine what counts as beneficial or harmful, a code of professional ethics must take respect for patient's autonomy as a central principle. This requires physicians to inform patients of relevant facts, thus enabling them to make free and rational decisions about their health. Patients now have the right to refuse treatment they believe to be unnecessarily burdensome or invasive. This approach also absolves physicians from the responsibility of making difficult moral decisions and decreases the fear of litigation.

In Chapter One I examine these three shifts (namely, the transformation of medicine from an art into a natural science, the replacement of a virtue-based ethical system by a principle-based system, and the more recent rejection of medical paternalism in favour of the view of the patient as an autonomous and rational agent) in more detail, focusing specifically on the role of the physician in each society and on the different attitudes toward death and suffering. This tour through history is by no means comprehensive. It merely aims to demonstrate that there can be no single answer, for all times and places, to questions surrounding the morality of euthanasia. By examining the dramatic changes that have occurred in medical practice over the centuries, one can better appreciate the unique dilemmas facing us today.

One of the central aims of this book is to provide a critique of the principle-based approach to medical ethics, using as a vehicle the moral issues surrounding end-of-life decision-making. Principle-based approaches seek to discover a principle and set of rules that will allow us to clearly separate acts that are permissible from those that are not. They rely on the assumption that all actions that are morally right share a common characteristic – for example, that they maximise utility – whereas all wrong actions lack this magical ingredient. We often find that what opponents and supporters of euthanasia disagree about is whether the rule 'It is always wrong to intentionally end the life of innocent human beings' adequately expresses the demands of morality. Perhaps the more specific rule, 'It is always wrong to kill innocent persons unless they explicitly ask to be killed', better expresses the demands of morality. In Chapter Two I argue that this approach does not allow us to meet the demands, challenges and ethical dilemmas that face medicine in multicultural and pluralistic societies. One of the main problems for principle-based theories is that secular moral philosophy, which has no use for the idea of divine law-giving, cannot make meaningful use of the idea of moral obligation. Although we have given up the idea that God commands us to do certain things and not to do others, we still formulate moral questions as if they could only render one of two answers – that the action is right, or that it is wrong – and as if the answer is 'out there' waiting to be discovered (see Anscombe 1997).

I shall use Aristotle's teleological account of the virtues as a starting-point for developing an ethical framework that permits us to deal more adequately with the moral problems involved in end-of-life decision-making. My current undertaking forms part of a more general movement that has taken place over the last few decades and that seeks to re-evaluate and develop the Aristotelian ethics of virtue. Some of the prominent figures in this movement are Elizabeth Anscombe, Alasdair MacIntyre, Rosalind Hursthouse, John McDowell, Philippa Foot and Martha Nussbaum. Whereas these writers have sought to develop versions of Aristotelian virtue ethics, my aim is more limited in scope. I focus specifically on the role of the virtues in medical practice, particularly with regard to end-of-life decision-making. In Chapters Three, Four and Five I develop an account of the virtues of compassion, benevolence and respectfulness, and defend this approach against charges that are commonly brought against an ethic of virtue. This pursuit is Aristotelian in method but not in content. Whereas Aristotle makes interesting and thought-provoking comments about specific virtues, much of what he says is of little relevance to modern readers. Instead of being left feeling nostalgic about what we, as members of liberal Western societies, have lost – a common goal, a shared conception of virtue and of the good life (or good death) – we should ask questions and seek answers that are relevant to our current situation.

One reason for the perceived failure of virtue ethics to provide moral guidance is, I believe, that virtue ethicists have been expected (and, foolishly, have sometimes attempted) to answer the same kinds of question raised by principle-based theorists, such as 'Is *x* right or wrong?' For instance, following the example of Kantians and utilitarians, Hursthouse identifies a criterion of rightness that reads: 'An action is right if and only if it is what an agent with a virtuous character would do in the circumstance' (1991:225). This 'criterion' has, quite justifiably, been criticised as being too vague to guide our actions. More importantly, the attempt by virtue ethicists to formulate a criterion of rightness loses sight of one of the central features of virtue ethics; namely, that its focus is on moral agents and their lives, rather than on discrete actions. We therefore need to reformulate the moral questions surrounding euthanasia in terms of the virtues. The ethical problems that arise with regard to the treatment of terminally- or incurably-ill patients are by no means peculiar to their situation. Instead, they are representative or indicative of a number of more general challenges facing contemporary medical practice. I shall focus specifically on three issues.

*Compassion*

The first issue concerns the role of compassion in medical practice and ethics. A popular argument in favour of euthanasia is that it is an act of mercy; it is a compassionate response to the suffering of a fellow human being. *Compassion in Dying*, a physician-staffed organisation in the state of Washington, claims to provide sympathetic counselling, advice on drugs, support and companionship for patients who choose an assisted death. Against this, supporters of the hospice movement have argued that that it is only a perverse kind of compassion that kills the suffering person. This raises the following question: 'Is euthanasia ever the appropriate expression of compassion or mercy?'

Although this question is often debated in the popular media, it is not seriously considered within the principle-based ethic. The heart-breaking stories of dying patients related in family magazines are frowned upon as presenting a threat to the responsible ethicist, who attempts to convince through rational argument and not through appeals to pity. For instance, in *Thinking Clearly About Death,* Rosenberg claims that morality is not 'a question of feelings but a matter of principled conduct'. While a patient's suffering might indeed be a terrible thing, and our inability to alleviate it may be deeply unfortunate, we should not allow ourselves to be 'blinded by (understandable) humane and sympathetic impulses' or to be moved by 'momentary impulses of pity or sympathy to abandon our reasoned moral convictions' (Rosenberg 1983:144). Under Kantian influence, compassion or pity has been rejected as a morally appropriate motivation for acts of benevolence. We are now required to act impartially and consistently according to certain universal and rationally determined duties.

The same attitude pervades medical law. In the South African Law Commission's (SALC) discussion paper on euthanasia and the artificial preservation of life it is stated that '[t]he jurist must however inevitably follow a more sober, certain and accordingly more clinical approach – just like the medical scientist' (SALC 1997:4). Although mercy-killers are usually found guilty of murder, they tend to be given very light sentences on the grounds of 'overwhelming extenuating circumstances'. Their motives for ending another's life are described as 'temporary insanity', 'an emotional state which renders them not accountable for their actions' or 'criminal incapacity' (SALC 1997:28-30). The light sentences reflect the view that emotions may give rise to acts of euthanasia, so that the *agents* cannot always be held legally accountable, but that this does not mean that such *acts* can be seen as either lawful or morally appropriate.

Medical law and ethics have followed the example set by the natural sciences by attempting to discover principles that have the same degree of objectivity, rationality and universality characteristic of scientific laws. In the process of transforming medicine from an art into a science the requirements of rationality and objectivity seemed to necessitate a rejection of compassion both as a means of understanding and as a motive for alleviating the patient's suffering. To diagnose correctly and treat effectively, the physician is now required to maintain an objective distance, to refrain from being emotionally affected by a patient's suffering, and to be impartial in the exercise of his duties.

In Chapter Three I shall argue that an important shortcoming of technological medicine, as guided by the principle-based ethic, is that it neglects the patient's emotional, psychological or existential suffering. Medical science focuses on explaining the origin of *physical pain*, on benefiting the *biological organism* and on respecting the autonomy of the patient as a *rational being*. I develop an account of the virtue of compassion as a response to the patient's sense of solitude, which is the first feature typical of human suffering. This virtue has played an important role in the establishment and development of medical practice, but has been rejected or neglected by enlightened scientists and ethicists. We have heard countless appeals for a more humane medicine, but when faced with the choice between compassion and science, physicians and patients understandably opt for the latter. I will argue that we need not make such a choice, that compassion is compatible with the scientific approach. Against the view held by philosophers such as Plato and Kant, I will show that compassion is not only (or merely) an emotion but contains both cognitive and moral elements. Insofar as it is a means of understanding a person's suffering, compassion offers a valuable corrective to the purely scientific, distanced mode of explaining physical conditions. This understanding also makes it possible to appropriately respond to – and hence alleviate – the suffering of a specific individual. The Aristotelian account of compassion differs significantly from the Christian virtue of pity. The association of pity with guilt, shame and divine forgiveness lies at the basis of the Nietzschean view that a person can only maintain his dignity and self-respect through an affirmation of his solitude, and by rejecting the pity and benevolence of others. I argue that the Aristotelian view of compassion may serve to strengthen or restore a person's sense of self-respect, since it is based on the recognition of the seriousness and undeservedness of the suffering of a fellow human being.

*Benevolence*

A second group of questions that arise when deciding on the treatment of terminally- or chronically-ill patients concerns the ends or goals of medicine: 'Is prolonging the life of a patient always a benefit?', 'Is death the greatest harm imaginable?', and 'Can one ever be better off dead?' If the purpose of medicine is conceived of as being the restoration and maintenance of health, the death of a patient under one's care can only be considered a failure. To prolong life would at least be a partial success. But when the quality of the life that is saved renders life more of a burden than a benefit to the patient, we have to question whether *effective* or successful treatment is always *beneficial* to the patient. While there seems to be no end to the growth of medical powers, the interests of the patient require that a limit be placed on efforts to prolong life. If we accept that life is not always a benefit, the further question arises as to whether ending life is ever a benevolent act: 'Is it ever in the best interest of a patient to follow a course of treatment with the deliberate intent to shorten life?'

To ask these questions is to question the role of medicine in furthering the human good, which includes a good life and a good death. In earlier centuries this question was answered by interpreting the notion of 'a good death'. The appropriate role for physicians and other caregivers was defined relative to the prevailing conception of a good death. In ancient Rome, for example, the difference between suicide and assisted suicide was considered trivial. It was more important whether it was a good time to die, and whether the person had good reason for hurrying death. By contrast, a substantial portion of the contemporary debate has focused on whether there is a morally significant difference between active and passive euthanasia, withdrawing and withholding treatment, or between bringing about death as an 'intended' and as a 'merely foreseen' effect. This focus on rules of right action is characteristic of principle-based ethical theories. Given the variability and subjectivity of other factors, such as the patient's suffering and quality of life, or the agent's motives and intentions, it is thought that it would allow for more objectivity and consistency if a set of rules is formulated regarding which sorts of treatment may or may not be withdrawn. Deontological ethicists, in particular, have attempted to specify moral principles without reference to ends or consequences. Characteristic of this approach is the view that negative duties, such as duties of non-maleficence, are absolute, or at least more stringent than positive duties, such as duties of beneficence. Accordingly, it is often considered wrong to actively kill patients, regardless of the consequences, since such actions violate duties of non-maleficence. On the other hand, it is sometimes permissible to allow a patient to die, since this amounts merely to a failure to benefit him or her. Against this, consequentialists have argued that one is morally responsible for the consequences of one's omissions as well as one's actions, and that there is no essential moral difference between active and passive euthanasia. Despite the increasingly complex and technical nature of this debate, the fundamental question has not been answered: 'What role should medicine play at the end of life?' One shortcoming of the principle-based approach is that it aims to *discover* the answers to moral questions, putting forward historical events as examples of how universal principles operate in seemingly diverse cultural contexts. In opposition to the view that the essence of medicine and medical ethics can be discovered, I will argue that we have to *create* our own answers to questions concerning the goal of medical treatment. Given our current circumstances, how much power do we want medicine to have, and what kind of role do we want it to play?

Chapter Four starts by examining a second feature of suffering, namely the patient's helplessness and dependence on others. This leads to a re-examination of the principle of beneficence by tracing its development through the history of Western philosophy. I examine Kant's rejection of Hume's philosophy – which sees in sympathy the appropriate motivation for benevolence – in favour of duty as the only morally-appropriate motivation, as well as J.S. Mill's rejection of the Kantian focus on motivation as the basis of moral judgement in favour of the consequences or utility of the act. I discuss the shortcomings of both the Kantian and utilitarian conceptions of the principle of beneficence within the medical context. I then develop a teleological account of the virtue of 'responsible benevolence', which is motivated by compassion and guided by the Aristotelian virtue of *phronesis* (practical reason, wisdom or intelligence). *Phronesis* is distinct from, but compliments, *episteme* (scientific knowledge) and *techne* (technical skills). The ethical problems surrounding the treatment of terminally- or incurably-ill patients necessitate a re-evaluation of the appropriate goals of medical science and technology and a reconsideration of the role of medicine in man's search for happiness and freedom from suffering. The concept of 'responsible benevolence' allows us to reconsider the morally-appropriate goals of medical practice without lapsing into a principle of beneficence which establishes goals of treatment in accordance with universal reason or overall utility.

*Respect*

A third question that arises with regard to the predicament of terminally- or chronically-ill patients is whether euthanasia allows them to *die with dignity*. Perhaps the most frequently heard argument in favour of legalising active voluntary euthanasia is based upon the notion of patient autonomy and the right to self-determination. Contemporary medical ethics was largely born out of an attempt to rescue the patient's dignity from the gross manipulation and dehumanisation of a technologically-driven clinical science. The discontent that seemed to underlie all the various criticisms stemmed from a concern for patient autonomy, the moral notion most easily extrapolated from the legal precepts of our political culture (Tauber 1999:28). To a certain extent, the increasing emphasis on patient autonomy over the past few decades has allowed many people to make decisions about their own deaths. Whereas the debate on active and passive euthanasia was largely focused on the agent's role in bringing about death, some of the attention has shifted back to the patient whose death is concerned. Patients are now entitled to information about their diagnosis and prognosis and may refuse any or all forms of medical intervention. The call for a right to physician-assisted suicide is the most recent attempt to enable people to become creators or directors of their own deaths. As Battin writes, 'dying is no longer *something that happens to you* but *something you do*' (1998:66, emphasis in original).

There are two main reasons why it has been difficult to apply the principle of patient autonomy in end-of-life decision-making. The first has to do with the physical and mental state of these patients. Since serious disease or injury typically serves to decrease a patient's ability to think, decide and act freely and rationally, it is not always clear whether their decisions meet the requirements of free and informed consent. (Indeed, critics disagree as to what these requirements are.) Similarly, surrogate decision-makers may be overwhelmed by fear or grief, rendering it difficult for them to make such important decisions.

The second problem in applying the principle of patient autonomy to the question of euthanasia involves the content of the patient's request. It is not uncommon for physicians and patients to disagree about treatment, but such conflicts become particularly intense when it is a matter of life and death. For instance, a patient may refuse treatment when there is a good chance of recovery, or request assistance in dying while the physician believes that she has a duty not to end life. A surrogate decision-maker, interpreting the notions of 'due care' as respect for the sanctity of human life, may refuse withdrawal of treatment regarded by the physician as futile and unnecessarily burdensome. The question is therefore whether 'respect for persons' requires a recognition of their *right to self-determination* – which does not necessarily ensure a promotion of their best interest or a preservation of their lives – or a recognition of the *sanctity of human life*, which might require a physician to disregard the patient's wishes.

In Chapter Five I begin by discussing the third feature of suffering, namely the patient's loss of self-respect. I then re-examine the principle of respect for patient autonomy, which is recognised in an attempt to restore to the patient some measure of self-respect through letting him participate in medical decision-making. I critically examine the Kantian and utilitarian defences of individual autonomy, and argue that they lie at the basis of the difficulties experienced in attempting to apply the principle of patient autonomy to end-of-life decisions. In response to the shortcomings of the principle of patient autonomy I develop a teleological account of respect for persons. In contrast to the principle of respect for patient autonomy, the virtue of respectfulness is not based on the view that humans are (or should be) rational and autonomous beings, but neither does it require that human life should be preserved at all costs, as proponents of the sanctity-of-life ethic often claim. This account of the virtue of respectfulness allows us to develop an alternative model of decision-making aimed at reaching consensus, rather than consent.

In Chapter Six I undertake what is perhaps the most important challenge for virtue ethicists, namely to apply the theoretical findings to the moral issues surrounding euthanasia. Over the past few decades there has been a remarkable revival of virtue ethics. Numerous writers have developed virtue-based ethical theories and analysed specific virtues, some of them dealing specifically with the virtues in medicine.[1] However, surprisingly few attempts have been made to apply these theoretical findings to actual moral issues. Philippa Foot's paper on euthanasia (1977) and Rosalind Hursthouse's book on abortion (1987) are among the very few exceptions. Opponents of virtue ethics often argue that this should come as no surprise, since virtue ethics cannot provide us with specific answers to the question, 'What ought we to do?' In response to this charge I argue that the demonstrated impotence of virtue ethics to make much of a contribution in this regard is due to the fact that the virtues are applied, in almost deductive fashion, to questions formulated in the language of rights, duties and principles, for example, 'Do we have a right to an easy death?' and 'Do we have an obligation to be merciful?' I argue that in order to appreciate the significance and implications of the virtues for the euthanasia debate, we must begin by restating the moral questions involved. I then outline a procedure for making decisions about the treatment of terminally- or chronically-ill patients that can be used as the basis of policy-making.

---

[1] See, for example, Pellegrino and Thomasma (1993), Shelp (1985) and Spiro *et al.* (1993).

# Chapter One

# Medicine, Death and Disease: A Historical Perspective

## Introduction

Apart from being mildly entertained by the ignorance and queerness of past cultures, what can we possibly learn from a journey through the history of Western medicine? Some find in history an affirmation of their own values, a reassurance that those who dared do otherwise paid dearly – Baumrin thinks the lesson from Nazi doctors in World War II is that 'a physician is to be always a champion of life and health in every context' (1998:179). Others use historical facts to show that things could be otherwise, that our current opinions are not the common sense of humankind – Rachels points out that the ancient Greeks, whose culture, philosophy, art and political institutions we so much admire, habitually and without scruples practised infanticide (1986:7). Yet others use historical facts to support their view of the essence of medicine – in his version of *The Story of Medicine* Victor Robinson writes:

> The first cry of pain through the primitive jungle was the first call for a physician. Early man... was rubbed or stroked when in pain, his broken bones were splinted with branches, and when bitten by a venomous animal he sucked the poison from his body or his fellows did it for him. Medicine is a natural art, conceived in sympathy and born of necessity; from these instinctive procedures developed the specialized science that is practised today (1943:1).

To say that every culture has devised ways of responding to and managing the 'cry of pain' is almost a truism, but to suggest that there is something natural or necessary about the goal and motives behind the development of medical science is to rely too much on the power of eloquent speech. Few would take this view seriously if it were simply expressed as 'medicine is still essentially the same, just much better'. It is this harmonious picture of historical development that lies behind the assumption that we can discover the essence of medicine, its true nature, motive and goal, and eventually demonstrate that practising euthanasia is (or is not) reconcilable with the true nature of medicine.

Medical practice arises within, and responds to the needs of, a particular society. This fact is obvious but often overlooked. We look disapprovingly at medicine for treating us in ways that are 'alienating' or 'dehumanising', not realising that medical practice merely presents us with a mirror image of ourselves: our values and attitudes, our beliefs and expectations. We complain about the medicalisation of dying, but we have no other way of responding to suffering than to call for a doctor, or to visit a pharmacy. Just as a journey to a foreign country adds to the understanding of one's own culture, my aim in tracing the historical development of medical practice is to develop a fuller understanding of the state of contemporary medical science and ethics. To this end I will focus on three interrelated shifts: (1) the changing paradigm of health and disease; (2) the movement from a virtue- to a principle-based approach to medical ethics; and (3) the combined effect of these changes on the physician's involvement in the dying process.

## Graeco-Roman Antiquity: The Hippocratic Response to Suffering

The Homeric poems, our earliest literary source of evidence for Greek medicine, depict a fantastic world where gods inflict disease and suffering upon humans as punishment, or simply out of anger or spite. In the *Iliad*, Apollo sends a plague to decimate the army invading Troy as punishment for Agamemnon's arrogant treatment of a priest who comes to ransom his captured daughter. Perhaps the most reasonable part of mythical thought is the belief that the gods, having the power to cause disease, also have the power to heal. The sick could go to temples and sanctuaries where a wide range of gods and demigods practised the art of healing. Initially Apollo was the most important, but he was subsequently outshone by his son Asclepius.

The sixty or more treatises of the Hippocratic *Corpus*, the main body of which was written by a number of physicians between 420 and 370 BC, provide a striking contrast. For the first time in the history of medicine, complete treatises survive which embody a relatively consistent doctrine of medical theory and practice, virtually free of magic, superstition, supernatural intervention and speculative philosophy. The treatises attempt to account for the causes and symptoms of disease in purely natural terms, explicitly rejecting the view that disease – even epilepsy – is caused by supernatural agencies. Until fairly recently historians assumed that Hippocrates had learned medicine from studying the case histories on display at Asclepius's temple at Cos. The following case – representative of the Asclepian approach to disease – should demonstrate the untenability of the assumption that Hippocratic medicine developed from religious medicine:

> A man had his toe healed by a snake. The man, in a terrible state because of a malignant ulcer on his toe, was carried outside in the daytime by the attendants and he sat down upon a seat. When sleep overcame him, a serpent came out of the Sanctuary and healed his toe with its tongue. When the patient awoke, he was healed. He had seen a vision: it seemed that a beautiful youth was spreading a potion upon his toe (*Inscriptiones Graecae*, IV.1, nos. 121-2, pp. 70-73, ll.113-119).

Historical evidence suggests that the cult of Asclepius and its temple healing reached Cos when the island was already famous for its secular medicine, and it is more likely that religious medicine was itself influenced by secular medicine than *vice versa*. The emancipation of medicine from magic and superstition was the outcome of the same attitude that the natural philosophers from the Ionian city of Miletus first applied to the world around them. Their attempts to give rational explanations of the world in terms of its visible, natural constituents, and without recourse to supernatural intervention or mythological conjecture, inspired Hippocratic physicians to account for sickness and health in the same way. Apart from the similarities in style and content, the clearest evidence of the close relationship between Ionian philosophy and Hippocratic medicine is that medical literature was written in the Ionian dialect, regardless of the fact that they practised mainly in Dorian settlements. The cult of Asclepius continued to exist alongside scientific medicine; indeed, under the impact of the plague in Athens it dramatically expanded throughout Greece during the fifth century Enlightenment (see Longrigg 1993:6-25).

Even though many attained heroic status, the Great Physicians of antiquity played a relatively minor role in society. This was the consequence of the strong competition that came from exorcists, midwives, surgeons, gymnasts and other 'experts' in health and disease at the time. Many members of the public remained sceptical of scientific medicine and distrusted the motives and abilities of physicians. Some scholars believe that this was the main reason why most ancient physicians refused to treat terminally-ill patients – a dead patient was the worst imaginable advertisement, providing clear evidence of the disutility of medicine (see Bodemer 1979:827-828). But in *The Art* the author defends the profession against this very objection by arguing that a competent physician would realise when the disease was stronger than the means at the disposal of medicine. To recognise terminal disease is already to show some expertise at diagnosis and prognosis.

The *Epidemics*, which has come to be looked upon as the very model of empirical observation, does show the physician in close proximity to dying patients. Indeed, of the 42 case histories, 25 end in death. The passivity of the physician is striking – he does little more than to carefully record the detail of each case. This passivity can be explained, in part, by the fact that the prevailing conception of disease did not encourage aggressive treatment. Disease was not understood as caused by an independent entity but was the result of an imbalance in the constituents of the body. The author of *On Regimen* thought that the whole body was in a perpetual state of flux, and that health consisted in keeping the flux within certain limits. Illness was caused when something occurred, either externally or internally, to disturb the balance. The physician's role was to understand the imbalance and to remove all that may hinder the natural tendency of the body to restore balance. The goal of medical practice was not to *combat* disease, but to act as an assistant to nature. The keynote of Hippocratic medicine was gentleness: no extreme measures, no harsh drugs, and no surgical intervention.

In one sense Greek medicine had a much broader focus than modern medicine. According to Plato, Hippocrates believed that a disease could not be treated without knowledge of the whole. The most common form of treatment was to attend to a person's 'diet', which encompassed his or her entire life-style. Besides prescribing food and drink, advice was given on sleep and dreaming, baths, massage, exercise and changes in climate. The focus was on preventing disease, rather than heroic attempts at cure. In this way the discipline of 'pathophysiology' was established, which is the attempt to seek the causes of a patient's suffering by examining his life-style, dietary habits, environment, etc. *Physiologia* means 'an inquiry into the nature of things', and *pathos* means 'suffering'. Literally, the quest of the Hippocratic doctor was to make an inquiry into the nature of suffering.

Most contemporary physicians find it easy to distance themselves from the simplicity and often-misguided nature of Hippocratic medicine. Yet surprisingly many appeal to *The Oath* to support their moral objections to euthanasia and physician-assisted suicide. Perhaps this reflects a belief that while our knowledge of scientific facts may change, moral values are universal and unchanging, independent of historical context. Baumrin sums up his (slightly more sophisticated) version of this argument as follows:

> [P]hysicians alive today are the beneficiaries of a two-and-a-half-millennia-old tradition that abjured assisting patients in suicide and killing people at the behest of others. None alive today has the right to betray the public trust that that tradition has endowed them with (1998:177).

Apart from the argumentative weakness of such appeals to tradition, it appears that the truth of his claim is dubious. Far from being the touchstone of medical ethics in antiquity, *The Oath* is rarely mentioned by contemporaries, and may not have been generally sworn until the sixteenth century. The five ethical works in the *Corpus* – *The Oath, Law, The Physician*, *Precepts* and *Decorum* – are sometimes referred to as the 'deontological works', but only for *The Oath* is this description appropriate. It begins by invoking the gods, and largely consists of specifying the duties of physicians towards each other and the profession: A pupil must regard his teacher and the teacher's relatives as if they were his own, and keep the secrets of medicine within this family. It defines ethics in terms of a specific set of obligations involved in belonging to a profession, and makes the physician foreswear involvement in abortion, surgery, and providing deadly drugs on request.

The other ethical writings in the *Corpus* paint a very different picture. The physician is depicted as a public figure that debates and consults with others, often in the presence of the patient. One of the few certain facts about the historical Hippocrates (c. 450-370 BC) is that he taught medicine for a fee to anyone who could pay, and not only to a select few. The presence of gynaecological treatises in the *Corpus* suggests that, instead of forming an isolated group of professionals, physicians co-operated with midwives and other women who treated female disorders. As far as relations with patients and the public were concerned, the ample advice about dress, behaviour and etiquette shows that, more than anything, the Hippocratic physician was eager to win public favour. But no attempt is made to formulate specific rules of action or compile a list of moral obligations. Most of the ethical writings are concerned with demarcating the good physician from the bad by applying a simple criterion: whatever is best for the case in hand. For the most part, medical ethics was equated with effective practice. Treating patients with compassion and respect, comforting and pleasing them were, at one and the same time, to benefit them.

From the *Epidemics* it is clear that there was no stigma attached to non-intervention or leaving the patient to die: 'As to diseases make a habit of two things – to help, or at least, to do no harm'. This maxim is sometimes mistakenly attributed to *The Oath*, and is often seen as similar to the statement found there: 'I will use treatment to help the sick according to my ability and judgement, but I will never use it to injure or wrong them'. But there is an important difference, not always appreciated, between notes jotted down among case studies about 'making a habit' of certain behaviour, and swearing before the *gods* that one will benefit and never harm the sick. As we have seen, religious explanations of disease are rejected throughout the *Corpus*, with the notable exception of *The Oath*. This, together with the fact that Hippocratic physicians acted as philanthropists rather than as contracted professionals, means that there was no proscribing authority, and without a lawgiver, there can be no laws. Nowhere in the Hippocratic *Corpus* do we find any mention of, even less an argument for, *The Oath*'s prohibitions against abortion or assisted suicide. We also know that many physicians did participate in these practices without a qualm. Coupled with the generally religious language of *The Oath*, these facts have suggested to many scholars that it was devised for a small, and perhaps unusual, group; others believe that *The Oath*, or parts thereof, had a later, probably Christian source.

That *The Oath* is not representative of Hippocratic morality also accords with what we know of Milesian culture and natural philosophy. There was no true religion expounded from a common sacred book by universally-recognised spokesmen and supported by an organised religious authority. The Milesians were not constrained to adhere to any inviolable dogmatic code, but participated in regular political debate, had an irreverent attitude towards traditional authority, and believed that any citizen was entitled to voice his opinion on any subject (see Longrigg 1993:29).

There is wide disagreement as to the character and motives of the ideal Hippocratic physician. Whereas some would have it that he was a kind and compassionate philanthropist, others think that self-interest and a concern with his reputation were his primary motives. A familiar quotation from the *Precepts* VI reads, 'where there is love of man, there is also love of the art'. Sir William Osler, an influential nineteenth century Christian physician, proclaimed this to be the height of medical idealism, and Jones says that the great lesson of the Hippocratic writings is that medicine is an art which is 'inseparable from the highest morality and the love of humanity' (1923, vol. I:296). Against this, others have argued that this phrase is nothing more than advice about good advertising. The injunction against harming a patient, in Jonsen's view, did not express the moral view that human life is sacred (as the later Christians would have it), but had as its aim the improvement of the dubious status of physicians. Indeed, he says, studies of Greek medical literature turn up very little altruism in the ethics of Hippocratic physicians, who were mainly concerned with promoting their own interests and improving their reputation and status as healers (Jonsen 1990:8-9).

The truth probably lies somewhere between these two extremes. It is obvious that ancient physicians were greatly concerned with their reputations, but self-interest need not exclude altruistic motives. Doctors were often honoured for their treatment of both rich and poor, slaves and free men, and for their concern with the general welfare of society. The fact that many physicians died while treating those sick with the plague that struck Athens in 430 BC, is evidence that self-interest was not the sole motivating factor for physicians of the day. We are told of one Xenotimus who, when most of his colleagues were overworked and ill, 'of his own free will, constantly rendered assistance to those who needed it; intent upon bringing recovery to all the sick indiscriminately, and toiling for all citizens equally... saved many'. The Athenians bestowed honour upon him for his benevolence and competence, his 'good will and care', and his readiness 'to serve gratis as public physician'. The authors of the first century AD took the presence of compassion among doctors for granted. The Roman encyclopedist Celsus thought that the surgeon should be 'filled with pity, so that he wishes to cure his patient', while not being moved by the patient's cries to too great a hurry (Temkin 1991:18-35).

We therefore need not think of self-interest and altruism as two mutually-exclusive motives. It is only with the Christian demand for selfless dedication to the good of others that altruism and self-interest come to be seen as mutually exclusive. The virtuous person of Graeco-Roman antiquity was concerned not only with the well-being of others, but also with his own reputation, honour and dignity. Both of these attributes were considered central virtues or constituents of the good life, as seen from the statement in the *Precepts* VI: '[I]t is well to superintend the sick to make them well, to care for the healthy to make them well, but also to care for one's own self, so as to observe what is seemly.' Hence their concern with reputation should not be seen as an attempt to gain riches by good advertising. Few physicians of this time could have been motivated primarily by greed or selfishness. In *Breaths* I we read that 'the medical man sees terrible sights, touches unpleasant things, and the misfortunes of others bring a harvest of sorrows that are peculiarly his; but the sick by means of the art rid themselves of the worst of evils, disease, suffering, pain and death'. There must have been easier and more pleasant ways of gaining riches.

Although many Greeks seem to have had considerable confidence in their medicine, they were largely distrustful of the character and competence of individual medical practitioners. The livelihood of the ancient physician as craftsman thus depended upon improving his reputation as a healer. To gain a reputation as a good physician, it was necessary for him not only to obtain greater knowledge and skills in medicine, but also to be of good character, trustworthy, honourable and benevolent. Recognising the fact that the physician's knowledge and skills gave him the power not only to heal, but also to harm, he had to demonstrate his integrity, compassion and benevolence to establish and maintain public trust. The following passage taken from *The Physician* I conveys the Hippocratic attitude more accurately than *The Oath* does:

> The prudent man must also be careful of certain moral considerations – not only to be silent, but also of a great regularity of life, since thereby his reputation will be greatly enhanced; he must be a gentleman in character, and being this he must be grave and kind to all. For an over-forward obtrusiveness is despised, even though it may be very useful.... In appearance, let him be of a serious but not harsh countenance; for harshness is taken to mean arrogance and unkindness, while a man of uncontrolled laughter and excessive gaiety is considered vulgar, and vulgarity especially must be avoided. In every social relation he will be fair, for fairness must be of great service. The intimacy also between physician and patient is close. Patients in fact put themselves into the hands of their physician, and at every moment he meets women, maidens and possessions very precious indeed. So towards all these self-control must be used. Such then should the physician be, both in body and in soul.

It is clear from this passage that the skills of a good physician included both altruism and a concern for their own interests. He had to display characteristics such as generosity, compassion and kindness, and had to make sure that others recognise these traits in him. Public trust was a necessary requirement for being a good physician.

The same attitude prevailed among Greek and Roman philosophers. Although they disagreed as to the moral acceptability of suicide and mercy-killing, they all approached these issues in terms of the virtues. The question they sought to answer was not: 'Is it ever morally justifiable to end life?', but rather, 'What does it mean to live and die virtuously?' Plato, for example, who was a contemporary of Hippocrates, criticised 'this modern medical technique of pampering illness' (*Republic* 406a). He thought that the proper task of physicians was to treat those who had a good constitution and led a healthy life, but who had contracted an isolated disease. After being treated by a physician, he thought, a patient should not be confined to bed but be sent off to continue with his normal tasks. Then, 'if his body isn't up to surviving, he gets rid of his troubles by dying' (*Republic* 406e). In this way an unhappy and unproductive life will not be prolonged, which would also prevent the production of equally unhealthy children. Plato thought that life is not worth living if one's health does not allow one to live well and to contribute to the welfare of the community. He compares the good doctor to the good judge, and concludes that the ideal state 'will leave the unhealthy to die, and those whose psychological constitution is incurably corrupt it will put to death' (*Republic* 410a). The difference between letting die and killing is not considered relevant – it just so happens that poor physical health naturally ends in death whereas criminals have to be put to death. The important point to note is that, in both cases, death is not considered a punishment but instead 'the best thing both for the individual sufferer and for society'. Death is not to be feared, according to Plato, since it is not an evil but rather the release of the rational soul from its imprisonment in the body and earthly existence. In the *Phaedo*, Plato's Socrates says that the philosopher can only achieve pure knowledge once he divorces the body – true wisdom can only be attained in death, when the soul is separate and independent of the body. In Plato's account of the trial of Socrates the wise man chooses death in order to convince his followers that the fear of death is irrational. He thought it infinitely more important to face death with courage and self-control, to maintain his integrity as a truly wise and virtuous person (*Apology* 17a-42a). In his *Memorabilia* the journalist Xenophon gives a less high-minded, yet similar account of Socrates's uncompromising attitude before his judges. In his view, Socrates was satisfied with the life he had lived and realised that death would permit him to avoid the disabilities and miseries of old age. Xenophon cites Socrates as saying: 'Have you not known all along that from the moment of my birth nature has condemned me to death?'

Aristotle, unconvinced of the immortality of the soul, did not seem quite as eager to take leave of this life. However, he shared Plato's concern with dying virtuously. According to Aristotle one has good reason to fear death, 'for it is the end, and nothing is thought to be any longer either good or bad for the dead' (*Nicomachean Ethics* III. vi). But he is quick to add that a virtuous person would not fear death in all circumstances. In battle, for instance, it is better to die a noble death than to gain safety from danger in a disgraceful fashion; and when sick, one should endure suffering with courage. A virtuous person would not commit suicide, for 'to die to escape from poverty or love or anything painful is not the mark of a brave man, but rather of a coward.... [Courage] chooses or endures things because it is noble to do so, or because it is base not to do so' (*N. Ethics* III. vii). Yet elsewhere he comes out strongly in favour of infanticide: 'With regard to the choice between abandoning an infant or rearing it, let there be a law that no cripple child be reared' (*Politics* VII. xvi). To the modern reader this might seem inconsistent with his opposition to suicide. Yet it is important to note that Aristotle's concern here is not primarily with the morality of the act of killing; he uses these examples to illustrate the virtue of courage. Suicide is wrong only because it shows a lack of courage. He could therefore quite consistently support infanticide for defective infants by arguing that it is unacceptable to allow such infants to endure suffering since they lack the capacity and potential to live and die with courage.

In his tragic dramas Sophocles portrayed death as morally neutral; in certain circumstances it was preferable to life, at other times not. Even premature death is bearable when life is filled with misery and moral conflict. For instance, Antigone decides to give her brother a decent burial regardless of the fact that she will have to pay for it with her own life. She explains her decision as follows:

> That death would come, I knew
> Without thine edict; – if before the time,
> I count it gain. Who does not gain by death,
> That lives, as I do, amid boundless woe?
> Slight is the sorrow of such doom to me.
> But had I suffered my own mother's child,
> Fallen in blood, to be without a grave,
> That were indeed a sorrow. This is none (*Antigone* ll. 461-470).

Antigone makes it clear that some things are more important than preserving life when she asks Creon: 'Wouldst thou aught more of me than merely death?' (*Antigone* l. 497). Sophocles was perhaps the first to advocate suicide as a general cure for life's burdens, and his lead was enthusiastically followed by most of the ancient Stoics. The Stoic philosopher Seneca saw death as the liberation of the immortal soul. Since the gods did not forbid suicide, the only thing that could hinder man from seeking out freedom from earthly sorrows was his own lack of courage. Most of the ancient Roman philosophers agreed with him, and it was not uncommon for physicians of the time to provide or administer poisons upon request. For Seneca, it was not pain itself that provided a good reason for suicide, but the fact that disease or senility would prevent him from living a good life. In his 58th *Letter to Lucilius* Seneca writes:

> I will not relinquish old age if it leaves my better part intact. But if it begins to shake my mind, if it destroys its faculties one by one, if it leaves me not life but breath, I will depart from the putrid or the tottering edifice. If I know that I must suffer without hope of relief I will depart not through fear of the pain itself but because it prevents all for which I would live.

At the same time, Seneca warned against the risk of idealising death:

> The brave and wise man should not beat a hasty retreat from life; he should make a becoming exit; and above all, he should avoid the weakness which has taken possession of so many – the lust for death.

For the ancient Greek and Roman philosophers the question was not 'Is it permissible to commit suicide or to assist someone in his or her suicide?' The questions concerning the morality of suicide were far more complex: 'When is life no longer worth living?' and 'How can we live and die virtuously?' As we shall see in the following section, it is only during the Christian period that the morality of suicide and euthanasia came to be discussed in terms of principles, rules and prohibitions.

## The Middle Ages: The Christian Response to Suffering

With the advent of Christianity in 313 AD the ancient world was de-secularised. Areas of life previously independent of religious cult and belief were annexed through the claims of Christianity to universality. Medical assistance was rejected in favour of the divine. Skin diseases in particular were associated with God's punishment for sin and were curable by Him alone. Instead of seeking out physicians, the sick prayed to God for forgiveness and salvation. Recovery from disease was a miracle, an undeserved bonus. Since there was little respect for the sick, tending to the physical needs of the sick was not an honourable job – it was left to widows (who had no other use), fallen women (who had already lost their dignity) and unemployed peasants (who had nothing better to do). Although it was universally acknowledged that disease and sin were closely connected, theory and practice did not always concur. Most writers in late antiquity and the early Middle Ages ascribed their own or their friends' sufferings to physical causes, and that of others, especially their enemies, to sin.

During the Middle Ages health care slowly regained respectability when the Christian church adopted care of the sick as one of the duties of charity and self-sacrifice. Christ's order to his followers to care for the sick, the poor, and the needy was given institutional form by the creation of a 'deacon' charged with the distribution of alms. Many wealthy Christians set aside a room in their house to provide food and shelter as part of a missionary outreach. Medicine was not a branch of science or even geared towards curing disease; it was oriented towards caring for the sick and thus provided one with an opportunity to display certain virtues. The virtue of compassion figures strongly in Christian ethics, where it is associated with notions such as selflessness, forgiveness, mercy and kindness. Perhaps the most celebrated example of compassion is found in the New Testament parable of the Good Samaritan, told by Jesus in response to the question 'What must I do to receive eternal life?' In this parable, a man travelling from Jerusalem to Jericho was attacked by robbers who left him 'half dead' at the roadside. Two other travellers, a priest and a Levite, passed by the injured man without rendering help. A Samaritan who saw him had compassion for him, took him to an inn and bandaged his wounds. He left money with the landlord, telling him to take further care of the man. The parable of the Good Samaritan was used in the first centuries of the Christian era and throughout the Middle Ages to exemplify the duties of the good physician and Christian. Acting like the good Samaritan accorded with Jesus' promise of the kingdom of Heaven to those who had visited 'the least of my brethren' (Luke 10:25-37).

Whereas self-interest was acknowledged as a proper motive of physicians in the Hippocratic tradition, the caregiver was now expected to be selfless and humble, to pay tribute to God as the true (and only) Healer. Physicians were the instruments of God, expected to emulate the Good Samaritan by giving the same impartial attention to all their patients, regardless of their economic status, racial identity or political affiliation. They were admonished to remember the words of the Lord: 'I was sick, and you took care of me.... I tell you, whenever you did this for one of the least important of these brothers of mine, you did it for me!' (Matthew 25:36, 40). Serving the sick – 'the least important' – became the ideal in modesty. The epitome of these selfless healers can be found in The Knights Hospitallers of the eleventh century, who provided hostels for pilgrims and care for the sick among them. They were said to live in celibacy and poverty, vowing to 'serve our lords, the sick, with zeal and devotion, as if they were serfs to their Lords' (cited in Jonsen 1990:70).

No medical knowledge or skills were required to be a Good Samaritan. The emphasis was on care, protection and charity, not cure. For the most part, there was little concern with the body in early hospitals. The Hippocratic idea of balance went out of favour during this time, since it was hard to combine with the Christian praise of asceticism and the mortification of the flesh, and with the notion of illness as a trial of sanctity. Nutton describes the conflict between these two paradigms of health and disease as follows: 'A religious rhythm of fasting and vigil was no harmonious counterpoint to the ordered progression of the humours. The more the body appeared a mere temporary habitation of an immortal soul, the less the need to attend to it' (in Conrad *et al.* 1995:76-77).

People of the Middle Ages became increasingly obsessed with death, which was often depicted as a cloaked skeleton hovering by the bedside of the dying. The Hereafter became a source of terror for most people. Yet nothing was done to avoid or postpone death. The faithful were warned not to put their final trust in physicians and medicines (see Psalms 103:2-4), and a popular code for physicians between the ninth and fifteenth centuries advised them 'never [to] become involved knowingly with any who are about to die or who are incurable'. If suffering is seen as God's punishment for the primal sin, the only way it could be removed was by Christ's grace. The act of dying was a religious event, and dying suddenly, without the opportunity to confess one's sins, came to be dreaded above all else. Versions of a treatise entitled *Ars Moriendi*, or *The Art of Dying*, was elevated to great prominence. Roman Catholics and Protestants considered the last hours of mortal existence a time for the individual to confront death with steadfast resistance against temptations to infidelity, despair, vanity and materialism. In a deathbed scenario the physician was not only unessential, but also unwelcome. The idea of sending for a 'bodily leech' before a 'spiritual leech' was actively condemned as a sign of 'this worldliness' and a weakening before satanic temptation. When the physician finally did assume a role at the deathbed, it was only to counteract the depressing influences that deprive the dying person of consolation. Thus De Sorbière, a seventeenth century physician, wrote in his *Advice to a Young Physician* that it is appropriate to give an 'elixir to wake people from a deep lethargy, which serves to prepare them for death by putting them into a condition to think of salvation' (cited in Bodemer 1979:829-830).

During the early Christian period moral views were expressed in the language of virtue. Christians were expected to possess certain character traits, and to emulate Christ. With the growth in power and influence of the Church, the language of virtues gradually made way for the language of absolute principles and prohibitions. The Hippocratic 'do no harm' came to be seen primarily as a rule against abortion and euthanasia. One of the cornerstones of Christian morality is the notion that it is always wrong to kill innocent persons. The sixth commandment states 'Thou shalt not kill' and the traditional Catholic view has been that the proper object for the verb is 'innocent human beings'. This became the supreme moral duty, grounded in religious authority, which medical professionals were required to adhere to. Infanticide was prohibited, for it was thought that all human beings were created in God's image. The value or sanctity of human life did not derive from individual experience or joy in being alive. Following the teachings of St. Augustine, one's life was viewed as a trust from God, and only He had the right to take it. Humans had to endure life until that time came, whether they liked it or not. To kill a person (including oneself) was not simply to deprive that person of life, but to sin against God. In this way religious faith provided people with a reason to keep on living, even in the face of the most horrible suffering, and with a way of giving their suffering meaning. The close relationship established between Church and State in the Middle Ages meant that suicide was not only prohibited and punished by God, but also legally prohibited and subject to heavy penalties. Those who committed suicide were denied the rites of Christian burial, and secular laws were passed in many countries requiring the forfeiture of the property of such persons.

## Modernising Medicine: The Erosion of Paternalism

Religious explanations for plague and madness, and the religious emphasis on dying virtuously gradually declined during the seventeenth century. The Enlightenment slowly replaced supernatural reasoning with reasoning based upon an ordered, mechanical nature. God initially created the world but allowed it to work according to causal laws, without any other direct interference. Descartes, the great philosopher of the Age of Reason, believed that the human mind is capable of achieving objectively true explanations of the material world, including the human body, in terms uncontaminated by spiritual or emotional qualities. This separation of the human mind and the natural world from God and from each other enabled the rapid growth in knowledge of anatomy, physiology and pharmacology. The phenomenal success of the scientific method created great expectations. Descartes himself, keenly interested in medicine, was convinced that it would eventually be possible to extend the human life span to several centuries. Science would make man the master and possessor of nature. Nature repossessed Descartes in 1650, at the tender age of 53.

Despite the liberating influences of the Age of Reason and the consequent growth of medical science, it appears that the physician was little more than an idealised father figure, a priest, whose main task at the bedside of the sick was to exhibit Christian faith, hope and kindness. The doctor-patient relationship was viewed in paternalistic terms – benefiting the sick served as the primary motivation and justification for the physician's behaviour. Patients were expected to comply with 'doctor's orders', and the physician had the authority to override their wishes if he considered it in their own best interest. The Hippocratic *Oath*, which was taken as the foundation of medical ethics for centuries, represents the relationship between physician, teacher and patient in terms of a family. Students relate to teachers as parents, and to colleagues as brothers. Patients are viewed as children, dependent on the kindness of the strong and wise father.

Verdi captures the ideal physician of the nineteenth century in his famous opera, *La Traviata*.[1] In the closing act we find Violetta suffering from the terminal stages of tuberculosis, abandoned by her friends and mourning the loss of her lover, Alfredo. Then her good and faithful friend, Dr. Grenvil, comes to visit

---

[1] This opera was originally entitled 'Love and Death', a title that well-suited an opera which had as its theme the love affair between Violetta and Alfredo, and her untimely and tragic death. Before its first performance in 1853, sensors requested that the title be changed to 'The Fallen Woman' ('Traviata') because of the adulterous nature of the love affair. The opera became a lesson in Christian morality; Violetta is punished for her sins.

her. He sits quietly next to her, displaying the character traits of a true gentleman. But he also does what any experienced physician of the time would do – he takes her pulse and realises that his patient is dying. He does not share his bleak diagnosis with Violetta. Instead, he whispers to the attendant: 'Her consumption leaves her only a few hours to live'. He encourages Violetta to be brave, telling her that 'convalescence isn't far off'. In the final moments of her life, Dr. Grenvil sits passively by, observing her reconciliation with Alfredo and listening as she speaks her last words. Violetta gives a great cry of 'Oh! I shall live again! Oh joy!', collapses, and dies.

Set in the early nineteenth century, Verdi's opera represents a stage in the development of medicine where it was conceived both as an art and a science. The *science* concentrated on objective description of the disease processes, discovering universal laws that are mechanistic in nature and which exclude the humanistic dimensions of the ill person from consideration. His knowledge as a scientist allowed Dr. Grenvil to correctly diagnose his patient as suffering from tuberculosis and to predict the course of this disease. But his greater knowledge did not enable him to affect a cure. Until the early twentieth century physicians could do very little to affect the disease process. If they wanted to help a patient, to make any kind of contribution to his or her well-being, they had to do more than give accurate diagnoses and prognoses. They had to be able to practice the *art* of medicine, which involved relating to patients as human beings, trying to understand their suffering, comfort them, and reassure them that 'all will be well soon'. The art of medicine was never clearly defined, since it was not a question of scientific knowledge but of practical wisdom, something the physician could only gain from experience and by following the example of his mentor. The ideal physician was the Christian gentleman; someone who was medically knowledgeable but also educated in morality, religion and psychology. Although medical science was clearly separated from religion, the art or practice of medicine maintained its religious significance. Medical skills were seen as a gift from God, designed to be used for human benefit, to affect a change in a physical state or process that distresses, debilitates, or destroys human life. The basis of the art of healing was not knowledge, but a way of interacting with individual patients. Its goal was to establish a fiduciary relationship in which the doctor was entrusted with the power necessary for benefiting the patient. To possess medical skills was to be able to *care* for the sick, to be troubled by the other's trouble.

Within the paternalistic model of the doctor-patient relationship the analogy between the roles of physician and father rests on the father's authority to make certain decisions on behalf of his children. This analogy gained added significance with the Christian view of the physician as an instrument of God, the true Father and Healer of mankind. His authority was based, in the first place, on the father's superior knowledge and insight. The Christian physician was a wise man, a well-educated and respected member of the community. He knew the patient's medical history better than anyone else, having treated her for the whole or most of her life, and understood all of her fears and desires. As a well-read member of the Christian community, he also knew what the patient's wishes *should* be. The second basis of authority is the father's (presumed) benevolence.

The Christian physician had a sincere desire to act in the patient's best interest. Dr. Grenvil's lie was rooted in compassion and aimed at protecting Violetta against the awful truth of approaching death.

During the 1960s and 1970s people became increasingly dissatisfied with the paternalistic model of decision-making, claiming a right to participate in decisions about their health as part of the more general right to self-determination. The rejection of the physician's authority was, however, only the last step in a gradual erosion of the analogy between physician and father that occurred with the modernisation of medicine.

*From Art to Science*

Modern science and technology have dramatically altered the nature and basis of the paternalist's authority. As the explanatory power of scientific theories and the effectiveness of medical technologies grew, the physician became less like a father and more like a scientist. The human dimension of the clinical encounter gradually lessened in significance as a result of being viewed as subjective and not capable of measurement or verification, and hence as unscientific. The distinction between the science and the art of medicine disappeared, and the clinical situation came to be interpreted almost entirely from the perspective of the natural sciences. The physician's ways of benefiting also changed significantly – the aim was no longer simply to comfort, but to cure, to combat disease.

Were one to rewrite *La Traviata* to suit our age, one would first have to explain how it came about that, despite the ready availability of antibiotics, the patient's tuberculosis was allowed to progress this far. (Perhaps she was a missionary in Africa.) Then we would find Violetta in a hospital bed with our hero, Dr. Grenvil, masterfully outwitting the disease by placing her on the latest in life-saving technology, coupled with an impressive regimen of drugs. Violetta might not sing, but we wouldn't have to sit through the tormenting final scene of her death either. To make up for the lost romance of the final scene, we could witness the joyful affair of her marriage to Alfredo. Dr. Grenvil will probably not be invited – it is unlikely that the couple would know him very well.

To fully appreciate the shift in medicine from (witchcraft to) art to science it is necessary to highlight some of the most important developments in the Modern era. Whereas some developments occurred gradually, others happened almost accidentally, their meaning and significance often escaping the individuals who received credit for them. One such figure is Thomas Sydenham (1624-1689), a physician and intimate colleague of John Locke, who was given much credit for the transformation of the medical perception of disease. Sydenham was sometimes called the 'English Hippocrates', since he rejected supernatural explanations of disease and thought of healing as a natural process which the physician could assist. He did not see disease as a purely local process, but as a reaction of the whole organism. The doctor had to treat, not a single organ, but the sick person as a whole, and for this it was necessary to understand the lives of patients. When asked by an eager student which books he should read to qualify him for medical practice, Sydenham replied: 'Read *Don Quixote*, it is a very good book. I read it still' (cited in Reiser 1993:121). Literature, he believed, could provide the young physician with a better understanding of the complexities and ambiguities of life.

It is ironic that Sydenham's greatest clinical achievement, his concept of illness as disease, would begin the process of removing from medicine a concern with personal experience. His radical wish to improve medicine for the benefit of all led him to study epidemic fevers rather than individual patients and their constitutions. In the Hippocratic tradition, illness was interwoven with the patient's own life history. The patient and his illness were inseparably connected as a unique event, one which the physician did not expect to recur. While Sydenham followed this tradition of writing cases from the patient's perspective, he discovered that diseases were discrete entities that could be classified by their predisposing traits and characteristic symptoms. The illnesses of different individuals could be named and identified and transformed into specific disease-histories. Whereas Hippocrates wrote the histories of sick persons, Sydenham wrote the histories of diseases.

In this way Sydenham laid the foundations for the science of pathology – the study of diseases. The term 'pathophysiology' lost its meaning as 'an inquiry into the nature of suffering', and became simply 'the science of diseases', the study of the set of symptoms and other clinical findings with the aim of identifying the disease which causes the symptoms. Sydenham's success convinced other physicians to study particular diseases in an attempt to establish order in the vast ocean of symptoms. Although Sydenham himself did not favour aggressive therapies, his work established in physicians the belief that diseases are entities that can be dominated and conquered by those who have the medical knowledge and skills to recognise and explain their nature and existence. Atypical cases were often encountered, but these were seen as deviations from a standard type or norm. The type or norm existed, even though it was sometimes difficult to understand why divergences took place. In this way the symptoms that combine patients into populations have become more significant than the symptoms that separate patients as individuals. This hallmark of modern medicine was a major step in physicians' growing detachment from the unique traits of their patients. While greatly enhancing the accuracy of diagnoses and the effectiveness of treatments, it diminished physicians' ability to understand and be able to identify with the individual patient's suffering.[2]

The Newtonian mechanistic philosophy had profound implications for medicine. Most influential was Descartes' image of the body as a machine and his separation of the spheres of mind and body. He argued that the body worked mechanically like the rest of the natural world; it was subject to scientific laws and its behaviour was therefore entirely predictable. J.O. de la Mettrie (1709-1751), a French physician and author of *L'Homme Machine*, interpreted the mechanistic view of the human organism in medical terms. La Mettrie questioned whether any aspect of human behaviour could reasonably be assumed to be distinct from

---

[2] For more detailed discussions of Sydenham's contribution, see Sigerist (1933:175-182), Jonsen (1990:84-89), Nuland (1993:89-90) and Reiser (1993:121-125).

physiology. He consistently emphasised the physiological sources and causes of complex human behaviour, and reinforced the correlation between human behaviour and the actions of animals. The implication of this philosophy was that the patient came to be treated as a biological machine that will continue to function normally, even if there is no mind or consciousness at all. Disease came to be understood as a purely physical phenomenon, a mechanical failure requiring medical intervention to restore physiological harmony. The patient's conscious interpretation of pain was irrelevant to the restoration of his health. In the medical sphere the Cartesian dualism lapsed into a materialistic monism: Humans were reduced to machines.

Physicians such as Georg Stahl (1660-1734) denounced this materialism, advocating instead an 'animism' that postulated the existence of a God-given, non-mechanical soul as the essential quality of human beings. Co-ordinated and purposive human actions could not, he argued, be explained in terms of mechanical chain-reactions, like a stack of tumbling dominoes. Wholes were greater than the sum of their parts. Human activity presupposed the presence of a soul as a constantly intervening and guiding power. The soul was an agent of consciousness and physiological regulation, and a bodyguard against sickness. Disease was caused by a disturbance of vital functions provoked by misdirected activities of the soul; to cure disease, one had to understand the soul. This anti-mechanistic movement did not, however, succeed in recovering the humanity of medical practice. Instead, it laid the basis for the establishment of psychiatry as a separate discipline from physiology. Physiologists sought to maintain a barrier between the study of vital functions and the study of mental phenomena, both in method and practice. Stahl's attempt to maintain the humane aspects of medicine therefore served to create a further division between body and mind.

During the eighteenth century physicians for the most part relied on the use of the five senses to make their diagnoses; they would feel the pulse, sniff for indications of decay, taste urine, listen for breathing irregularities, and observe skin colour. Although the invention of modern diagnostic equipment is sometimes seen as the beginning of the 'loss of the personal touch', it had obvious benefits for both physicians and patients. Apart from allowing more accurate diagnoses, diagnostic equipment had the function of decreasing the need for direct physical contact between doctor and patient. In eighteenth century Britain, physicians rarely performed physical examinations, choosing to rely on the patient's detailed narration of their own history. They maintained, in stark contrast to physicians in other countries, that little could be learnt through physical examinations. It is more likely, however, that this approach stemmed from their dislike of touching the bodies of sick strangers. The stethoscope, invented in 1816, soon became an essential piece of equipment for any health-care professional. The stethoscope is a relatively simple device for transmitting sound more accurately than the human ear, but physicians of the time no doubt found it very useful as a distancing mechanism. Technology also reduced the extent to which physicians relied on history taking, personal experience and intuition. Physicians used the findings provided by new technologies to create portraits of disease.

By far the most significant impact of technology was on the methods used to pursue certain goals. Technology is not simply a collection of machines, but involves the application of the scientific method to production processes. It requires a disciplined, systematic mode of thinking and is aimed at replicating specific results in a reliable fashion. The science of statistics became an indispensable part of clinical medicine in the 1830s, when Pierre Lois devised his 'numerical method' of determining the efficacy of a procedure. Before then, the only statistics available to physicians were birth and mortality rates. These made it possible to detect growth and decline in the size of a population, but not to affect public health in any way. But the Enlightenment project brought home the belief that what could be enumerated could also be expressed in terms of natural laws, even if they were only laws of probability. This made it possible for science to master the natural world. The advantage of the introduction of sound statistical methods for controlled trials was that the safety and efficiency of medicine could now be determined statistically, rather than by personal experience or intuition.

With the growth of medical science and technology came a closer specification of the role of the physician and the goal of medical treatment. As we have seen, the Christian physician, like a good father, brought love and compassion to the bedside of the sick, and sometimes even helped to secure their religious salvation. In contrast, the proper end of modern medicine became the physical health of the patient, not the alteration of the patient's conduct, his moral goodness, happiness or salvation. The goals of medicine were confined to what medical science and technology could produce. Hence Lasagna, a professor in medicine, writes: 'Is medicine primarily a "moral enterprise"? I doubt it, any more than plumbing or auto repair is' (1977:44). Dr. Richard Cabot (1868-1939), a distinguished member of the Harvard Medical School faculty, played an important part in delineating the goals of twentieth century medicine. Cabot laid the basis for the 'ethics of competence' – the mastery of the science and skills of diagnosis, therapy, and prevention of disease. He specified competence as primarily *clinical* competence, as the mastery of diagnostics and therapeutics, requiring that the 'benefits' and 'harms' be translated into specific clinical effects for the presenting patient. In the assessment of professional propriety it was no longer important whether the practitioner went to church on Sunday, swore the Hippocratic *Oath*, or was law-abiding and loyal to the codified rules of his society. What counted for Cabot was whether a practitioner understood specific diseases, their causes, symptoms, prognoses and effective treatments. It is therefore the possession of medical skills, not moral and religious beliefs, which has become the standard to which all physicians are held by both the medical profession and the general public. The 'ethics of competence' finds its expression in statements such as 'I'd rather have a competent bastard do my surgery than a bumbling humanist' (Jonsen 1990:124).

### *From Virtue to Duty*

The first change in the doctor-patient relationship, then, was that the physician's authority came to lie in the superiority of his scientific knowledge and technological expertise, rather than in any fatherly wisdom. Further erosion of the parental analogy occurred with the shift from a virtue- to a principle-based ethic. The ideal Christian physician, like a good father, was motivated to act by his benevolent concern for his patients. He was an independent philanthropist who felt himself obliged to do his best to help the patient, but the patient had no corresponding right to such treatment. Today the clinical encounter is more commonly perceived as a transaction between individuals in which their respective rights and responsibilities stem from contracts or agreements. For instance, Beauchamp and Childress argue that in contrast to the Hippocratic physician, health-care professionals are today deeply indebted to society for their education and other privileges, as well as to patients for research, 'practice' and financial reward. This indebtedness creates an obligation of general beneficence both to patients and society, so that the role of medical professionals is misconstrued if modelled primarily on philanthropy, altruism and personal commitment. Their care is rooted in the 'reciprocity of giving and receiving' (1994:270).

This contractual relationship could only arise because the demonstrated success of modern medicine restored public faith in the powers of medicine. Public scepticism and hesitance to call for a physician gave way to a demand to share in the benefits of scientific medicine. This placed physicians in a position to determine the nature and terms of the contractual relationship, which is very different from the doctor-patient relationship in previous eras. The livelihood of the Hippocratic physician depended on his reputation, and having as he did only his random experience and untested intuition to count on, he was understandably concerned with winning public confidence. In early Modern Europe the practitioner was often criticised by the patient's relatives and friends, who offered their own advice and suggested alternative treatments. Learned physicians borrowed and used popular remedies from wise women and lay people, and medicine was popularised in a number of vernacular books. Because medical knowledge, terminology and treatment were not so esoteric that the patient could not understand it, the doctor-patient relationship was more equal. In contrast, the twentieth century physician became a detached authority-figure, his competence rooted in experimental science and the elaborate methods of clinical evaluation and patterns of clinical care. Whereas he could support his claims with the results of clinical trials and studies in epidemiology, patients possessed neither the knowledge nor the vocabulary to question or engage in debate with the learned man. They understood that they could only gain the benefits of medicine within the context of a transaction in which they entrusted themselves to the physician and complied with his orders. Whereas the Christian physician thought that medical skills were given to him by the grace of God for the sake of the suffering, the enlightened physician slowly lost his modesty. Drawing on John Locke's conception of rights as property rights, they came to think of medical knowledge and skills as property over which one might have dominance, giving them the rightful authority to specify the terms of the contract.

Sydenham's conception of disease as a natural entity lies at the basis of the frequently-heard objection that 'doctors tend to treat diseases and not patients'. Proponents of the medicalisation critique take an overwhelmingly negative view of doctors as attempting to enhance their position by presenting themselves as possessing the exclusive right to define and treat illness, thereby subordinating the opinions and experiences of the patient. Jonsen argues that physicians of the Modern period came to perceive themselves not only as having a right over medical expertise, but also over disease itself. Discovered by them, and often named after them, disease came to be seen as the property of physicians which they aimed to dominate and destroy in order to make the body healthy. Although the disease may be in the patient, it belonged to physicians. The contract was perceived as giving the physician right of way to go through the patient in order to get to the disease: 'Even though the physician must get access to the disease through the patient – he cannot trespass – he almost has an independent right over the disease itself' (Jonsen 1990:91-94). In this view, the contractual relationship consists of the patient handing over certain freedoms in order to obtain the benefits that the other effects.

However, it is both unfair and over-simplified to suggest that individual physicians had the authority to control the terms of the contract and the nature of their obligations to patients. As individuals, physicians are subordinated to a professional body that demands certain patterns of behaviour. Dr. Sherwin Nuland, a twentieth century surgeon and medical writer, admits that the driving force of modern medicine is the quest to solve 'The Riddle' – to make a correct diagnosis, and to design and carry out the cure. As a young student he wanted only to care for the sick, and saw himself as bringing hope and comfort to patients and their families. Yet he became 'the embodiment of a biomedical problem-solver'. The drive to solve 'The Riddle' will sometimes be at odds with the best interest of the patient, but by giving up the quest, by admitting defeat, he would risk the scorn of his peers. Although Nuland laments some of his heroic attempts to cure disease, he admits that he would probably repeat his behaviour, since 'the code of the profession of surgery demands that no patient... be allowed to die if a straightforward operation can save her, and we who break that fundamental rule, no matter the humaneness of our motive, do so at our own peril' (Nuland 1994:247-249).

Nuland here touches on an important feature of the shift from a virtue- to a principle-based ethic. It is not simply that physicians are no longer as compassionate and humane as in 'days gone by', but that virtuous ideals cannot form the motivation for morally-appropriate behaviour. As a member of a professional organisation he is *obliged* to follow a specific ethical code. He could have a very compassionate understanding of the patient's emotional and existential suffering, but this compassion is (and must be) irrelevant when responding in a way that is both professionally and morally appropriate. The full significance of professionalisation is not always appreciated. *It is not simply that the patient is treated as an instance of disease rather than as an individual; it is also that the physician no longer reacts as an individual but as a representative of a profession.* The professional duty of care demands that everything possible be done for the patient, despite the costs, burdens or consequences for any involved. Sir William Osler states: 'If a life is worth living at all, it is certainly worth living to the very end, a position from which the conscientious physician has no possible escape in the care of the cases which he is called upon to treat' (cited in Keown 1997:76). Unlike his predecessors, the modern doctor cannot simply refuse to treat terminally-ill patients; he is 'called upon'. Unlike the prudish British doctor of the eighteenth century, he cannot decide that physical examinations are not worth the effort. He cannot escape his professional duties.

Side-by-side with the development of modern scientific medicine with its emphasis on objectivity, rationality and value-neutrality, a shift has taken place in medical ethics from a virtue-based morality to a principle-based ethic. The Enlightenment philosophy, exemplified by the work of Kant, lies at the basis of the principle-based ethic adopted in the medical field. The contemporary physician is no longer expected to have the virtues of benevolence and non-malevolence; instead, he is required by law to act according to the principles of beneficence and non-maleficence.

A significant advantage of reformulating virtues in terms of professional duties is that the latter are codifiable and thus more readily enforceable. Hippocrates laments the fact that many physicians have gained the reputation of healers through false demonstrations of virtue and competence. He ascribes the low esteem in which the art of medicine is held to the fact that there were no penalties for malpractice in the Greek states. The physician who transgressed risked only dishonour, and 'dishonour does not wound those who are compacted of it' (*Law* I). In pre-modern societies, the sick person who sought the help of a physician was left to rely on his judgement of the character and trustworthiness of the physician. Since the latter's private life was usually transparent to his local community, he would soon earn a bad reputation if he abused their trust. In modern societies, however, a patient may not see the same doctor even during the same illness on any two successive occasions; different doctors attend to different members of the family and to different parts of the body. The patient now approaches the physician as one stranger to another, so that the basis of trust cannot be sought in the virtuous character of the physician. The impersonal standards of a professional organisation are intended to ensure that when we confront any individual who fills a given role within that profession, we can expect exactly the same outcome. The individual is trained to fulfil a specific function, and can be substituted for any other individual with the same training. When consulting doctors one can feel assured that they are bound by a clear set of obligations to respect one's rights, and that fear of litigation, if nothing else, would keep them from intentional harm.

A closely-related advantage is that physicians can now be held accountable for their failure to perform the duties specified in the professional code. In traditional structures authority always is, and is known to be, fallible. The traditional physician's mistakes were not really his own errors, but instead derived from the very nature of his activity. Everyone understood that disease was often stronger than the means at the physician's disposal. It was more important for the physician not to abuse patients' trust. An occasional honest error was not culpable and never ground for doubting or dispensing with the physician's authority: 'Intellectual error is tolerable within the context of a trust that has not been abused; it provides no ground for accusation of breach of contract precisely because the relationship of patient to physician is not merely or even primarily contractual' (MacIntyre 1977:207-209).

By contrast, the Cabotean ethic of competence is far less tolerant of errors in judgement. Because the doctor-patient relationship is a contractual one, physician error does provide a ground for accusations of malpractice. Advances in medical knowledge, in particular the science of statistics, have made it possible to formulate a standard of due care in more specific terms. Professional codes protect patients from the careless or unreasonable imposition of risks or harm. It is no longer enough to have good intentions; physicians are required to perform the duty of benefiting patients, and may be held accountable for failing to do so.

Even if the physician's motives are pure, it can be argued that good character and intentions do not guarantee that the agent will succeed in accomplishing the desired goals. Being a *benevolent* person does not ensure that one will perform *beneficent* actions. An agent may, through ignorance, undue emotional involvement or lack of competence fail to benefit someone, or may even end up harming her, despite his good intentions. Virtue-ethics, it is often claimed, is not action-oriented. The basic moral question for virtue-ethicists is not 'What shall I do?', but rather, 'What shall I be?' Furthermore, since it focuses only on the goodness (or badness) of the agent's character and intentions, virtue ethics is seemingly unable to provide a means of holding people responsible for their actions. Perhaps being a kind and compassionate physician was sufficient in previous decades when there was very little that medicine could accomplish. But physicians today are required to be skilful and knowledgeable, to be able to do more than provide comfort and reassurance.

The virtues have also been criticised as being too vague in guiding decision-making and action. Louden argues that the virtue-ethicist, when asked 'What should we do?' can only answer 'Do what a good person would do' (1997:205-210). By contrast, duty- or principle-based ethical systems have the advantage that they focus on formulating rules of conduct or moral imperatives. Central to Kant's moral philosophy is the principle of universalisability, according to which the rules of morality, if they are rational, must be the same for all rational beings. The answer to the question 'What should I do?' must be derived from a conjunction of premises consisting of (1) a rule or universal imperative enjoining all actions of a certain type in situations of a certain type, and (2) a statement to the effect that the particular situation is of the type specified in the applicable universal imperative.

A final reason for favouring a principle-based ethic derives from the Kantian argument that virtues typically contain an emotional element, and may therefore hamper the agent in making rational and objective decisions that would enable him to succeed in benefiting patients. Compassion – placing oneself in the position of the sufferer, *imagining* what he is going through, sharing his *feelings* – simply does not provide sufficient insight into the person's disease or illness. A much more accurate understanding, it is argued, may be gained through the rational, distanced and scientific approach to disease and illness characteristic of the post-Enlightenment era.

*From Patient to Agent*

The analogy between father and physician gradually eroded with the modernisation of medicine. The physician's authority to make decisions on behalf of his patients no longer rested on his fatherly or priestly wisdom, but on his scientific knowledge; his decision-making power was no longer legitimated by his altruistic motives, but by his professional duty to benefit patients. The final phase in the decline of (the acceptability of) paternalism occurred when Western societies began to challenge the physician's authority to make decisions on behalf of his patient. The relationship between doctor and patient is now construed as one between equals, which requires a recognition of the right of patients to make free and informed decisions about matters concerning their own health.

Contemporary bioethicists often phrase the central moral issue arising from this shift in terms of a conflict between the principles of autonomy and beneficence: 'When, if ever, is it justifiable to override a patient's decision for the sake of his own welfare?' I will deal with issues surrounding patient autonomy, informed consent and medical paternalism in Chapters Two and Five. In what follows I examine the socio-political context within which the conflict between autonomy and beneficence originated and which resulted in the rejection of medical paternalism.

The adoption of the principle of patient autonomy was the outcome of the critique of the process of medicalisation in the 1960s and 1970s. The critique emanated from social movements that took a Marxist or liberal humanist perspective. Despite their differences, both these groups were characterised by their emphasis on individual freedom, human rights and the necessity of social change. They criticised the process whereby 'normal' or 'natural' physiological processes are defined as pathological and in need of treatment, arguing that this objectifies human beings who come to be treated as medicalised bodies. The rejection of the existing structure of medical decision-making formed part of a revolt against the dehumanising effects of the process of modernisation, and was a clear statement of mistrust in the medical profession. Patient autonomy was meant to be part of the solution to the medicalisation of Western societies but, as will become clear later on, insofar as the notion of autonomy is itself a modern one, it cannot function as a cure for the maladies of modernity.

A central concern was with the dependency that scientific medicine was seen to encourage. The tremendous growth of the power of Western medicine has made people dependent upon strangers for the most intimate of their physical needs, leaving them vulnerable and exposed. Having little or no understanding of scientific medicine, yet with a naive trust in their medical fathers, patients could easily become victims of modern medicine. In its weakest form, this critique holds that paternalists, although they may be well-intentioned, could still fail to benefit (or perhaps even harm) patients. Since people hold different views of what is harmful or beneficial, and since there are usually diverse treatment possibilities, each with its own expected effects, the physician can no longer assume that all reasonable patients would have the same values and preferences. Thus Irving Zola (1972) argued that medicine had begun to take on the role of social regulation traditionally performed by religion and the law: Doctors decided what counted as disease and then proceeded to decide on the appropriate treatment. The most radical form of this critique came from Ivan Illich (1975). He argued that scientific medicine undermined rather than improved health, both through its iatrogenic side-effects and by diminishing people's capacity to deal autonomously with their own health. A feminist version of this critique maintains that the increasing power of scientific medicine has detrimental effects for traditionally disempowered and exploited groups, insofar as such a change deflects questions of social inequality into the realm of illness and disease, there to be treated inappropriately by drugs and other medical therapies.

The answer, according to these critics, was for patients to challenge the right of medical practitioners to make decisions on their behalf. They advocated the empowerment of patients, encouraging them to regain control of their own health by refusing unwanted treatment and/or seeking out alternative treatment. The acknowledgement of the patient's right to autonomy, including the physician's duty to obtain informed consent prior to proceeding with treatment, is an attempt to rectify the power imbalance, and thus to protect the patient from exploitation and other unwarranted or unwelcome intrusions. The kind of freedom that matters for liberals is 'negative' freedom, the freedom from undue interference by government or other institutions. In the medical field, the rights to self-determination and individual freedom translated into, among others, the right to refuse treatment, the right to non-interference, and the right not to be used as a research subject against one's wishes. It was under the banner of negative freedom that appeals were made to legalise passive euthanasia: Individuals have the right to refuse life-prolonging treatment.

Attempts to justify some degree of paternalistic decision-making often rely on the very same aspects of the doctor-patient relationship. It is pointed out that patients are typically sick and medically ignorant, often overwhelmed by fear, depression, trauma and so forth, while physicians are typically fit and medically knowledgeable. Instead of claiming a right to self-determination as a corrective to the power imbalance, the patient's relative powerlessness is cited as a justification for paternalistic decision-making. Dependency is reason for abandoning, not demanding, the right to make decisions for oneself. Dr. Oliver Sacks dwells on his own experience as a patient:

> [T]hough as a sick patient, in hospital, one was reduced to moral infancy, this was not a malicious degradation, but a biological and spiritual need of the hurt creature. One had to go back, one had to regress, for one might indeed be as helpless as a child, whether one liked it, or willed it, or not. In hospital one became again a child with parents (parents who might be good or bad), and this might be felt as 'infantilising' and degrading, or as a sweet and sorely-needed nourishing (1991:128).

What lies at the basis of the dissatisfaction with paternalism is not an imbalance of power as such, but mistrust. One's experience of and response to dependence is shaped by one's trust (or lack of trust) in the caregiver. However, this is not the type of mistrust exemplified by Illich's work – it is not lack of faith in the effectiveness of medical treatment. People would not seek out medical help, and the medical enterprise would not be as powerful and as influential as it is today, if people did not believe that medicine holds a promise or possibility of benefit.

Another, closely related, concern that underlies the medicalisation critique is that dependency is undignified. This objection focuses not so much on the potential for harm through the abuse of power, but on the indignity of being a patient in the modern hospital. This is clearly illustrated in the *Oxford English Dictionary (OED)*, which contains the definition of 'patient' as 'a person or thing that undergoes some action, or to whom or which something is done'; 'that which receives impressions from external agents', 'as correlative to agent, and distinguished from instrument; a recipient'. It illustrates its use with a statement by Wesley (1791): '*He that is not free is not an Agent, but a Patient*'. Apart from protecting against exploitation and harm, the autonomy model of decision-making is supposed to recover the dignity of patients by recognising their claims to privacy, self-direction, the establishment of their own values and life plans based on information and reasoning, and the freedom to act on the results of their contemplation. In this view, the fundamental responsibility of the physician is to respect and to facilitate patients' 'positive' freedom of self-determination by adequately informing them of alternative modes of treatment, so that they are able to make informed and reasoned decisions about their own treatment (Pellegrino and Thomasma 1988:12).

In response to the view that the primary duty of physicians is to benefit patients, autonomists claim that a physician often cannot heal a person just by curing a disease, especially if the physician systematically ignores or disregards the patient's view. In assuming that 'the doctor always knows best', it is said, the paternalist position denies the freedom and autonomy of individual patients by assuming that they are incompetent to participate in decisions affecting their health and lives. By thus violating a patient's autonomy, the paternalist does not heal the patient, which is the primary aim of medicine, but wounds his dignity (Pellegrino and Thomasma 1988:23). Becoming 'medicalised', it is felt, denies rational, independent human action by allowing doctors to dictate how patients should behave.

This view is rooted in the Kantian ethic, where respect for autonomy is not considered a means to promoting human welfare, but as a requirement deriving from the nature of rational beings. According to Kant, it follows logically from the principle of universalisability that respect for autonomy is a necessary feature of being a rational agent, and that this is only possible within the context of respect for the autonomy of all rational agents. In medicine, the recognition of the principle of patient autonomy was an attempt to safeguard the freedom and dignity of the human being as a *person*, as someone who has goals of his own. To violate a person's autonomy is to treat him as a means to an end, and hence as a non-rational or heteronomous being, a being that is not self-determining but determined by external causes.

One cannot deny the necessity nor the value of the almost universal acceptance of the principle of patient autonomy in Western medical practice over the last few decades. Being informed of one's diagnosis, having access to one's medical records and having the final say in one's own treatment have obvious empowering and liberating effects. But the adoption of this principle has not been effective as an answer to the dehumanising effects of modern medicine. As much as ever, people complain that they are 'objectified by the medical gaze', that they are not 'respected as persons', or simply that 'doctors do not understand'. I will explore the weaknesses of the autonomy model in more detail in the chapters that follow. At this stage a few brief comments will suffice.

The failure of the autonomy movement to re-humanise medicine, I suspect, lies in the very notion of autonomy. Autonomy originated as a scientific ideal in the seventeenth century Enlightenment, that of gaining objectively-true knowledge of the external world, uncontaminated by prejudice and subjectivity. From the laboratory the problem of autonomy migrated to the political arena. John Locke, inspired by his scientist friends, saw autonomy as a crucial tool for a society struggling to transform itself from the subject of the divine rule of monarchs to democratic self-government. In this way the scientific ideals of rationality, objective experimentation and autonomous observation translated into the political and moral ideals of English liberalism: Man became the proprietor of his own person, in control of his own destiny. During the 1960s liberal humanists called into question the social role played by members of powerful and high-status groups such as the legal and medical professions. They put forward as an ideal the notion that individuals should not have their autonomy constrained by those more powerful. The notion of autonomy therefore has its foundations in the Lockean ideals of rationality, objectivity, and independence. However, the appeal to patient autonomy also emerged as a *rejection* of the Lockean-inspired view of medical expertise as the property of physicians that gives them a right to specify the terms of the clinical transaction. The counter-movement responded to medicine's dehumanising effects by joining the Modernist's club. This movement, I believe, cannot fully counteract the problems of medicalisation since it employs an impoverished conception of 'personhood' as requiring independent, rational thought and agency, unconstrained by emotional and spiritual qualities. As such, it responds to, or attempts to rectify an impoverished conception of what 'dehumanisation' or 'depersonalisation' involves, namely a loss or denial of such rational, independent human action.

## Conclusion

The basis of the dissatisfaction with medical authority, I think, can be found in the process of modernisation itself. First, it lies in the tendency of scientific medicine to focus on the elimination of disease, physical pain and disability while denying or disregarding patients' emotional and existential suffering. Indeed, for a patient to be taken seriously, to be respected as an autonomous person, he or she has to demonstrate an ability to think rationally, to reach judgements that are uncontaminated by emotional and spiritual qualities and independent of the opinions of family and friends. Secondly, it lies in the principle-based ethic adopted by the medical profession, which has as an implication that physicians themselves no longer decide and act as individuals, but as members of a profession. They cannot allow themselves to be taken in by a patient's suffering, to feel her pain, or to act on compassion. In the following chapter I examine the shortcomings of the modernistic ethic in more detail by focusing on the principle-based approach to moral problems surrounding euthanasia.

# Chapter Two

# Euthanasia and the Principle-Based Ethic

## Introduction

In the last few decades a number of steps have been taken to ensure greater respect for the needs and rights of patients. Most modern hospitals have a ready supply of brochures and pamphlets informing patients of their rights and responsibilities. In stark contrast to previous decades, patients now have a right to be adequately informed about their diagnosis, prognosis and available medical procedures, and a right to participate in medical decision-making. Patients are entitled to have their need for dignity and privacy respected, and to receive competent, considerate and confidential care in a respectful and culturally-acceptable manner. They also have a right to refuse treatment, even when such treatment is deemed necessary to prevent or remove harmful conditions. This right has also been extended to incompetent patients in the forms of advance directives and surrogate decision-making.

Yet various studies conducted in recent years show that, despite steps taken to protect the rights of patients, many people still endure extreme suffering at the end of life. A major study conducted in the USA revealed that 50 percent of patients in the five major tertiary-care hospitals it studied were reported to have suffered moderate to severe pain at least 50 percent of the time during the last two or three days of their lives (SUPPORT 1995). It has also become clear that advance directives have failed to protect the wishes and interests of vulnerable patients. Despite the legal requirement of informed consent, many patients are ill-informed or lack an understanding of their condition and of the options available to them. Medical professionals frequently misunderstand their patients' preferences or refuse to respect their wishes. Terminally-ill patients are often of dubious competence to make decisions about their own treatment. As a result, many suffer unnecessarily before dying.

These problems, I will argue, are symptomatic of a more fundamental shortcoming of the dominant approach to ethical issues in medicine. The language of rights and principles is ill-suited to dealing with the problems and questions surrounding the treatment of terminally- or chronically-ill patients. I shall focus on three such questions. The first is whether compassion can ever be seen as the appropriate motive for ending a patient's life. The second concerns the goals of medical practice, more specifically, what limits should be placed on the competence of physicians to prolong life, and whether death ('treating to die') can ever be seen as the appropriate goal of medicine. The third question is whether euthanasia can ever be justified as a means of respecting a person or preserving his dignity. Having rejected the virtues as morally irrelevant, there is very little that principle-based theories can provide in response to these questions. Their focus is on justifying old rules or formulating new ones, and subjective terms such as compassion, mercy and dignity are of no use if one's aim is to develop a set of rules that is universalisable, impartial and objective.

## The Argument from Mercy and the Death of Compassion

One of the oldest arguments in favour of euthanasia or 'mercy-killing' is that it is cruel or inhumane to stand by without helping a suffering person to end his miserable existence. In the *Journal of Pediatrics* Dr. J.M. Freeman expresses his frustration brought about by the conflict between his compassion for suffering infants and a medical ethic which demands of him not to end life. He writes:

> Having seen children with unoperated meningomyeloceles lie around the ward for weeks or months untreated, waiting to die, one cannot help but feel that the highest form of medical ethic would have been to end the pain and suffering.... Should society not allow physicians to alleviate the pain and suffering and help nature take its course – quickly? (1972:905)

After the appearance of this editorial Freeman was criticised by various physicians who pointed out that one should not rely on sentiment and emotion when making moral decisions. The responsible physician maintains a rational and objective distance. Freeman's appeal for legalising euthanasia is clearly clouded by emotion: It is simply not true that infants with unoperated meningomyeloceles 'lie around the ward' – they are kept as comfortable as possible – and neither are they 'waiting to die' – they have no conception of what is happening to them.

The Scientific Revolution and the Era of Enlightenment, having freed rationality from the yoke of emotions, intuition, superstition and other irrational restraints in practising medicine as a science, have had a significant impact on the practice of medicine. Western medicine has come to rely on a strict opposition between reason and emotion. It is characterised by its focus on explaining physiological disorders, as opposed to understanding a person's suffering. Whereas the physician of previous eras had very little scientific knowledge and technological means to help him in his attempts to benefit patients, and relied for the most part on intuition, empathy and random experience to be able to understand the nature of a patient's suffering, the modern physician has at his disposal advanced forms of scientific knowledge and technical skills. This has allowed for more accurate diagnoses and effective treatment of diseases, with a consequent faith in the powers of science over the powers of intuition. The belief that all medical problems are soluble by scientific research and technological innovation has also brought about a loss of compassion. The physician of the early twentieth century achieved very little, but was highly esteemed for his compassion and care. The modern doctor can achieve infinitely more, but is often regarded as a cold, impersonal technocrat whose primary aim is personal enrichment.

However, critics who call for a more humane medicine tend to be overly pessimistic in their assessment of the character of contemporary physicians. It is true that the Cartesian-Newtonian paradigm of disease has expelled emotional and psychological factors from the domain of medical science and education, with the result that physicians are often ill-equipped to deal with the suffering of their patients. Yet this problem cannot be fully attributed to physicians as individual persons – it is also rooted in the expectations of patients. Modern society in general tends to view disease as a purely medical problem, which is to be solved by physicians and medication. The general feeling among patients is that medical competence is infinitely more valuable than compassion. Enduring the treatment of a 'cold, impersonal technocrat' for a time is, after all, worthwhile if we have the assurance that we will leave the hospital with regained health and vitality. We need no longer rely on the doctor's character, his compassion and benevolence, but can be assured that he is under an obligation to benefit us or, at least, not to harm us.

The plight of terminally- or incurably-ill patients requires us to re-evaluate the virtue of compassion as a means of understanding and responding to suffering. The call for a more humane medicine does not only challenge the rationalistic bias shown by medical scientists in their approach to disease and injury, but also the general tendency of the public to view disease and suffering as problems to be dealt with by medical professionals alone. It has become necessary to confront the questions, 'How do we respond to a person's suffering when it is no longer possible to cure the disease?' and 'Can compassion ever be seen as a morally-acceptable motivation for ending or shortening a person's life?'

Since the 1960s a number of organisations have been created in response to the perceived failure of medicine to deal with the suffering of the terminally ill. All of these organisations state their mission as offering humane aid-in-dying, but they differ widely as to what this involves. A prominent organisation, *Compassion in Dying,* aims to provide support for the right of terminally-ill patients to choose to die without pain and suffering, which includes the right to receive personal assistance to intentionally hasten death. To be eligible for their help, patients must be terminally ill (which is taken to mean having less than six months to live) and must make a voluntary request to this effect. In 1993 it made public that it had performed its first actual case of assisted suicide. The cover story of the *New York Times Magazine* related in detail the story of Louise, who suffered from a degenerative neurological disease and wished to die peacefully. After her death many objected that doctors have a duty not to kill and that the right to life cannot be waived. Herbert Hendin adopts a different perspective, questioning whether much compassion was conveyed in the way Louise was helped to die and whether she truly died with dignity:

> Compassion is not an easy emotion to express in the context of an imminent loss. It requires that we look beyond our own pain to convey the power and meaning of all that has gone before in our life with another. Although the mother, the friend, Mero, and the physician may have acted out of good intentions in assisting the suicide, none appears to have honored Louise's need for a 'peaceful' parting (Hendin 1998:56-57).

Hendin supports the approach of the Hospice movement, which he sees as gradually re-humanising death by addressing the dying patient's emotional, social, spiritual and physical needs. The Hospice movement was initiated in the 1960s in England by Dame Cicely Saunders, and became a major force in protecting terminally-ill patients from medical treatment that serves only to prolong suffering. Its 'philosophy' is to combine sophisticated palliative medicine with compassionate care. In reaction to the ineffectiveness of standard medical methods of relieving pain, it pioneered techniques of preventing pain and emphasised the importance of providing comfort to people suffering from 'psychological and spiritual pain'. Hospice joined the right-to-life groups and the Catholic Church to oppose aid-in-dying initiatives, arguing that there are other, more humane or compassionate ways of dealing with and responding to the pain and suffering that accompanies terminal illness. They also believe that, if active euthanasia became a legal option, many patients would feel pressured into choosing death and would not be able to die peacefully (Menard & Perrone 1994, Campbell 1993).

The question for ethicists, then, is whether mercy-killing can ever be justified as an act of kindness, motivated by the compassion one feels for the suffering person and performed for the sake of that person. In recent ethical and philosophical literature on euthanasia we find very little discussion of this question. Indeed, the term 'mercy-killing' is hardly ever used, and 'euthanasia' is also becoming less fashionable. The preferred term has become 'assisted suicide' or 'physician-assisted suicide', and the debate is now between those who think that killing or assisting in the killing of innocent persons is always wrong and those who believe it is sometimes permissible or even obligatory. The ethical tools used by both sides are principles (beneficence, non-maleficence, utility and patient autonomy), rights (to life, death and dying) and rules (such as 'It is always wrong to kill innocent persons' and 'Respect the wishes of competent persons'). Sissela Bok, after summarising the argument from mercy, concludes that the presence or absence of compassion is irrelevant when deciding the morality of euthanasia. Even if euthanasia does not always represent the most merciful act for patients, and even if it precluded some from recovery, it could still be argued that those who choose to die ought to have the right to decide for themselves how to weigh their continued suffering against such odds (1998:110-112). Whether or not euthanasia is an act of mercy does not, it seems, make a moral difference.

By contrast, a glimpse through the indexes of a number of books on euthanasia published in and around the 1970s reveals a far greater concern with the virtues of mercy, kindness, charity and compassion. For example, Trubo's *An Act of Mercy: Euthanasia Today* (1973) investigates the reasons for considering euthanasia a merciful act. Kohl examines the attributes necessary for an act to be kind in *The*

*Morality of Killing* (1974) and argues that failure to give help in the form of beneficent euthanasia is a failure to live up to the Good Samaritan ideal. In his essay 'Beneficent euthanasia and benemortasia: Alternative views of mercy' (1975) Dyck responds to Kohl by providing an analysis of 'mercy', his vision of the ideal of the Good Samaritan, and a view of what it means to die a 'good death'.

Most of these writers argue from, or respond to, a Christian perspective on the morality of killing. As we saw in the previous chapter, the transition from a virtue- to a principle-based ethic is most apparent in Christian ethics, where there is an emphasis on – and a tension between – virtues and principles. Alongside God's commandments that take the form of absolute rules prohibiting certain kinds of action, the Christian has in Jesus Christ the perfect ideal of a good or virtuous person. Accordingly we find that, apart from their discussion of particular virtues and views on what constitutes a good death, a central concern is with the Biblical Commandment against intentionally killing innocent persons. Some defend this rule as an absolute prohibition, whereas others argue that we need to replace it with another, more specific rule that would permit euthanasia in certain circumstances. Joseph Fletcher, unlike most Christian moralists, does not only dispute this prohibition, but rejects the principle-based ethic altogether. He argues that Christian ethics is love-oriented, not law-oriented, and that human needs validate human rights, not the other way around:

> Legalists and moralists claim that the good consists in obeying rules and following abstract principles; they are duty-bound and speak grandiosely of human rights. But agapism seeks the good, in a purposeful effort to optimize human potentials; it is goal-linked and either respects or rejects alleged rights according to whether they do or do not meet human needs (Fletcher 1975:45).

Ethical theories that aim to formulate and apply abstract, absolute rules or 'universal negatives' such as 'To end an innocent life is murder' or 'We may never interrupt a pregnancy' are, in Fletcher's view, simply embracing the clichés of an irrelevant ideology. Instead of approaching decisions with prefabricated *a priori* solutions, he advances a 'situation ethics' where a decision is made on the basis of the specific circumstances of an individual case:

> [T]he rightness or wrongness of euthanasia, or easy death, whether direct or indirect, depends on the situation. Neither form is intrinsically or invariably good or evil: Sometimes mercy killing is right; sometimes 'letting the patient go' is wrong. It depends (Fletcher 1975:50).

For Fletcher, love and concern should be our ideals, not moral laws and rights. In his view, the moral acceptability of euthanasia depends on whether we prefer quantity or quality of life, and on when we think a life is no longer worth living. The implication of this approach is that the answers to questions about the morality of euthanasia are not to be *discovered* in the precepts of an already existing, universal law. The answers are yet to be decided. We cannot resort to the answers of previous generations and cultures but have to *create* them. Fletcher writes:

> Ethics deals with the preferable, as science deals with the possible and probable. Do we prefer personal or human being, or do we favor biological life at any cost to personality and humanity?... The crucial business of ethics is decision-making, not the adumbration of abstract principles (Fletcher 1975:48-49).

These questions – whether and when euthanasia enables a person to die a good death, and whether it is an appropriate expression of compassionate concern – were never settled. This should not surprise us – philosophical and ethical debates are seldom concluded – but it is interesting and important to note why most philosophers and ethicists chose to discuss a different set of questions.

*The Battle between Virtues and Principles*

In his influential paper entitled 'Neither for love nor money: Why doctors must not kill' (1989), Leon Kass launched a full-blown attack on the argument from mercy. His paper reveals the reasons one might have for rejecting the virtues in favour of principles. Gerald Dworkin (1998:6-16) has already revealed some of the straw men, inconsistencies and rhetorical devices in Kass's arguments, and I will not repeat his critique here. However, a brief discussion of Kass's approach to morality, in particular his treatment and interpretation of the notions of compassion, mercy and human dignity, allows some insight into the reasons one might have for rejecting a virtue-based approach to morality.

Following the Christian tradition Kass makes room in his approach for virtues and principles, both of which are intimately linked to what he claims to be the nature or essence of medicine. Within the limits of medicine, Kass says, no fixed rules of conduct apply; the wise physician will find and adopt the best outcome of action in the light of the specific circumstances, and will be guided by the virtues of moderation and self-restraint, gravity, patience, sympathy, prudence and discretion. But the outer limits of medicine are fixed and non-negotiable; the boundaries are set by absolute rules or prohibitions, among which are the rules that forbid killing patients, breaking patient confidentiality, and seducing patients. Despite his attempt to incorporate both in his medical ethic, the tension between these two approaches – the discretion incorporated into a virtue ethic, and the strictness of an absolutist morality – is evident throughout his work.

Kass considers two kinds of reason in support of the view that physicians may or ought to kill under certain circumstances. The first kind of appeal is based on the principle of patient autonomy, and need not concern us here. The second is advanced by what Kass calls the 'school of general benevolence and compassion', according to which,

> death is to be directly and swiftly given because the patient's life is deemed no longer worth living, according to some substantive or 'objective' measure. Unusually great pain or a terminal condition or an irreversible coma or advanced senility or extreme degradation is the disqualifying quality of life that pleads – choice or no choice – for merciful termination.... It is not his autonomy but rather the miserable and pitiable condition of his body or mind that justifies doing the patient in...; not the will of the

> patient, but the humane and compassionate motive of the physician – not as physician but as *human being* – makes the doctor's actions ethical.... All acts – including killing the patient – done lovingly are licit, even praiseworthy. Good and humane intentions can sanctify any deed (1989:27-28).

Kass rejects this approach on the grounds that it cannot make sense of some specific duties and restraints long thought to be absolutely inviolate under traditional medical ethics: 'Must we now say that sex with patients is permissible if... the doctor is gentle and loving and has a good bedside manner?' (1989:28). He argues that physicians, in order to resist the temptations to which they are most vulnerable – breaching confidentiality, having sexual relations with patients, and dispensing deadly drugs – impose limits on their own conduct by pledging to adhere to certain absolute rules: not to breach confidentiality, not to have sexual intercourse with patients, and not to kill patients. The goal of medicine further requires the physician to take a detached stance towards patients and not to become emotionally involved with them. The physician necessarily objectifies, reduces and analyses: '[M]edical nakedness is not erotic nakedness; frank speech is not shared intimacy and friendship; giving out diets and drugs is not hospitality' (Kass 1989:37). Compassion is here presented as a feeling that may tempt the physician into doing wrong, much like sexual feelings may lure him into mischief, and hence is treated as a vice. But further on Kass does acknowledge that compassion has some value in the doctor-patient relationship, yet he thinks it irrelevant when assessing the morality of the physician's behaviour: 'For a physician, to be sure, things go better when the patient is freely willing and the physician is virtuous and compassionate. But the physician's work centres on the goal of healing, and he is thereby bound not to behave in contradiction to that central goal' (1989:43).

Like every other profession, Kass claims, medicine has an essence that can be discovered by examining its tradition. The core of medicine is revealed in the Hippocratic *Oath*: 'I will apply dietetic measures *for the benefit of the sick* according to my ability and judgement. I will keep them from harm and injustice' (cited in, and emphasis added by, Kass 1989:38). He follows the Christian physician of the nineteenth century in his reading of *The Oath*. It is not simply that the physician should refrain from harming the patient. Kass has much more in mind: '[B]ecause a body possessed of reason is a body whose "possessor" may lead it astray through ignorance or self-indulgence, the physician, as servant of the patient's good, must teach, advise, and exhort to keep him from *self*-harm and injustice' (Kass 1989:38-39, emphasis in original). The physician should keep his patient on the path of virtue. He is in charge of 'promoting the wholeness of the one who is ailing' (1989:39). If the patient wished for something contrary to the essence or goal of medicine, the physician would be obliged to lead the patient back to 'wholeness': '[I]t is as true today as it was in the days of Hippocrates that the ill desire to be whole' (1989:39). The physician, we are to understand, is to further the goal desired by all patients, regardless of the patient's current wishes. His main argument against euthanasia, then, is that it conflicts with the role traditionally afforded to medicine.

In the final section of his paper Kass turns to the objection that adhering to an absolute rule against mercy-killing may seem inhumane, cruel or unkind. He agrees that when animals suffer, the humane response is to put them out of their misery. Since they cannot make sense of their suffering, and thus cannot live out a fitting end, 'compassion for their weakness and dumbness is our only appropriate emotion'. Given our responsibility for their well-being and care, we do the only humane thing we can by killing them. But with human beings, he continues, things are altogether different. When a human being asks us for death, he displays by that very action the presence of something that precludes us from regarding him as a dumb animal: 'Humanity is owed humanity, not humaneness. Humanity is owed the bolstering of the human, even or especially in its dying moments, in resistance to the temptation to ignore its presence in the sight of suffering' (1989:44). Although Kass steers clear of religious arguments in this paper, he clarifies his thoughts on human dignity elsewhere: 'There is, in man, something god-like. Man shares in reason, freedom, judgement, and moral concern' (1990:169). We are therefore made to believe that, although euthanasia is a compassionate and humane response to suffering, it is also disrespectful of man's godliness. Compassion is portrayed as being no different from pity, a feeling provoked by the pathetic sight of a weak and dying patient. Compassion appears once more as a vice.

Finally, Kass presents his concept of what it means to die virtuously. In order to die a good death, he says, a person needs the virtues of courage, pride, and dignity. Kass believes that the medicalisation of dying has already robbed man of his dignity and moral agency by casting people who were once proud and independent into the roles of 'passive, obedient, highly disciplined children'. If we care for dignity and autonomy, he claims, we should reverse the dehumanisation of the dying process by rejecting its medicalisation and institutionalisation. Giving in to the 'desperate plea for poison' is to give dehumanisation its final triumph. Thus, we put animals out of their misery but insist on compelling fellow human beings to suffer to the bitter end because to face death and endure suffering with courage is dignified, is worthy of Man (1989:44-45). Paris and Moreland clarify the Catholic perspective on killing by pointing out that the view that a life may be so devoid of dignity that it should be destroyed runs counter to the Catholic understanding of life as a divine gift, over which we exercise stewardship and not domination: 'The Christian finds death's meaning in the example of the suffering Savior who abandoned himself in perfect obedience to the Father's will' (1998:331-332). We do not only have a right to life but a duty to live, whether we like it or not.

It is obvious that Kass's personal vision of a good or fitting death does little to support the *absolute* rule against mercy-killing, which he sets out to defend. For some human beings it is not (or is no longer) possible to die with dignity, if dignity is seen to reside in the god-like qualities of man (consciousness, rationality and freedom). And even if one shares his admiration for people who die courageously and proudly, there is no reason why one cannot believe other ways of dying to be equally virtuous. In the final analysis, Kass's account of a courageous death reads as a personal manifesto, a dedication to his mother-in-law 'who exemplified with her last breath the noblest possibilities of the human soul' (1989:25n). It is therefore understandable that most Christian moralists rely on rules and principles to support their views on euthanasia.

We can list a number of problems one could expect to encounter when trying to formulate a virtue-based approach to euthanasia, which can also be seen as reasons why, after hovering between a virtue- and a principle-based approach to moral decision-making during the Christian era, the latter found more support in modern cultures.

1. *A virtue could well turn out to be a vice.* One's sympathy may render one incapable of making an objective, rational decision. Being at least partially constituted of brute feeling, the virtues cannot be trusted to allow just and impartial decision-making. Virtuous people find themselves 'drawn', 'swayed', 'inclined', 'disposed' to do what they believe is appropriate. One can never know what to expect from them.
2. *The virtues provide no safeguard against slipping down slopes.* If we base our judgements on mercy, Kass argues, we will begin by killing those who suffer intolerable pain and eventually kill those whose lives we no longer value: '[I]t would be difficult – if not impossible – to develop the requisite calculus of degradation or to define the threshold necessary for ending life' (1989:33). We may begin by granting mercy to those who request to be killed, but will soon commit involuntary euthanasia, claims Kass: 'It is easy to see the trains of abuses that are likely to follow the most innocent cases, especially because the innocent cases cannot be precisely and neatly separated from the rest' (1989:34). (It is strange that Kass should write of 'innocent cases' while arguing that there is something essentially or intrinsically wrong with doctors killing patients.) The virtues do not provide a method for drawing a line between right and wrong, which leads us to a third problem:
3. *The virtues cannot be used as a basis for formulating clear moral rules.* Despite the fact that the virtues feature prominently in Kass's paper, they appear to be little more than window-dressing. His defence of the rule against killing has nothing to do with virtue. At best, the virtues are chameleons that take on the characteristics of whatever moral position one already holds. They are called in (and reinterpreted) to add a personal touch to a moral view that otherwise might seem harsh and bossy.
4. *Finally, an ethic of virtue cannot tell us what to do.* If we ought to do what the virtuous person would do, we would end up speculating, rather than reasoning. 'What would the Good Samaritan do?', for instance. According to Kohl (1975), failure to give help in the form of beneficent euthanasia is a failure to live up to the Good Samaritan ideal, a failure to be kind. But according to Dyck (1975), killing is cruel, and contrary to the ideal of the Good Samaritan. Both Dyck and Kohl ultimately resort to principles to answer the question of whether mercy-killing is ever morally acceptable. Dyck defends the traditional principle that prohibits killing. Kohl thinks we should formulate a better rule, rather than dogmatically adhering to a rule that serves to protect innocent life but also allows needless suffering to occur. He suggests that we reformulate the

> prohibiting killing as follows: 'Do not do *k* except in circumstances of the sort *c*', where *k* denotes the killing of innocent people and *c* denotes the voluntary inducement of a painless and quick death, the intention and actual consequences of which are the kindest possible treatment in the actual circumstances for the recipient of that act.

Over the past few decades the euthanasia debate has largely consisted of attempts to discover a general principle and formulate a more specific rule (or set of rules) that can be used to distinguish permissible from impermissible forms of killing. In the remainder of this chapter I discuss three different principle-based approaches to the ethical questions surrounding end-of-life decisions. The first emphasises the principle of beneficence as the primary duty of the physician, while the second gives priority to the principle of non-maleficence. The third approach, one that has become increasingly prevalent in recent years, emphasises respect for patient autonomy as the most fundamental duty of the physician. I argue that the principle-based approach does not allow us to deal with the most significant questions faced by physicians and patients at the end of life.

## Unbridled Competence and Absolute Beneficence

The principle of beneficence asserts a positive duty to benefit patients. It supports an array of more specific rules such as 'Prevent harm from occurring to others', 'Remove conditions that will cause harm to others' and 'Rescue persons in danger'. As we have seen in the previous chapter, the Cabotean ethic of competence takes the principle of beneficence as the primary duty of health-care professionals, which often requires them to take heroic measures in an attempt to 'save' patients' lives.

Lasagna voices the dominant view held by medical professionals in the 1970s when, in response to those who claim that the first duty of physicians is not to harm patients, he argues that the proper medical and moral stance is to optimise treatment. In ancient times, when the therapeutic cupboard was relatively bare of excellent remedies, yet brimming with measures of questionable merit and with indubitable capacity for harm, it was certainly proper for a physician to see the duty of non-maleficence as his first and foremost obligation. However, since modern physicians possess infinitely more power for good than their forebears, their role is misconstrued if viewed primarily in terms of the negative goal of non-maleficence. They can now more accurately predict and weigh the risks and benefits pertaining to treatment and should therefore not avoid risk-taking at all costs. Physicians are obliged, for example, to use penicillin to treat pneumococcal pneumonia, despite the fact that this antibiotic sometimes causes death, because the untreated disease is even deadlier (Lasagna 1977:43-46).

Many opponents of euthanasia support the view that the primary duty of the physician is to benefit patients. They typically argue that intentionally letting a patient die by withholding or withdrawing life-prolonging treatment (passive euthanasia) is to violate one of the central rules of beneficence. Gay-Williams

(1979) for instance argues that medical professionals are and should be totally committed to saving lives. It is for this reason that they often experience the death of a patient as a personal failure, as an insult to their skills and knowledge. He thinks that allowing euthanasia would have a corrupting influence so that in any case that is severe, physicians might not try hard enough to save the patient.

We cannot deny that advances in modern science and technology, together with the admirable dedication and commitment of medical professionals to preserve life, have produced enormous benefits for many people. The specification of the goal of medicine in terms of *clinical* effects is also an attractive alternative to the way Christian moralists such as Leon Kass define it. Yet the marriage between the principle of beneficence and medical competence has not always been a happy one. Some of the children born of this union include the brain dead, the irreversibly comatose, those who die a prolonged and agonising death, and those whose lives are saved, only to be doomed to a life of subhuman quality. Whereas modern technology has made it *possible* to keep these patients alive, the duty to benefit them *requires* physicians to do so. Hence the question arises as to whether physicians ought to do everything they are competent to do, that is, whether attempts to prolong life are always morally praiseworthy. Jonsen cites the case of a woman whose husband was in an irreversible coma and who complained: 'It's not that he's being poorly treated – he's being *too well treated*' (1990:29, emphasis in original). *Effective* treatment may not always be *beneficial* to the specific patient.

The breakthrough in treating brain-dead patients by Japanese doctors in the 1980s offers a particularly good example. At the time the Japanese did not accept the brain-death definition of death. They continued to treat these patients, but asystole (and death) inevitably occurred within a few hours or days of brain death. The doctors then discovered that the reason this happened was that brain-dead patients lacked an antidiuretic hormone normally made by the brain. They decided to administer this hormone to their brain-dead patients by means of a drip, which was an enormous success in the sense that brain-dead patients could now be maintained almost indefinitely. However, I fail to see how any of the patients were benefited by this breakthrough, and I am sure that the physicians who made the breakthrough did not suffer any delusions to the contrary.

How is it possible, then, that the very *adherence* to the principle of beneficence, together with the *successful* performance of medical procedures can still lead to a failure to benefit patients? The sanctity-of-life ethic, which elevates the virtuous ideal of helping patients to a universal, absolute or perfect duty of beneficence, is often criticised. But the objection is usually that *it requires too much from the benefactor*, not that it harms or fails to benefit the recipient of such beneficent acts! The answer to the above question can partly be found in the way in which the content of the term 'benefit' is determined. The principle of beneficence is seen as supporting more specific rules, for example that one should prevent death, cure disease and alleviate suffering. As such it declares the prevention of death to be a universal good, and assumes that one cannot harm someone by saving or prolonging his or her life. Ethics thus follows the scientific method, insofar as the ethic of competence measures medical competence in terms of certain universally-desirable clinical effects (and death is surely the worst possible 'clinical effect' of treatment).

At this stage one might want to respond by pointing out that the problem does not lie with the principle-based approach as such, but with specific rules. Clearly, the rule 'Always prolong life where possible' is too broad to be universalisable. It commits us to the view that to prolong life is also to benefit someone, which is not true in all circumstances. A simple solution to this problem, it seems, would be to take Kohl's advice and modify the rule to read 'Always prolong life, except in circumstances of the sort *c*', rather than to discard the principle-based approach altogether. There seems to be no reason why a principle-based ethic should embrace a specific rule – different rules can be made to suit different circumstances. It is for this reason that Kant was wise enough to refrain from committing himself to any specific rule. The Kantian ethic is based on the principle of universalisability, namely that 'I am never to act otherwise than so that I could also will that my maxim should become a universal law' (Kant 1988:27). This principle is purely formal in that it describes the form that moral obligation must take rather than its content. Substantial moral rules have to be worked out by asking in the case of each particular action 'What is the maxim I am following here?' and 'Can the maxim be universalised?'.

Over the past few decades a number of attempts have been made to specify the rules of beneficence more closely, so as to justify withholding life-sustaining treatment under certain circumstances. It is now generally accepted that the rules of beneficence are not as stringent as the rules of non-maleficence, so that it may sometimes be permissible to allow a patient to die. The couplet by A.H. Clough is often cited to express this view:

> Thou shalt not kill: but needst not strive
> Officiously to keep alive.

Many ethicists have rejected the requirement, supported by both Christians and utilitarians, of acts of positive beneficence towards others. Following Kant they argue that the rules of beneficence are not positive obligations but virtuous ideals or acts of charity. Whereas rules of non-maleficence are generally seen as perfect duties that allow no exceptions, beneficence cannot be a perfect obligation, simply because of one's limited resources and abilities. According to this line of reasoning it is *sometimes* morally permissible to allow harm to befall someone but *always* wrong to harm her.

The attempt to specify the rules of beneficence by stating under which circumstances it is permissible to allow someone to die has met with a number of difficulties. Firstly, drawing attention to the fact that the principle of beneficence is an imperfect obligation is already a very precarious starting-point for discussing the problems surrounding euthanasia. As we have seen, it is not simply a shortage of resources that necessitates a limitation of positive duties, but the fact that prolonging someone's life does not always serve the patient's best interest and hence may not be a virtuous ideal. The claim is not merely that one *need* not, but that one *should* not strive officiously to keep alive. A failure to prolong life may sometimes be obligatory or praiseworthy, and not simply permissible.

Secondly, it is extremely difficult to change rules that have been endorsed by religious institutions and accepted by health-care professionals for centuries. Building exceptions into the formulation of a rule is seen as undermining the moral force of the rule. Perhaps the best illustration of the sanctity of some moral rules is the debate surrounding the status and treatment of patients who have suffered whole-brain death. During the 1960s advances in technology made it possible to sustain the vital functions of brain-dead patients. Despite the fact that it was impossible to restore consciousness in these patients, physicians were obliged to keep them alive since it was argued that every person has an equal right to life, regardless of the quality of his or her life. It subsequently proved easier to change the definition of death, than to simply refine the rule that obliges physicians to prevent death. In 1970 a redefinition of death in terms of whole-brain death was proposed and subsequently accepted by most hospitals in the Western world. The main reason for the widespread acceptance of the whole-brain definition of death is, I strongly suspect, its perceived implications for the moral acceptability of certain modes of treatment. Changing the status of people who suffered whole-brain death from 'patients' to 'corpses' meant that rules governing the treatment of patients no longer applied to them. Physicians no longer felt obliged to do everything possible to prolong their lives, and were no longer required to obtain the family's consent before terminating treatment. They could also remove organs from the body while blood still circulated, hence improving the success rate of organ transplants. Although I agree that such treatment of brain-dead patients is morally justifiable, I have deep reservations about the redefinition of death in terms of whole-brain death. I cannot develop my argument here, but suffice it to say that the attributes ascribed to these patients – for instance, that they are in a hopeless condition, totally dependent upon machines for sustaining their vital functions, that they have no quality of life, that they will soon die, and so forth – are features more readily attributable to living organisms. Following the Japanese breakthrough it has even become possible for pregnant women who suffer brain death to carry their infants to term.

A third difficulty appears when trying to formulate a more specific version of a rule in a way that allows for consistency and objectivity in application. A rule stating that one should 'usually' or 'often' prolong life is of no use unless it specifies what counts as a legitimate exception. Various efforts have been made to specify the sort of circumstances in which providing life-sustaining treatment is no longer obligatory. In the celebrated case of Karen Ann Quinlan the distinction between 'ordinary' and 'extraordinary' means of life-support was invoked to justify withdrawal of treatment. Quinlan was in a permanently vegetative state but was maintained on a respirator and received tube feeding. It was subsequently decided that a surrogate decision-maker might request 'extraordinary' means of treatment to be withdrawn, but that the patient was still to receive 'ordinary' treatment. The respirator was withdrawn because it was considered extraordinary treatment, but the patient was still to receive artificial nutrition and hydration. Providing food and water, it was believed, even if it came from a tube and was administered by a machine, is ordinary treatment. Doctors expected her to die soon afterwards, and no doubt relatives hoped she would. Yet Quinlan surprised everyone by continuing to breathe on her own. She survived in this state for ten years until she died a 'natural death' in 1986.

The main problem with reformulating rules through the specification of obligatory and non-obligatory modes of treatment is the apparent disregard for the consequences of treatment for individual patients. To specify in advance that extraordinary treatment may legitimately be foregone, without knowing what the treatment would yield in a particular case, is to lose sight of the obvious point that the principle of beneficence requires one to benefit patients. The focus on means of treatment is an attempt to find an objective standard or criterion for decision-making – a rule is of little use if it contains concepts that are wide-open to interpretation. Quality-of-life judgements are too subjective, it is believed, and they deny the view that all human beings have an equal right to life. Yet it is highly questionable whether the proposed alternative avoids either of these problems. As Peter Singer (1995:70-73) argues, labelling a means of treatment as 'extraordinary' serves to disguise a judgement about the quality-of-life of the patient on whom the means of treatment is being used. In the Quinlan case, for example, the very description of the respirator as 'extraordinary' treatment depended on an already formed judgement to the effect that it is not worthwhile to prolong the life of a patient in her condition. If the patient were only in a temporary coma and did have reasonable hope of recovery, the use of a respirator would be regarded by everyone as essential.

While the development of medical science and technology has raised the question of the limits to be placed on competence, asking us to re-evaluate the view that prolonging life is always beneficial, a deontological approach to moral decision-making is unable to meet this need. Duties are often blind to consequences. Doctors should do what is 'the right thing to do', which is to obey the principle of beneficence, according to which one should cure disease, save life and prevent death. Kant makes it clear that 'the basis of obligation must not be sought in the nature of man, or in the circumstances in the world in which he is placed, but *a priori* simply in the conceptions of pure reason' (1988:11-12). But when effective treatment is no longer in the patient's best interest, or when adherence to the rules of beneficence no longer benefits a specific patient, the medical enterprise becomes highly dubious. I will discuss the Kantian approach in more depth in Chapters Four and Five, which will allow us greater insight into the theoretical shortcomings that lie at the basis of the difficulties experienced when trying to apply this approach to actual dilemmas in health care. In the following section I examine the principle of non-maleficence in the context of end-of-life decision-making. I also show that consequentialist theories, whether rule- or act-based, do not provide a satisfactory alternative to deontological approaches.

**Non-Maleficence and the Sanctity of Life**

There is a long tradition in medical ethics that has taken the principle of non-maleficence – the obligation not to inflict harm intentionally – as the fundamental obligation of physicians. This principle supports more specific (negative) rules such as 'Do not intentionally end the life of an innocent human being', 'Do not cause pain or suffering to others' and 'Do not incapacitate others'. The first of these rules forms the cornerstone of the sanctity-of-life ethic and has its origin in the Biblical commandment 'Thou shalt not kill'. During the early centuries of Christianity the commandment was seen as absolute, and interpreted as applying to all human beings. The early Church fathers condemned suicide, euthanasia and infanticide, as well as participation in warfare, killing in self-defence and capital punishment. Gradually, however, the rule against killing came to be specified more closely as it became apparent that a resolutely pacifist stance was unsustainable. The Church came to accept capital punishment and killing in a just war, subsequently changing the rule to read 'The intentional killing of *innocent* humans is always wrong'. To explain how killing in war was consistent with the prohibition against killing, St. Augustine argued that moral goodness was not a property of actions but of the attitude with which one performs them, with what one is trying to accomplish by an action. The rule ultimately developed by the Church was that *the intentional killing of innocent persons is always wrong*.[1]

But why should the process of refining the prohibition stop here? If Christians allow exceptions to the Sixth Commandment in wartime and for capital punishment, why don't they also allow an exception for killing to alleviate pain and suffering near death? Fletcher (1960) observes that the Hebrew in which the Sixth Commandment is written was incorrectly translated as 'Thou shalt not kill'. In the *Episcopal Book of Common Prayers* we find the correct translation: 'Thou shalt not murder'; and 'murder' of course means 'to kill wrongfully'. To end the lives of those who are sick and suffering, Fletcher argues, does not constitute wrongful killing, and hence is not a violation of the Sixth Commandment. But what help, one might ask, is a rule that merely states the obvious, namely that one should not do what is wrong? We can imagine that Fletcher would respond as follows: 'That is just the point. Rules can only affirm the outrageously obvious. But in difficult and complex cases, there is no simple answer to the question "What ought we to do?" There can be no simple set of rules that can be applied to all cases. It is naive to think that one can, with a single rule, draw a line between right and wrong cases of killing. Does anyone consistently abide by the rule that it is wrong to lie? Most people, Christians and heathens alike, think that there are times when it is permissible or even obligatory to tell a lie, even though we all agree that honesty is a virtue and still teach our children that they should tell the truth. Why should the rule against killing be any different?'

In response to this kind of position many Christian moralists resort to a slippery-slope argument, not very different from the one often advanced by

[1] For a detailed account of the specification of the rule against killing, see Rachels (1986).

consequentialists. They accept that euthanasia might be the kindest way of ending the relentless suffering of an individual, but nevertheless hold that it is wrong to kill an innocent human being. They fear that legalising active euthanasia or physician-assisted suicide would be detrimental to the well-being of society in general through bringing about an erosion of the sanctity-of-life ethic. In a report issued by The British House of Lords in 1994 it is stated that:

> [W]e do not believe that these arguments are sufficient reason to weaken society's prohibition of intentional killing. That prohibition is the cornerstone of law and of social relationships. It protects each one of us impartially, embodying the belief that all are equal. We do not wish that protection to be diminished and we therefore recommend that there should be no change in the law to permit euthanasia.

Many rule-utilitarians support the view that weakening society's prohibition against killing would have adverse effects for society as a whole. Once such a law is accepted, they maintain, we would be unable to set secure limits on euthanasia, and we would soon accept Nazi-type exterminations of the 'socially degenerate'. Although they agree that euthanasia is sometimes the most beneficent alternative for the individual concerned, they reject the institutionalisation of euthanasia as an acceptable medical practice. Allowing physicians to sometimes end the life of a patient is to open the door to abuse: '[T]he risks of such institutionalisation are so grave as to outweigh the very real suffering of those who might benefit from it' (Potts 1988:504).

A familiar objection to the slippery-slope argument is that it allows for the sacrifice of the few for the sake of the many. It is acknowledged that some patients would be better off dead, but they are denied this escape for fear of the consequences it might have for others. This points to a more fundamental problem with principle-based ethics, namely that it does not take kindly to exceptions to its carefully formulated rules and maxims. It is felt that once we allow exceptions to rules, or once a policy is made discretionary, the danger arises that they would come to be applied expediently and arbitrarily. This holds true for both deontological and rule-utilitarian theories. For Kant, a rational morality is one that lays down principles, such as the rule against killing, which can and ought to be held by everyone, independent of circumstances, conditions and consequences, and which could consistently be obeyed by every rational agent on every occasion. Although the rule-utilitarian, by contrast, sets out by examining the types of consequences that would usually follow some form of treatment or action, the rules and principles formulated in this way are regarded as universal, aimed at maximising overall social utility. The utilitarian will therefore not be convinced to change a rule because it *sometimes* leads to adverse consequences for *some* people, nor would he be willing to make exceptions to a rule, fearing that in the long run such rule-meddling would have disastrous consequences for the well-being of society.[2] While duties that stem from principles have the advantage of being

---

[2] For a comparison of deontological and rule-utilitarian attitudes to exception-making, see R.M. Hare (1977:49-61).

enforceable, they are also characterised by a certain rigidity, by a failure to consider the specific circumstances of every individual case within a changing context. The duties of medical professionals are often treated as if they were scientific truths – universal, objective and impersonal – whereas in fact they are only the fossilised proceeds of tradition.

*Finding Ways Around the Rule*

The fear of allowing exceptions accounts for the frequent attempts to find a way around a rule so as to allow for the justification of certain kinds of action that appear to violate the rule yet are intuitively thought to be morally acceptable. A number of arguments have been put forward in an attempt to show that certain instances of euthanasia do not violate the absolute rule against intentionally killing innocent people. These arguments work by taking advantage of the ambiguity of the concepts 'intentional', 'persons' and 'killing'.

*Intentionality* The doctrine of double effect, developed over hundreds of years in the Catholic Church, has brought relief to many patients suffering from extreme pain. According to adherents of this doctrine there is a significant ethical difference between administering a lethal injection with the aim and intention of ending someone's life, and treating a patient with the intention of relieving suffering, but where death is a 'merely foreseen effect'. For instance, it is held that the act of injecting a cancer patient with morphine, which has the double effect of alleviating pain (the primary intention) and of shortening life (the merely foreseen effect), does not constitute the intentional termination of life and hence is morally acceptable. By contrast, if one administered the morphine with the intention of ending life it would count as a violation of the rule against killing.

*Personhood* Another strategy has been to argue that there is a significant difference between 'persons' and 'human beings', and that the prohibition against killing applies only to persons. Human beings who lack characteristics such as consciousness, self-consciousness, rationality or the potential for becoming autonomous are not persons, and hence do not have a right to life.

*Killing and letting die* It is widely held, in both medical and legal circles, that there is a significant ethical difference between active and passive euthanasia. Passive euthanasia is morally (and legally) acceptable since it does not involve killing patients. The cause of death is the patient's illness or injury; the physician simply allows nature to take its course. In many cases the patient is allowed to die after he refuses to consent to further efforts to sustain his life. By contrast, in cases of active euthanasia the agent is directly responsible for causing the patient's death, and there could be no question that she intends to terminate the patient's life.

The distinctions between intended and merely foreseen effects, persons and human beings, and between killing and letting die have provided ethicists with an affinity for the analytical style of argumentation with a seemingly endless supply of stimulating material. For our present purposes it is unnecessary – and impossible – to examine these debates in any detail, thus I limit the following discussion to a few comments on the distinction between active and passive euthanasia.

The debate was initiated by James Rachels in his 1975 paper entitled 'Active and passive euthanasia', in which he argues that there is no morally significant distinction to be drawn between the two (a position often referred to as the 'equivalency thesis'). He uses the (by now) famous example of the vicious uncles (Smith and Jones) and their six-year-old cousin to illustrate his claim that the moral acceptability of both killing and letting die depends on the agent's motive (his reason for acting as he did) and intention (the end he had in view). This argument, if it is sound, does not imply that we must also accept the conclusion that active euthanasia is sometimes morally permissible (and Rachels is well aware of this). It only requires us to choose between two alternatives:

1. *Both active and passive euthanasia are unacceptable.* This position is not as untenable as it might appear, since it does not prohibit doctors from ever withdrawing or withholding life-sustaining treatment. As Steinbock (1979:59-64) has pointed out, letting die is not equivalent to passive euthanasia. With the latter, the intention for withdrawing treatment is to hasten death, but this is not necessarily the case when letting someone die. Doctors can cease treatment to respect the wishes of the patient, because continued treatment is painful and has little chance of success, or because of a shortage of resources. In none of these cases is the patient's death intentional. In this view, then, it is always wrong to intentionally bring about death, whether by act or omission. A separate argument is needed to show why both forms of euthanasia are always wrong.
2. *Euthanasia, whether active or passive, is acceptable under certain circumstances.* The tenability of the claim that active euthanasia is morally acceptable is often made to rest on the assumption that passive euthanasia is already accepted. It is pointed out that most hospitals already allow physicians to practise passive euthanasia and have done so for a long time, and that to be consistent we also have to accept that active euthanasia is also morally acceptable. This position clearly stands in need of support – that a practice is already accept*ed* does not imply that it is also accept*able*.

The implication of the equivalency thesis is that the moral acceptability of euthanasia does not depend on the means used to bring about death, but on a combination of two factors: the agent's intentions, and the desirability of the consequence. Neither of these factors alone is sufficient for determining whether euthanasia is ever acceptable. The mere fact that the agent intended the patient's death does not in itself make his actions immoral – one also has to show that his actions brought about an unfavourable result or consequence. And simply knowing that the agent brought about or hastened the patient's death does not make his actions right or wrong – we also have to know that he intended the death to occur to be able to ascribe moral praise or blame.

Most prominent bioethicists have rejected the view that there is an essential moral difference between active and passive euthanasia,[3] arguing instead that the morality of euthanasia depends on an evaluation of consequences and/or intentionality. Yet they have had very little effect on medical professionals and policy makers. The reason for this lack of impact is not to be found in their arguments against the traditional distinction – for these, I think, are sound – but in the difficulty of finding a satisfactory alternative. If we play by the rules of a principle-based ethic, we have to formulate a new rule before we can discard the old.

*Reformulating the Rule Against Killing*

It seems plausible to suggest that, instead of focusing on the *means* of bringing about death, we should focus on the *ends* that are desirable and attainable in the patient's specific situation, and then try to determine which mode of treatment would best promote those ends. This raises the question of whether an act or omission that results in death can ever be seen as a way of benefiting (or not harming) a patient. If we were to formulate a new rule about the acceptability of intentionally killing and letting die, it would be necessary to specify clearly in which circumstances death would be a benefit.

A number of views have been advanced on this matter. From a clinical perspective the goal of medicine is health, so that death is always a greater harm than life, whatever its quality. (If biology students were assigned with the task of tending to a beanstalk in conditions of extreme drought, the student who handed in a dead plant would always receive a lower grade than the one who ended up with a living beanstalk, no matter how miserable its state.) A popular version of this position is that active euthanasia is always harmful since it leaves no room for miraculous recovery and excludes the possibility that a hitherto untried technique will save the patient's life. Against this, some proponents of euthanasia hold that death is not a harm to someone whose life has become a burden to him because of extreme and unrelievable pain or incapacity, and that life is not in itself a good which it is always rational and reasonable for a person to want more of. Others have even suggested that death can sometimes be counted as a *benefit*, so that active euthanasia may be considered as actively benefiting a person, and passive euthanasia as 'refraining from preventing this benefit' (Nesbitt 1993:255). Dr. Jack Kevorkian, who has become (in)famous for assisting patients to commit suicide, has described his actions not only as benefiting individual patients, but as a service to the well-being of mankind. Kohl develops his argument in favour of 'beneficent euthanasia' on the basis that euthanasia is often the greatest kindness that can be shown to someone in dire need (1977:75).

Whatever the merits of these viewpoints, their differences draw our attention to the lack of consensus in contemporary societies over what is to be considered

3 See Rachels (1975 and 1986), Singer (1995) and Beauchamp and Childress (1994) for detailed discussion and criticism of this distinction.

beneficial or harmful (and we have not even begun to ask more specific questions, such as 'Under which circumstances is death a benefit?'). Based as they are on religious belief or views about the meaning of life, these opinions can only be highly subjective. The fact is that no living person knows, nor can they know, what it is like to be dead. It is impossible to weigh harms such as pain, discomfort and disability, all of which are harms suffered *in life*, against *death*, which is not a state of being that can be described in terms of the goods and evils experienced in life. There can be no objective (or even inter-subjective) standard for determining whether death is to be considered the greatest harm imaginable, a lesser evil than prolonged and extreme suffering, or as a benefit. Despite the attempts to specify and delineate the appropriate and desirable goals of medicine, no universal or generally-accepted concepts of 'harm' and 'benefit' can be found. Seneca still has the last word: 'Death is sometimes a punishment, often a gift. To many it has been a favour' (cited in Potts 1988:493).

*The Utilitarian Alternative*

The pluralism of values and preferences stands in the way of any rule-consequentialist attempt to formulate a rule or set of rules about when it is in the patient's best interest to die. Another route followed to determine when and whether death can be seen as the appropriate goal of treatment (or non-treatment) is the one taken by Peter Singer. Singer's act-utilitarian approach has the advantage that we need not formulate a rule for determining when death is a lesser harm than continued suffering. Instead, we can judge each case on its own merits. His approach also includes two elements found lacking in deontological approaches, making it an attractive alternative: A consideration of consequences, and an inclusion of quality-of-life judgements.

Singer argues that we should admit the fact that the sanctity-of-life ethic has suffered irreparable damage. Instead of trying to find ways around the prohibition against intentionally killing innocent persons, we should make decisions on the basis of a utilitarian calculation of the consequences of the act or omission for all parties concerned. He proposes that decisions about life and death should be guided by a quality-of-life ethic, which is based on the recognition that the value of human life varies. All human beings do not have an equal claim to life. The mere fact that a being is a human being, that is, a member of the species *homo sapiens*, is not relevant to the wrongness of killing it; instead, it is characteristics such as rationality, autonomy and self-consciousness that make a moral difference. His position on the status of the foetus further leads him to conclude that it is actual, rather than potential characteristics and abilities that form the basis of one's moral status. In this way he distinguishes between the appropriate treatment of 'personal' and 'non-personal' sentient beings.

With regard to our dealings with *non-personal beings* (such as infants and most animals) the classical utilitarian principle of maximising pleasure or happiness applies. Singer argues that beings that are conscious but lack self-consciousness, rationality and autonomy do not have as strong a claim to life as persons because they have no preference for continued life. The reasons it might be wrong to kill such beings do not derive from the intrinsic value of their lives. Rather, under normal circumstances infanticide is wrong because it decreases the aggregate of happiness, insofar as there would be one less happy being in the world. A second kind of objection to killing non-personal beings concerns its side-effects; for instance, the bad effects that infanticide would have on the parents, or the fear and mistrust that could result if it is known that a hospital allows non-voluntary euthanasia.

Where these objections do not pertain, non-personal sentient beings could be killed with full moral justification. The wrongness of killing an infant that is accepted and wanted by its parents derives from the parents' emotional suffering. Singer argues that infanticide would be justifiable in the case of infants suffering from spina bifida (which involves various degrees of mental retardation, paralysis and incontinence, depending on its severity). Since their lives include more pain than pleasure, the objection from decreasing happiness does not apply. And if the parents do not want the child, the objection from side-effects does not apply either. With regard to less serious abnormalities such as haemophilia or Down's syndrome, Singer agrees that people suffering from these conditions do generally find their lives worth living. But infanticide would nevertheless be justified in cases where this would increase the sum-total of happiness in the world; for instance, where the parents replace the defective infant by another child with better prospects of a happy life, but who would not have existed if the defective infant were not killed (Singer 1979:131-138).

One objection to Singer's position is that the adoption of it would place us on a slippery slope. His argument in favour of euthanasia for infants suffering from Down's syndrome applies equally to all normal infants not wanted by their parents, even those for whom good homes can be found with adoptive parents. Unless their circumstances do not allow for it, we usually frown upon parents who do not want to raise their infant. On Singer's reasoning, however, their not wanting to raise the child is not only morally acceptable; it also counts as a valid reason for not letting the infant live. Indeed, if one follows the logic of the utilitarian balancing game, the less they want the child to live, and the unhappier they will be made by the very thought of the child's existence, the more the scales are tipped in favour of infanticide. This entirely defies the intuition most people share, namely that parents, even if they are unable or unwilling to raise their child themselves, should want it to have the best life possible. Granted, it is unlikely that their preference to have the infant killed would ever outweigh other considerations of utility (such as the happiness of the infant, or the preferences of prospective adoptive parents), but most people would think that their preference should not even be counted as a consideration in favour of infanticide.

The main shortcoming of Singer's approach to infanticide is that he does not consider the agent's motive to be morally relevant but focuses only on the consequences of the action. As a result, he does not simply embark on a slippery slope; his very first step sends him on a backbreaking fall. With regard to infants suffering from severe forms of spina bifida I agree that their suffering and prospects for the future are such that continued life would be utter misery to them, but it is clear that Singer's support of infanticide does not rest on such considerations. As a utilitarian who has to calculate *aggregate* utility, he is primarily concerned about the threat to the happiness of the parents and any other children they might have. He uses the same method of valuing quality of life as was used in the 'euthanasia programme' in Nazi Germany, which started out by exterminating all those who were unable to work and considered non-rehabilitable for work. They included the mentally defective, psychotics (particularly schizophrenics), epileptics, senile or weak elderly persons, and people suffering from neurological disorders such as Parkinsonianism, multiple sclerosis and brain tumours; in short, all those considered useless or a burden on society. If based on such considerations, euthanasia would cease to be a dangerous practice that *might* lead to immoral practices. It would already be thoroughly immoral, since it involves a method of 'quality control'. Hitler's project all but had an 'innocent start' – it is clear that the concern was not with the suffering of the individuals in question but with their social utility. It is one thing to euthanise an infant with infantile paralysis to prevent her from suffering; it is quite another thing to kill her because she would impose a burden on society.

As far as the treatment of *personal beings* is concerned, Singer does recognise the need to secure them from being sacrificed for the sake of the utilitarian goal of maximising aggregate pleasure. It is to this end that he introduces a third objection to killing, namely a preference-utilitarian objection. In this view, killing a person is morally wrong because it thwarts that person's desire to go on living. In addition to pleasure and happiness, we should also consider the preferences of persons when determining the aggregate utility of an action. Since non-personal beings have no preference for continued life, preference utilitarianism applies only to our dealings with persons, and only insofar as our actions satisfy or frustrate their personal preferences.

The counter-intuitive implications of Singer's arguments do not solely follow from his position on the morality of killing non-personal beings. His adoption of preference utilitarianism with regard to our dealings with persons does not enable him to avoid the typical implications of classical utilitarianism, namely that all individuals with moral standing are mere replaceable receptacles of what is morally valuable in itself (i.e., happiness). Singer admits that personal preferences can be outweighed: 'Even for preference utilitarianism, the wrong done to the person killed is merely one factor to be taken into account, and the preference of the victim could sometimes be outweighed by the preferences of others' (1979:81). The implication is that persons have no intrinsic moral value as individual beings. A person's wish to live is a reason not to kill him, but it is not a *conclusive* reason since it may be outweighed by the preferences of others. In other words, the lives of persons cannot be given their due protection against the joint wishes of others. Despite Singer's objection to involuntary 'euthanasia', his approach allows for the justification of killing persons against their wishes if doing so would further the interests of others. (The fears of a few elderly patients would count very little on the utilitarian scales.)[4]

Although, as an act-utilitarian, Singer does not resort to the rules that tend to land other principle-based theories in trouble, the shortcomings of his approach are a direct implication of his taking utility as a universally-binding principle. A discussion of principle-based approaches to euthanasia would not be complete without examining the implications of accepting the principle of respect for patient autonomy for the treatment of the terminally ill. I shall now examine the third principle-based approach to euthanasia, which takes autonomy as the central principle in making end-of-life decisions.

**Respect for Patient Autonomy and the Problem of Incompetence**

Since the 1970s the notions of patient autonomy and informed consent have gained wide recognition in medical law and practice. Once the norm, physicians who refuse to respect a patient's autonomy are now labelled paternalists. In recent decades the principle of patient autonomy has formed the basis of many attacks on stringent euthanasia policies. One of the difficulties with specifying rules of beneficence and non-maleficence, we have seen, is that individuals have different views as to what counts as beneficial and harmful. A significant advantage of the autonomy model is that it allows every individual to decide this for herself, and to balance the perceived advantages and disadvantages of treatment with any other values and considerations she thinks relevant or significant.

Following a wave of popular sentiment in favour of the 're-humanisation' of the dying process in the 1970s, the right of patients to refuse treatment under certain circumstances has been acknowledged. The first 'Right to Die' legislation passed in the United States was the *California Natural Death Act 1976*. Courts have subsequently held that physicians may not substitute their judgement for that of the patient. Physicians are now required to withdraw from the case and turn it over to a colleague if they disagree with the patient's instructions to discontinue treatment. More recently it has been argued that the right to self-determination includes not only a right to *die*, but also a right to *death*, that is, a right to receive assistance in committing suicide or even to be actively killed (voluntary active euthanasia). It is typically argued that, since there is no significant difference between killing and letting die, it follows that if patients have the right to refuse treatment, they also have the right to receive 'treatment' that would end life. Singer proposes, for instance, that we substitute the sanctity-of-life commandment, 'Never take your own life, and always try to prevent others taking theirs', with the rule, 'Always respect a person's desire to live or die' (1995:196-198). The right to self-determination has also been extended to include incompetent patients through surrogate decision-making and advance directives.

---

[4] See Landman (1990:159-171) for a more detailed critique of Singer's position.

Though theoretically attractive, many difficulties appear when trying to apply the principle of respect for patient autonomy to end-of-life decision-making. Again, the obvious task facing us is to formulate a set of rules that clearly expresses the requirements of the principle of autonomy with regard to patients who wish to die. As was the case with the principles of beneficence and non-maleficence, this is a daunting task. Consider the following cases:

> April is a 25-year-old woman who suffers from depression and requests her physician to provide her with a lethal drug. He suggests she tries a course of *Prozac*, but April remains adamant that she has had enough of this life.

> Boris is a 50-year-old man who refuses to undergo surgery for a potentially fatal but fully treatable condition. He says he hates hospitals, and trusts his physician to cure him with medication alone.

> Cain, a 40-year-old man, requests his physician to end his life with a scalpel, since God requested Cain to join Him in heaven.

If the principle of autonomy is interpreted as an obligation to respect a patient's wishes, a physician who wants to remain consistently committed to this principle will have to comply with these patients' wishes or requests. A refusal to do so would indicate an admission of the paternalist's view that the obligations of beneficence and non-maleficence do sometimes override the obligation to respect autonomy.

Alternatively, one could argue that the rule, 'Always respect a patient's wishes' is too broad and stands in need of further specification. In its present form, the rule would oblige a physician to mow the patient's lawn every Saturday if this is what the patient wanted! To prevent physicians – who themselves have a right to self-determination – from becoming the puppets of their patients, the rule should be rephrased so as only to require them to obtain consent for medical interventions with patients. Accordingly, there would be no obligation to adhere to April and Cain's requests to be killed. The rule commonly accepted in health-care contexts adds a further qualification: 'A physician should always obtain consent for interventions with patients, *unless the patient is incompetent to refuse or consent to treatment*', and it is not difficult to justify this qualification. As Beauchamp and Childress point out, the principle of respect for patient autonomy is not so broad that it covers non-autonomous persons (1994:127). Most theories of autonomy agree that three conditions are essential for being considered autonomous, namely (1) liberty (independence from controlling influences), (2) rationality and understanding, and (3) agency (capacity for intentional action). If a patient does not meet these conditions he is considered non-autonomous, so that overriding his right to self-determination by making decisions on his behalf or refusing to conform to his wishes is both necessary and justified.[5] Thus it could be argued that our three

[5] Some have been reluctant to describe such actions as paternalistic, since overriding the wishes of non-autonomous patients is not an instance of disrespecting their autonomy.

patients are not sufficiently autonomous or competent for their decisions to require respect. In none of these cases can the wish to die be described as voluntary, freely formed or rational, since they are all impelled or controlled by their emotions or irrational beliefs. April's choice of a lethal drug over an anti-depressant is clearly not a rational choice, Boris lets his fears get the better of him and Cain suffers from religious delusions on a grand scale.

A crucial question now arises, namely 'What are the criteria for being found competent to participate in clinical decision-making?' or 'How much autonomy should a person have for his autonomy to require respect?' In medical practice it is not always clear whether the patient is, in his present state, competent to participate in decision-making that may affect his health or life. A person's ability to deliberate rationally or act freely may be hampered or limited, to a greater or lesser extent, either by external factors such as coercion, duress, undue influence or manipulation by others, or by internal constraints such as compulsion, drug addiction, mental illness, emotional factors, inadequate or incomplete information about various courses of action and their consequences. It is widely accepted that competence refers to the capacity to perform a specific task. In medical affairs the relevant task is that of deciding among alternative courses of medical treatment, each with its own expected benefits and risks. It is generally agreed that competence is not a simple case of 'all or nothing', but that there are degrees of competence. Yet different theories disagree on which capacities are to be the criteria for competence. The following criteria, listed by Beauchamp and Childress (1994:137) are currently in competition as favoured reasons for considering a patient incompetent to consent to or refuse medical interventions and therapies. The standards range progressively from that requiring the least ability to the other end of the spectrum:

1. Inability to express or communicate a preference or choice
2. Inability to understand one's situation and its consequences
3. Inability to understand relevant information
4. Inability to articulate a reason for decision
5. Inability to give a rational reason for decision
6. Inability to employ a risk-benefit calculus
7. Inability to reach a reasonable decision

If we are to apply the rule to respect the wishes of competent patients consistently and impartially it is necessary to reach consensus on the criteria for judging competence. This far, however, efforts to do so have not proved very successful. Obvious reasons for this are that the notion of competence is a complex

---

Others refer to instances where the physician overrides an incompetent patient's refusal of life-saving medical treatment as 'weak paternalism'. Whereas *strong* paternalism involves overriding the wishes and choices of the *competent* patient, *weak* paternalism involves an action taken that is considered by the physician to be in the best interest of the patient who cannot give fully informed consent for some reason.

one and that judgements about competence are very subjective and difficult to verify. For example, 'Can the desire to die ever be seen as *rational*?' or, stated otherwise, 'Is a person who wishes to die ever competent or autonomous?' For some, a suicidal person shows himself to be irrational by virtue of his very desire to die. Kant argues, for instance, that to maintain one's life despite the most adverse circumstances is the only rational decision and hence one's duty as an autonomous person. According to him, the maxim 'From self-love I adopt it as a principle to shorten my life when its longer duration is likely to bring more evil than satisfaction' is not universalisable and thus not rational (1988:50). Yet it is also plausible to argue that, when it is certain that continued life would bring relentless suffering, the only rational choice is to hasten death. Another question that needs to be asked is, 'Can we ever be sure that a person's consent is *voluntary*?' It could be argued that the circumstances surrounding most terminally-ill patients make voluntary consent impossible, since they are usually either pain-racked or heavily drugged. A doctor might not be certain that the tormented cries of a stomach-cancer patient to be put out of his misery is an expression of informed consent or one of profound pain and despair. Yet one may ask whether the presence of pain and emotion necessarily excludes voluntariness: Do not the very tormented cries of someone suffering from profound pain and despair pay testimony to the voluntariness, if not also to the rationality, of his wishes?

These difficulties surrounding the term 'competence' have been the subject of much discussion. What lies at the basis of the failure to reach consensus on criteria of competence is that the debate is still carried out between two opposing fronts – those who favour the principle of autonomy, and those who give priority to the principles of beneficence and non-maleficence. Once we admit that competence is a matter of degree for which there can be no objective measure, the search for criteria becomes a matter of reaching a compromise between two important values: respecting the patient's right to self-determination, and protecting and promoting the patient's well-being. The implication is that the more lenient the criterion for competence, the more common will be a failure with regard to the principle of beneficence, and the stricter the criterion, the more common will be the failure with regard to the principle of autonomy.

### *The Discreet Paternalist*

The more paternalistically-inclined critic or physician would favour a stricter criterion for competence. The most stringent test listed above, standard 7, bases judgements of competence on the outcome chosen (consent or refusal), rather than on the process by which the decision was reached. By using a 'reasonable person' standard, this criterion restricts the range of acceptable outcomes of a reasoning process. When one considers that, in practice, the physician is usually the judge of what most reasonable people would choose, a patient would in effect be found incompetent if her decision conflicts with that of the physician, but competent if she agrees with him. This could occur through the physician making a recommendation with regard to treatment, leaving the patient to sign the informed consent form. A refusal to sign would be taken to indicate incompetence, since the patient failed to choose what most reasonable people would choose under similar circumstances. The obvious shortcoming of this approach is that it merely pays lip-service to the principle of autonomy. Making the physician's judgement the standard against which the patient's decision is judged ultimately leaves the physician free to decide.

Although some would find it blatantly paternalistic, this position is not entirely unattractive. Do we not think someone has made a rational decision based upon the fact we agree he has chosen the best outcome possible? Our grounds for considering April, Boris and Cain incompetent appear not so much the reasoning processes which led them to their conclusions, but the fact that we do not agree with the terms on which they are not prepared to accept life. If, for example, God appeared to Cain in a dream and told him to quit smoking, few would declare him incompetent or try to convince him of the irrationality of his decision.

I suspect that many who support legalised euthanasia by making reference to the principle of patient autonomy are indeed discreet paternalists. The greater the fervour with which they promote their case for voluntary euthanasia the more apparent it becomes that they think death to be a desirable goal for those suffering relentless pain, discomfort or degradation. Concern with the content of the decision is clearly reflected in the way advocates of legalising voluntary euthanasia formulate their proposal. They have contended that provision should be made (legally as well as medically) for a person's desire to die to be satisfied (in some swift, painless and bloodless way) if a person is in fact: (1) currently incurable; (2) beyond the aid of any cure or restoration which may reasonably be expected to eventuate within his life expectancy; (3) suffering intolerable and unmitigable pain; and (4) of a fixed and rational desire to die (see Young 1976:265). This proposal clearly reflects the belief that under such circumstances it would be in the best interest of the patient to die. A fixed and rational desire to die is not sufficient – the patient must also be terminally-ill and suffer intolerable pain. Indeed, we wouldn't think his decision *rational* if this were not the case. In the same way, the reason we find involuntary euthanasia morally abhorrent is not so much the disrespect shown to a person's rational decision to continue living, but because we think that the desire to live makes life worth living.

If one accepts this reasoning, one will just have to grit one's teeth and bear the label of 'closet paternalist'. (This position might not be too uncomfortable since most patients would be satisfied that their autonomy is indeed being respected, not knowing they are only considered competent because they signed the informed-consent form.) It is important to note that those who judge competence on the basis of the outcome chosen are not absolved from taking a stance on the appropriate goals of medical treatment. As noted earlier, one of the perceived advantages of the autonomy model is that it seeks to avoid making judgements about what is harmful or beneficial by letting each patient decide for herself. But as soon as competence is judged on the basis of the outcome chosen we have to consider what counts as a reasonable or desirable outcome, and this once again burdens us with all the problems faced when trying to specify the principles of beneficence and non-maleficence. A further implication is that the rule 'Always respect the wishes of competent patients' cannot be used as grounds for justifying euthanasia, since the criterion for competence used by discreet paternalists requires us to judge whether and when the choice of death is a reasonable decision. Alternatively, we could insist that the judgement of competence not be based on the content of the decision, but on whether the choice is freely and rationally made.

*The True Autonomist*

The true autonomist would have to be less strict in judging decision-making competence, and should take care not to use a standard that bases judgements of competence on the outcome chosen. Gillon (1995), amongst others, shows himself to be a true autonomist when he argues that the level of competence required should not exceed that which is set in determining whether someone is eligible to vote. If standard 1 is used, for example, a patient who refuses amputation surgery necessary to save her life would be found competent simply because she *uttered* a refusal. Her motive for refusing treatment, whether it be fear, ignorance or stubbornness would not be considered relevant. In this view, April, Boris and Cain will all be considered competent to make decisions about their own treatment, even if a somewhat stricter standard such as 2 or 3 is employed.

The obvious danger with this approach is the avoidable harm that could come to patients who are in a vulnerable state and who may need the intervention of physicians and other caregivers to protect their welfare. Of course, the autonomist reply to this objection is that it is paternalistic to suppose that physicians know what is best for their patients, and that this is exactly what the autonomy model seeks to avoid. The core of liberal philosophy is that individuals should be free to make their own decisions, and this includes the freedom to make mistakes. Their right to freedom can only be legitimately overridden if they violate the rights of others. For our present purposes it is unnecessary to examine the aims and justifications for the principle of respect for patient autonomy in any more detail (I will do so in Chapter Five). At this stage it is necessary to point out that the principle of respect for patient autonomy is of little use when trying to justify euthanasia or physician-assisted suicide.

Advocates of *voluntary passive euthanasia* implicitly or explicitly challenge the traditional interpretations of the principle of respect for autonomy and the right to self-determination.[6] J.S. Mill, one of the fathers of liberalism, argues that we need to respect and protect individual freedom of thought and discussion because it is a requirement for intellectual growth. It is doubtful that he would have considered the freedom to die an appropriate expression of individual autonomy:

> As it is useful that while mankind are imperfect there should be different opinions, so it is that there should be different experiments of living; that free scope should be given to varieties of character, short of injury to others; and that the worth of different modes of life should be proved practically, when anyone thinks to try them (Mill 1985:20).

---

[6] See Feinberg (1978:93-123) and Young (1976:264-283).

The view that respect for a patient can be conveyed through complying to her wish to die is a significant departure from the concept of respect for freedom generally held within Western medicine and culture. But even if we accept that the right to refuse treatment can be used to justify withdrawing life-sustaining treatment, it does not follow that *voluntary passive euthanasia* is morally acceptable. The patient's right to self-determination imposes upon others a corresponding obligation of non-interference. For a physician to impose treatment on a patient who has refused her consent would be a violation of her rights to privacy and bodily integrity. However, if this patient were to die as a result of cessation of treatment it would not really be a case of passive euthanasia, since the physician's intention is not to bring about the patient's death. As mentioned before, not all cases of letting die amount to passive euthanasia. In this case the physician's intention was to respect the patient's right to refuse treatment. If she continues to live despite cessation of treatment the physician will not feel that he has failed to achieve his goal.

With regard to *voluntary active euthanasia* or physician-assisted suicide the principle of patient autonomy and the right to self-determination provide even less support for the view that these practices are morally acceptable. The right to self-determination, being a negative right, does not impose upon others a corresponding positive obligation to provide one with assistance in acquiring the desired goods or for reaching a set goal. It only imposes the obligation not to interfere in one's attempt to reach one's own goals. The right to self-determination thus supports a right to commit suicide, but not a right to receive assistance in one's suicide.

It can be argued that the contractual relationship between health-care professionals and the public does generate certain claims on behalf of patients. Whether it is through private insurance or government funding, patients have a legitimate claim to be provided with medical treatment on offer. Just as a shopkeeper cannot refuse to sell the wares on display in his shop to someone who is willing to pay the price, physicians have an obligation to provide their clients with medical services. However, this argument relies on an already-formed judgement to the effect that active euthanasia and physician-assisted suicide are (or should be) among the medical procedures on offer. One cannot demand to buy an item from a shopkeeper unless he already has this item for sale. In the same way, patients have a right to be informed of medical procedures available, but it is yet to be determined that euthanasia is one of these procedures. The implication is that advocates of voluntary euthanasia who seek to justify their position with reference to the right to self-determination or the principle of respect for patient autonomy *are not absolved from taking a stance on the question concerning the appropriate goals of medical treatment.* The right to self-determination does not entail a right to active euthanasia or a right to be assisted in one's suicide, unless euthanasia or assisted suicide has already been determined to be an acceptable medical procedure.

## Conclusion

The first question that arises with the treatment of terminally- or incurably-ill patients is whether euthanasia can ever be seen as the appropriate expression of compassion; in other words, whether 'mercy-killing' is indeed merciful. Yet in the modern era it appears that compassion has largely lost its relevance in science and ethics. The compassion for which the nineteenth century physician was known seems possible only in the comfortable surroundings of a patient's bedroom and within the context of a previously-established personal relationship. The progress of medical science seems to depend on a cultural context and scientific paradigm that reject subjective values, religious beliefs and emotions, all of which stand in the way of gaining knowledge that is universal, objective and impersonal. Adherents to a principle-based ethic have followed scientists in viewing compassion as an irrational and often dangerous force in human affairs. Morality is founded in reason, which in their view requires the acceptance of duties or principles that are universal, absolute and impartial. In Chapter Three I argue that scientific values and compassionate care do not constitute two incommensurate forces, and I develop an account of compassion which will allow us to answer the question of whether and when euthanasia is the appropriate expression of compassion.

A second problem complex explored in this chapter regards the ends of medicine, more specifically, whether death can ever be seen as the appropriate goal of treatment. Recent advances in medical science, together with the value pluralism typical of modern societies, have led to a crisis in ends, asking us to re-evaluate the proper goals of medical treatment. Medical science and technology aim to produce certain clinical results, yet these reliable results are not always in the best interest of individual patients. There are exceptions to the general rule that a successfully prolonged life is a benefit. We find a similar intolerance towards exceptions in the principle-based ethic. The focus on issues concerning the procedures or means used to bring about death reflects a typically-modernist attempt to define clear rules of conduct, to sharpen the soft edges of ethics to conform to the exactness of natural sciences. The application of universal rules of conduct to specific cases often results in a failure to achieve the best possible outcome for the individual in question. In Chapter Four I will examine the questions concerning the goals of medicine by re-examining the principle of beneficence and by developing an account of the virtue of benevolence.

Finally, the crisis of ends has led to the adoption of the principle of respect for patient autonomy, which has formed the basis of renewed attempts to justify voluntary euthanasia and physician-assisted suicide. However, these attempts fail to show that the right to die imposes upon physicians a duty to kill or to give assistance in suicide. If euthanasia were to be a morally-acceptable practice, it would be as an act of charity or compassion, that is, as a virtuous response to an individual's suffering. In Chapter Five I critically examine the principle for respect for patient autonomy and develop an account of the virtue of respect which overcomes the shortcomings of the autonomy model.

## Chapter Three

# Compassion and Reason

### Introduction

We often hear the complaint that medical professionals have become cold and impersonal technocrats who treat their patients as biological organisms or machines. Despite being quite eager to reap the benefits of medical science, people increasingly plead for a more 'holistic' and humane approach to health care. It is argued that the physician should respond to the patient as a person, and pay attention to both the physical and mental factors affecting a patient's overall well-being. One of the voices in this chorus of complaints is that of Buytendijk. He writes:

> The diagnosis of a doctor does rest, to a certain degree, on a generally accepted scheme of physical processes, the causes of their being interrupted and the means of restoring equilibrium. This knowledge is applied independently of personal factors affecting the sick person. At most the patient's life history, constitution and milieu, which can be gauged by objective examination, have a certain contribution to make. But when the patient calls for help in his *suffering*, then the doctor is no longer concerned with a 'case', but with a sick man, and more is required of him than could be expected from a scholar or technician. The doctor is now expected to understand man, in health and in sickness.... A doctor seeks from the natural sciences the basis of his professional treatment. But in addition he needs to have more intimate knowledge of the human personality than the layman has, and his experience provides him with some knowledge of human society (1961:39, emphasis in original).

In much the same way Sauerbruch and Wenke argue that, in trying to understand the suffering of patients, the physician should not focus exclusively on one aspect of the pain experience, but on the total experience of suffering: 'No interpretation of pain that fails to establish a relationship with the total personality of the individual in question can possibly do justice to the whole problem' (1963:141). More recently, Alfred Tauber has reiterated this viewpoint by arguing that, beyond technical expertise and performance, medical ethics must face the challenge of establishing the physician's identification with the patient. Medical science needs to be oriented back to its primary moral responsibility, which is 'the empathetic response to the call of the ill'. Without prioritising empathy, he argues, we doom ourselves to 'a myopic technocratic medicine' (1999:114).

This insistence by many contemporary critics of the Western medical paradigm that we need a more holistic understanding and treatment of patients has not, however, had much of an impact on medical practice. One reason for this is that Western medicine and culture have certain deep-seated suspicions about notions such as compassion, pity and empathy, reflected in the work of philosophers such as Plato, the Stoics, Kant, Spinoza, Nietzsche and others. For some of these thinkers, the rejection of compassion as a virtue forms part of a more general rejection of virtue ethics. Other figures in the anti-pity tradition object only to the view that compassion is a virtue, instead arguing in favour of virtues such as courage, self-sufficiency, pride, and the like.

Another reason for the lack of impact of the appeals for a more humane or holistic medical ethic is that, for the most part, proponents have failed to substantiate their appeals with well-reasoned arguments in favour of their position. This has added fuel to the objection that virtue ethicists rely on emotional appeals to promote irrational views. Louden argues, for instance, that contemporary accounts of virtue ethics have a 'negative rather than positive thrust', their primary aim being 'to criticize the traditions and research programs to which it is opposed rather than to state positively what its own alternative is' (1997:202).

In this chapter I develop an account of what I believe to be a central virtue in medical practice – compassion – in an attempt to show that scientific and humane values do not constitute two incommensurate forces.

## The First Feature of Suffering: The Solitary Patient

One of the shortcomings of principle-based ethical systems, as well as the Cartesian-Newtonian paradigm of disease, is their neglect of the emotional and existential elements of the patient's experience of disease: Medical textbooks say precious little, if anything, about the patient's personal experience and interpretation of his condition. The obvious reason for this is that, while diseases and symptoms are recurring and predictable, the patient's experience and interpretation of his medical condition are highly individualistic. Suffering is not subject to prediction and explanation, and hence not to treatment.

However, we should guard against over-estimating the degree to which experiences, values and interpretations are unique to individuals. A study of the vast number of literary texts on the nature of suffering, written in different times and places, reveals certain common themes. As I shall argue in greater detail later in this chapter, to understand and fully appreciate an individual's suffering it is necessary to focus on both the similarities and the differences in people's interpretation and experience of disease and disability. Next to personal experience, the best avenue for developing insight into suffering is through literature. I shall therefore illustrate my arguments using various examples from Western literature which deal specifically with the tragic dimensions of suffering, with particular focus on Sophocles's tragic drama *Philoctetes* (produced in 409 BC) and Leo Tolstoy's short story entitled 'The Death of Ivan Ilyich' (written in 1886).

In this chapter I focus mainly on the first aspect which typically forms a significant part of human suffering, namely the sense of solitude often experienced by patients who suffer from serious disease or illness.

Legend has it that Philoctetes, a good man and soldier, was on his way to Troy to fight alongside the Greeks, when he paid a visit to the temple of the goddess Chryse. There he was bitten on the foot by the serpent that guarded the shrine. His foot began to ooze with foul-smelling pus, and the pain made him cry out curses that are said to have spoiled the religious observances of the other soldiers. Consequently he was banished to the uninhabited island of Lemnos, a lame man with no friends and no resources but his bow and arrow, where he eked out a wretched and lonely existence throughout the ten years of the Trojan war. In Sophocles's tragedy, we meet Philoctetes after he has spent ten years on the island. He still suffers severe physical pain, but his physical affliction is not the only source of his misery. He suffers from a terrifying isolation, abandoned by his friends and removed from his family. Being alone on an island, there is little he can do to improve his situation, and during the ten years of his stay on the island he has barely managed to survive. The soldiers find the formerly virtuous and independent soldier in a helpless, desperate and dependent state that renders him vulnerable to exploitation and deception. Their arrival does not bring respite from isolation. Philoctetes remains separated by his dependency and helplessness, the offensiveness of his wound and, most of all, by the deceit of the soldiers. At the end of the play, he repeatedly expresses the wish to die. Ultimately, his only choice seems to be between an agonising but noble death, and accepting the help of his enemies at the price of his integrity.

In 'The Death of Ivan Ilyich' Tolstoy relates the story of the suffering of a dying man, a story which has been described by Nuland as 'terrifying in its uncanny accuracy' (1994:245). Although the nature of Ivan Ilyich's disease remains a mystery to the reader (as to Ivan Ilyich himself), the reader gains insight into the nature of his suffering, which in many ways is similar to that of Philoctetes. In a masterful way, Tolstoy brings home to the reader the dying man's frustration with his ailing and weak body, his sense of helplessness in not being able to defeat illness, and his reflection not only upon his physical state, but also on the meaning of his life as a whole. 'He wept at his own helplessness, at his terrible loneliness, at the cruelty of man, the cruelty of God, at the absence of God' (Tolstoy 1960:152). A central feature of Ivan Ilyich's suffering that strikes the reader is his terrifying isolation, stemming from his inability, as well as that of his family, to discuss the significance of his disease and impending death in an open and honest way, so that 'he had to live thus on the edge of the precipice alone, without a single soul to understand and feel for him' (Tolstoy 1960:132). It is often this feeling of solitude that, apart from physical pain and discomfort, constitutes a person's suffering.

By its very nature, physical pain tends to isolate the sufferer. The sensation of pain is an entirely subjective experience – no one can experience or share my pain. I can experience and observe pain when it happens to me, but not when it happens to anyone else. Analogy leads me to believe that other people have similar experiences, but this is an inference only. The implication is that 'sympathy', in its strictly literal sense of sharing another's pain, is impossible. For the person in pain, it is so incontestably present that 'having pain' may come to be thought of as the most vibrant example of what it is to 'have certainty'. At the same time, pain is so elusive for the other person that 'hearing about pain' may exist as the primary model of what it is 'to have doubt'. Thus pain appears at once as that which cannot be denied and that which cannot be confirmed (Scarry 1985:4). Medical contexts provide many instances of this phenomenon: To have pain is to have certainty, but to hear that another person has pain is to have doubt. This doubt may aggravate the suffering and isolation of those already in pain.

Language allows us to objectify an experience verbally, to make it an object of discussion. But it is difficult, if not impossible, to communicate one's pain accurately, to describe the sensation to someone who has not experienced a similar sensation. Pain remains one's own to deal with and to reflect upon. Sartre remarks:

> [P]ain-consciousness is an internal negation of the world; but at the same time it exists its pain – i.e., itself – as a wrenching away from self. Pure pain as the simple 'lived' cannot be reached; it belongs to the category of indefinables and indescribables which are what they are (1993:333).

But pain does not only resist language, it also has the ability to destroy language and finally consciousness itself. Scarry (1985:54) gives an illuminating account of pain in his discussion of the politics of torture. Pain first monopolises language by becoming its only subject; complaint becomes the exclusive mode of speech. Eventually the pain so deepens that the coherence of complaint is displaced by the sounds anterior to learned language. Severe and prolonged pain tends also to obliterate the contents of consciousness. It begins by annihilating the objects of complex thought and emotion and later destroys even the most elemental acts of perception (hence the expression 'blinding pain'). Finally, pain leads to a total loss of consciousness.

One of the implications of pain's tendency to resist language is that the same pain or disease appears fundamentally different to the patient who is suffering it than to the physician who has to diagnose and treat it. Sauerbruch and Wenke (1963:107-108) use the terms 'anthropological sickness' and 'medical sickness' to clarify the different perspectives of patient and physician. In the first case it is a question of 'being', the existentialist total state; and in the second case it is a question of a 'picture', an abstract construction of the inner-functioning relationships worked out by research according to medical indications. It is quite impossible to comprehend the latter form of sickness as though it were an experience; similarly, the physician himself cannot experience the condition of his patient.

Insofar as pain isolates the sufferer from the rest of the world and from all that is unconnected with his suffering, and in posing a threat to his health or life, it leads to an urge of self-preservation. The person may appear to be excessively preoccupied with himself. His suffering tears him out of his normal relationships and forces him into a special position. This preoccupation with his own pain may also limit his perspective or ability to interpret the meaning and significance of the experience. It is not only with regard to the explanation and management of physical pain that the sufferer may need the help of others. He or she may also be unable to answer the existential questions brought about by pain. For instance, a patient may wonder whether or why he is being punished or tested by God, he may consider how the illness will affect his life plan and inter-personal relationships, or how to deal with the limitation of freedom brought about by the illness. 'Tormented by pain', Buytendijk writes, 'the questioning bears the mark of a protest. Pain is painful in a double sense, since it is also a puzzle tormenting us' (1961:25-26). If the sufferer is unable to answer these questions about the meaning or significance of suffering, the sense of isolation and the reflection it brings about gives way to a feeling of abandonment, where he becomes aware only of his weakness and helplessness in the face of pain.

In the Modern period the motif of dying alone occurs more frequently than ever before. The most obvious cause of this isolation is the medicalisation of the dying process, which removes the patient from his home and places him into a foreign environment. A more fundamental cause of isolation is the fear of death, often accompanied by a denial of the inevitability or finality of death. A patient's acceptance of the reality of impending death is often frowned upon by bystanders as pessimism, a lack of courage, or sheer negativity. This accounts for the embarrassment people often feel in the presence of the dying. Having previously related to the person as a parent, friend or colleague, others now have to relate to a dying patient. The inability and unwillingness of people to communicate openly with a dying person perhaps stems from the fact that his or her dying reminds them of the inevitability of their own death. Modern man does not want to identify with the dying person. As John Donne writes in his *Devotions*: 'Any man's death diminishes me, because I am involved in Mankinde.' Whether consciously or unconsciously, people tend to resist the idea of their own ageing and dying as best they can.

## The Compassionate Response

Sophocles demonstrates two possible attitudes that one might have towards Philoctetes in his tragic circumstances. The first is that of Odysseus, who returns after ten years to fetch Philoctetes from the island. Odysseus knows that they cannot win the war without the invincible bow and arrows that Heracles gave to Philoctetes at his death. The leaders of the expedition know that Philoctetes will not surrender the bow and arrows to those who have betrayed him in the past, so they plan to trick him into returning with them.

A second response is that of the chorus of young soldiers. Even before they see Philoctetes, and never having met him before, the chorus vividly imagines what it is like to be him, and they enter a protest against the callousness of the commanders:

> 'Tis a pitiful life for a man, and no mistake. Lonesome. Not a living soul to talk to; no one to help him bear his pains; pitiful. Suffering like that. Pretty near out of his mind, I should say, with all he has to put up with. You'd wonder a man could stand it. To think the gods could send such mischief to man! 'Tis ever a curse for a man to be marked above the common lot. Son of a high-born house, likely as not, as good as the best; and now, lost and alone with the furred and feathered creatures, tortured with want and pain he can never cure; and no one to answer his cries but the echo in far-off hills (*Philoctetes* ll. 169-183).

As the members of the chorus imagine the suffering of a man they do not know, they stand in for the imaginative activity of the audience, for whom the entire tragic drama is a similar exercise in empathy. The chorus responds to Philoctetes's innocence in the terrible turn of fortune that has befallen him, and they recognise the fact that his affliction or misfortune is something that can happen to anyone, including themselves. This sentiment is eventually shared by Neoptolemus, one of the leaders of the expedition. Although he initially plays along with Odysseus's attempt at trickery by pretending to pity Philoctetes, in the end his compassion shows itself to be genuine.

Tolstoy captures the sentiment of compassion in the figure of Gerassim, a young peasant boy. Gerassim helps Ivan Ilyich with the most ordinary activities of daily living which he becomes increasingly unable to do for himself, such as moving him from the bed to a chair, cleaning and feeding him, and complying to his somewhat bizarre wishes. Ivan Ilyich discovers, for example, that he is most comfortable when his legs are raised, so that Gerassim often holds his legs up with his master's feet resting on his shoulders. For the most part, however, the dying man is alone in his room while his family goes about their daily business. The comforting presence of Gerassim is contrasted with the discomfort Ivan Ilyich's family feels in his presence. They avoid him, and when they do 'drop in' they shun the topic of his illness and his impending death. Tolstoy also contrasts Gerassim's response to that of the physicians attending Ivan Ilyich. Despite being the competent authorities on explaining disease, the physicians are unable to understand their patient's suffering:

> To Ivan Ilyich only one question was important: was his case serious or not? But the doctor ignored this misplaced inquiry. From the doctor's point of view it was a side issue not under consideration: the real business was the assessing of probabilities to decide between a floating kidney, chronic catarrh or appendicitis. It was not a question of Ivan Ilyich's life or death but one between a floating kidney or appendicitis (1960:127).

Compassion also forms a central part of the Christian response to suffering, which is captured in the parable of the Good Samaritan. Various thinkers in the history of Western philosophy, such as the Arthur Schopenhauer, Adam Smith, Jean-Jacques Rousseau, David Hume and John Hick have analysed compassion or closely related terms such as empathy, pity and sympathy, each ascribing to it a different role in moral decision-making and acting. I shall refer to some of these accounts in the course of this chapter, and demonstrate how they differ from the

Aristotelian account of compassion. At this stage it is only necessary to provide a general account of compassion.

Compassion is one type of emotional reaction to the fortunes that befall others. Following Ortony *et al.* (1988:92) one may distinguish four basic types of 'fortunes-of-others-emotions' on the basis of the relation between the object's feelings and the subject's emotional response:

1. being pleased about an event that is desirable for the other (e.g. delighted-for, happy-for, pleased-for, etc.);
2. being displeased about an event undesirable for someone else (e.g. compassion, pity, sympathy);
3. being displeased about an event that is desirable for the other (e.g. envy, jealousy, resentment); and
4. being pleased about an event undesirable for someone else (e.g. gloating, *Schadenfreude*).

Of these, the first two are forms of empathy, in that the subject reacts to the object with the same type of emotion. The word 'empathy' is derived from the Greek *empatheia*, 'in feeling' (German: *einfülung*). Compassion is, then, a form of empathy involving an imaginative dwelling on the condition of the other person. Empathy requires a person to understand or appreciate how another person must feel, given the situation the other is in, and it requires the empathising person to be in some related (but not necessarily identical) emotional state.

However, compassion is not only a 'feeling with' another. It is also, and more specifically, a 'suffering with' another, as suggested by the etymology of the word (Latin: *compassio*). Compassion and sympathy differ from other empathetic emotions insofar as the subject specifically focuses on the *suffering* or *negative state* of the other, and this suffering evokes a similar feeling of distress or suffering for the person who perceives this plight. But in contrast to sympathy, compassion also has a strong *cognitive* or *intellectual* element. It does not simply involve feeling the same but also understanding the nature of the other's plight. Compassion characteristically involves an identification with the other by imagining what the afflicted person is going through and coming to share in his feelings or suffering in this way.

Compassion involves three elements:

1. *empathy*, an understanding of and identification with the other's suffering;
2. *benevolence*, a concern for their welfare giving rise to attempts to alleviate their misfortune or suffering; and
3. *respect*, conveyed through one's concern for their welfare and the attempt to understand and help them.

As such, compassion is intricately related to the virtues of benevolence and respectfulness, which will be analysed in the following two chapters. My focus in this chapter is on the empathetic element of compassion.

## Two Objections to Compassion

The virtues of compassion and benevolence formed the basis of medical practice in the Hippocratic and Christian eras. However, the virtue-based ethic has gradually given way to a predominantly duty- or principle-based ethic, so that the virtues play a marginal role in contemporary medical practice. Nurses are still expected to be compassionate, while physicians – those who make the 'important' decisions – are expected to be rational and objective. These requirements, many believe, exclude emotions such as compassion. In one of the most widely used and frequently reissued textbooks on biomedical ethics, *Principles of Biomedical Ethics* (Beauchamp and Childress 1994), the four principles of medical ethics (beneficence, non-maleficence, autonomy and justice) form the focal part of the book, while the virtues, being of 'supplementary value', are briefly discussed in a separate chapter at the end of the book.

There has been a long tradition in Western thought of rejecting the claim that compassion is a morally valuable disposition. This tradition started with Plato and the ancient Stoics, and includes influential thinkers such as Kant, Spinoza and Nietzsche. The Platonic and Stoic criticism of compassion involves two central objections: the first being that compassion is irrational and rests on false beliefs; the second that compassion is disrespectful towards the sufferer. My central aim in this chapter is to develop an account of compassion that is immune to these objections. First, however, we need to examine the objections in more detail.

### *The Distant Onlooker: The Irrationality of Compassion*

The first form of criticism of the virtues has been made by some modern moral theorists – particularly liberal individualists – following the strict Kantian opposition between emotion and reason. This attack involves the claim that compassion, being an emotion and a form of empathy, precludes rational judgement and deliberation. A passionate (even a compassionate) engagement with others frequently blinds reason and renders partial what should be impartial reflection. The Platonic and Kantian traditions have thus treated compassion as an irrational force in human affairs, one which is likely to mislead or distract us when making moral decisions.

Liberal philosophy, grounded as it is in the independent and rational decision-maker, has established a hierarchical opposition between reason and emotion. The choice is portrayed as one between a compassionate community and the Enlightenment's commitment to reason and reflection. Emotions, being irrational, have nothing valuable to contribute to public reasoning. In economics, politics and law we find a similar contrast between emotion and reason, especially where appeals to compassion are involved. People's choices are only to be respected if they do not reflect the influence of emotional factors, that is, if they are fully autonomous. By contrast, communitarian critics of liberalism argue that sentiments such as compassion are important in moral decision-making and have rejected the liberal ideals of impartiality and universalisability. However, they grant that this will mean basing ethical judgement upon a force that is affective and instinctive rather than concerned with rational judgement and thought. In this way they affirm the simple opposition between the cognitive and the emotive.

The appeal for distance and the exclusion of partiality has a special relevance in the medical field. The modern medical paradigm necessitates scientific insight into disease, which demands that experience be obtained at a certain distance from the object studied. This in turn requires that the false perspectives due to emotional involvement be excluded. For this reason medical practitioners are discouraged from forming emotional ties with their patients, since this would impair and prejudice their medical judgement. The first task of the physician is to make a diagnosis of a patient's medical condition, which requires scientific insight. Their second task is to benefit the patient by restoring health, relieving pain and preventing death of the biological organism, and this requires technical skill. In this view, the tragedy of Ivan Ilyich's suffering consists solely in the fact that medical science of the time was not sufficiently developed to enable a correct diagnosis and adequate treatment.

The task of understanding a patient's suffering, and of helping him to overcome his sense of solitude and abandonment is therefore passed on to the family and friends of the patient. In modern hospitals, however, the patient is often refused even this escape from solitude. Modern medicine has greatly added to the isolation of the patient through removing the patient from the home and restricting visiting hours. Writing in the 1960s, Glaser and Strauss warns that the presence of relations at the bedside of a dying family member during the last days can pose serious problems for the doctors and nursing staff of the hospital, thereby reducing the efficiency of patient care. They appreciate that close relations offer comfort and care to the patient in economically less developed regions but point out that the crowding around the stricken person is not particularly hygienic. Family members bring in dirt from the street to the sickbed, and tend the patient with unwashed hands. For this reason modern hospitals rarely allow unhampered visits (Glaser and Strauss 1968:151-152). There seems to be a direct conflict between compassionate and effective treatment. In modern hospitals patients might receive the most advanced, scientifically-based medical treatment available, but this is only possible if the inconvenience of the presence of friends and family members is removed wherever possible, and if doctors maintain an objective distance to allow rational and objective treatment.

Over the last few decades we have seen a movement towards more humane health care, particularly in the fields of terminal and maternity care. Yet this movement has resulted in the establishment of separate institutions, leaving the medical sphere untouched. The Hospice movement, for instance, aims to provide compassionate care for the dying through the exclusion of technological intervention and by focusing on the development of palliative care. At the other end of life the call for more humane medicine has given rise to the establishment of maternity centres that aim to de-medicalise childbirth. Pregnant women today are faced with the decision between *either* the homely environment of a birth centre and a team of midwives (for uncomplicated births only) *or* the maternity ward of a hospital that provides specialist obstetric care and has facilities for epidurals, Caesarean sections and special care for premature and sick babies.

Some of those who do acknowledge the role of compassion in modern medical practice have attributed to it only a marginal role, as valuable in addition to reason. In their brief discussion of the virtues, Beauchamp and Childress (1994:467-468) argue that the expression of compassion makes a critical moral difference insofar as people feel assured and cared for by a person of compassion. The emotional tone displayed in the interaction is part of the assistance rendered. On the other hand, however, they accept Kant and Spinoza's objection that compassion may also cloud judgement and preclude rational and effective responses. They argue that constant contact with suffering can overwhelm and sometimes paralyse a compassionate physician or nurse. To prevent impartial judgement from giving way to impassioned decision, medical education should be designed to inculcate detachment as well as compassion. They conclude that when compassion appropriately motivates and expresses good character, it has a role in ethics alongside impartial reason and dispassionate judgement. Their position is based on a rigid distinction between the patient's physical pain and his emotional suffering. The physician's only serious task is to diagnose and treat a patient's disease, while his compassion is merely a display geared towards comforting and reassuring the patient as an emotional being. However, I think that the role of compassion is more central to medical decision-making than these writers would grant. Its value is not limited to the reassurance given to sufferers through the emotional tone displayed in the interaction. Before developing this argument it is necessary to examine the second objection to compassion.

### *The Lonely Hero: Compassion as Disrespect*

Various writers have argued that pain is existentially meaningful exactly because it isolates the sufferer from others. For instance, Buytendijk sees pain as valuable since it forces the sufferer to reflect on his condition, the seriousness of the threat posed by the pain, and its origin, meaning and significance in the context of his life. Pain in all its forms is conducive to reflection – in the words of Husserl, our pain sensations receive an objective 'interpretation' or 'taking-up'. The attempt to understand the nature and significance of pain reveals a capacity that is particular to human beings. Only human beings can make their experience of pain the subject matter of reflection. The possibility of a reflective attitude, of a personal reaction to pain, is given in the very form of helplessness which involves a 'destruction of self in the body of agony' (Buytendijk 1961:148).

In *Philoctetes* the deified Heracles presents a similar attitude when he says to Philoctetes: 'So you must win, it is ordained, through suffering glory in life. You are to go to Troy with him; you are to have your sickness cured; you are to be the chosen champion of that great army' (*Philoctetes* ll. 1426-1428). Philoctetes's escape from suffering is not made possible by the compassion and benevolence of any of the other characters. Instead, their compassion only insults him by implying that he needs their help. He achieves 'glory in life' as a reward for his relentless and independent struggle through misery and hardship. Despite his desperate situation and the relief that leaving the island with the soldiers would bring, he maintains his integrity by holding fast to his moral convictions.

The view that suffering forms a meaningful part of human life by separating the person from others is perhaps best exemplified by Nietzsche. Nietzsche's affirmation of the value of suffering, together with his rejection of pity,[1] forms a central part of his critique of Christian morality as an enterprise which preaches selflessness and self-sacrifice as central virtues. Fundamental to Nietzsche's view is the idea that individual responsibility for overcoming weakness in all its forms is the prime expression of man's biological nature. An individual succeeds only to the degree that he asserts his autonomy by separating himself from the community and shunning its help. Nietzsche's philosophy takes Modernism and the Lockean ideal of individual autonomy to its logical extreme. In many ways, his arguments in support of the view that pity is disrespectful of the worth and dignity of the sufferer are reminiscent of those expressed by Plato and the Stoics, yet as we shall see, he also explicitly distances himself from certain aspects of the Stoic tradition. It is possible to identify four arguments against pity in Nietzsche's writings.[2]

*Pity disregards the positive value of suffering by inappropriately inflating the value of worldly goods* Nietzsche's argument against pity is directed at the philosophy of Schopenhauer, whom he sees as being hostile to life. Schopenhauer views suffering as ultimately pointless and intrinsically abhorrent. Nothing could be more desirable than eliminating suffering. He insists that suffering is nevertheless inseparable from life: Human life is one of misery. This suffering can be rendered meaningful and bearable by establishing a community of sufferers through pity. Nietzsche argues, against Schopenhauer's profound pessimism, that pity persuades men to nothingness, for it fastens upon all that is miserable. By making suffering contagious it merely multiplies misery (1990:130-131).[3]

---

[1] The meaning of term 'Mitleid' as used by Nietzsche is the most accurately rendered by the term 'pity' as it is used today, that is, as a condescending attitude to the sufferer as one who suffers because of weakness or some fault of his own. In referring to Nietzsche's conception, I shall therefore use the term 'pity', while 'compassion' shall be used to refer to the Aristotelian conception.

[2] I am indebted much to Martha Nussbaum (1994 and 1996) for the analysis of Nietzsche's position on pity.

[3] This is the view expressed by Caravaggio in Michael Ondaatje's novel entitled *The English Patient*. Caravaggio finds Hana – the nurse who takes care of a patient suffering from severe and fatal burn injuries – half-naked and weeping at the kitchen table. When he asks her why she adores the patient so, she answers: 'He is a saint. I think. A despairing saint. Are there such things? Our desire is to protect them.' Caravaggio answers: 'You have to protect yourself from sadness. Sadness is very close to hate.... If you take in someone else's poison – thinking you can cure them by sharing it – you will instead store it within you.' He advises her instead to focus on her own survival and self-realisation: 'Those men in the desert were smarter than you. They assumed he could be useful. So they saved him, but when he was no longer useful they left him' (Ondaatje 1992:45).

Although Nietzsche agrees that human existence is one of suffering, the answer for him does not lie in the denial of the will to live, but in life's ecstatic affirmation. Our pains are no excuse for slandering the world (1974:256-257). It is the very inseparability of life and suffering which leads him to emphasise the necessity of coming to terms with suffering rather than avoiding the issue in one's philosophical moments. Against the strongly negative evaluation of suffering Nietzsche sees pain as giving us the opportunity for self-development exactly through experiencing and enduring it. He regrets that sufferers and pitiers alike disregard the positive value of pain. In an aphorism entitled 'Wisdom in Pain' Nietzsche writes:

> [T]here is as much wisdom in pain as there is in pleasure: both belong among the factors that contribute the most to the preservation of the species. If pain did not, it would have perished long ago; that it hurts is no argument against it but its essence. In pain I hear the captain's command: 'Take in the sails!' The bolder seafarer 'man' must have mastered the art of doing a thousand things with his sails; otherwise he would be done for in no time, and the ocean would swallow him. We must learn to live with diminished energies too: As soon as pain gives its safety signal the time has come to diminish them; some great danger or other, a storm is approaching, and we are well advised to 'inflate' ourselves as little as possible (1974:252-253).

Nietzsche's objection to pity stems from his view that the pain and suffering for which we pity people are usually not things that are bad for them. He shares with the Stoics the view that pity denigrates the sufferer's own efforts by inappropriately inflating the importance of worldly goods such as money, status, friendships and material comforts. Indeed, for Nietzsche, ill health should not be seen as an occasion for lamentation but as an opportunity for growth. He goes even further than the Stoics by claiming that the loss of external goods is actually good for us. In *The Will to Power* he writes:

> To those human beings who are of any concern to me I wish suffering, desolation, sickness, ill-treatment, indignities – I wish that they should not remain unfamiliar with profound self-contempt, the torture of self-mistrust, the wretchedness of the vanquished: I have no pity for them, because I wish them the only thing that can prove today whether one is worth anything or not – that one endures (1967b:481).

Unlike the Stoics, his rejection of pity does not form part of a more general rejection of passion and emotion. In *The Gay Science* he denounces the Stoic attitude to pain by asking whether our life is really painful and burdensome enough to make it advantageous to exchange it for a Stoic way of life and petrifaction. He answers: 'We are *not so badly off* that we have to be as badly off as Stoics' (1974:257, emphasis in original). Like Schopenhauer, he views *suffering* as inseparable from the qualitative enhancement of *life*; but instead of taking the former to warrant repudiation of the latter, Nietzsche takes the latter to sanction the former, and so to require a reversal of the basic intention of the morality of pity (Schacht 1992:461). Unlike the Stoic morality of apathy as well as Schopenhauer's contempt for human life, Nietzsche's philosophy affirms the value of life and suffering, which are intricately linked to each other.

*One cannot fully comprehend the other's suffering* Nietzsche argues that the essential subjectivity of the pain sensation and the isolation brought about by pain cannot be overcome by sharing one's pain and suffering with others. The other is not only incapable of feeling one's pain, but also of understanding one's suffering. Nietzsche's insistence that one should 'keep to one's own way' in bearing suffering with courage also stems from his view that true compassion is impossible:

> Our personal and profoundest suffering is incomprehensible to almost everyone; here we remain hidden from our neighbour, even if we eat from one pot.... [O]ne simply knows nothing of the whole inner sequence and intricacies that are distress for *me* or for *you* (1974:269-271, emphasis in original).

Because others cannot fully understand the nature of the individual's suffering, their attempts to do so through the supposed virtues of compassion and benevolence end in pity and a denigration of the sufferer's worth:

> But whenever people *notice* that we suffer, they interpret our suffering superficially. It is the very essence of the emotion of pity that it strips away from the suffering of others whatever is distinctively personal. Our 'benefactors' are, more than our enemies, people who make our worth and will smaller (1974:269, emphasis in original).

Nietzsche believes that attempts to feel compassion for someone inevitably end in pity and disrespect since it is impossible to form an understanding of the complexities of the other's suffering. The Christian conception of pity does not promote or convey respect for the sufferer. The cost to the individual of the comfort he gains from seeking out the pity and companionship of others, is his self-worth. The only way to maintain his self-respect is to affirm his individuality by not seeking to share his suffering and by rejecting the pity of others. In other words, the value of suffering – and thus also of life – can only be affirmed if one chooses the solitary route. Whereas the herd finds it a crime to 'go apart and be alone', Zarathustra welcomes solitude and the incomprehension of the crowd as necessary conditions of true creativity: 'Go apart and be alone with your love and your creating.... I love him who wants to create beyond himself, and thus perishes' (Nietzsche 1969:90-91). Courageous people do not want to be pitied, but instead prefer to deal with their pain alone:

> Their expression is never prouder, more warlike, and happier than it is when a storm comes up; indeed, pain itself gives them their greatest moments. This is the heroic type, the great *pain bringers* of humanity, those few or rare human beings who need the very same apology that pain itself needs.... They contribute immensely to the preservation and enhancement of the species, even if it were only by opposing comfortableness and by not concealing how this sort of happiness nauseates them (Nietzsche 1974:253, emphasis in original).

*Pity is based on a view of human beings as weak and shameful* According to Nietzsche, those who experience suffering and displeasure as evil, hateful, worthy of annihilation, and as a defect of existence know little of human happiness, 'for happiness and unhappiness are sisters and even twins that either grow up together or, as in your case, *remain small* together' (1974:270, emphasis in original). He believes that suffering has intrinsic value since it separates those who bear pain with courage, pride and nobility from those who adhere to the 'religion of comfortableness'. This is superior to a Christian attitude to suffering – the 'religion of pity' – that views and treats human beings as equals. In *Beyond Good and Evil* he writes:

> The spiritual haughtiness and nausea of every man who has suffered profoundly – it almost determines the order of rank *how* profoundly human beings can suffer... this spiritual and silent haughtiness of the sufferer, this pride of the elect of knowledge, of the 'initiated', of the almost sacrificed, finds all kinds of disguises necessary to protect itself against contact with obtrusive and pitying hands and altogether against everything that is not its equal in suffering. *Profound suffering makes noble; it separates* (1989:220, emphasis added).

Heroic endurance of suffering separates a person from 'the herd'; it defies the attempts of the weak to defile the sufferer to the inferior status of being their equal. Inherent in Christian pity is a view of human beings as low and pathetic, as beings whose shameful bodily nature and animal instincts lead them into sinfulness. Suffering is therefore an equally shameful and disgusting affair, punishment for humankind's innate sinfulness. Pity belittles not only the pitied but also the pitier. By feeling pity for another, we ourselves are defiled to the level of the herd by acknowledging our weakness and insufficiency. By *identifying* with the weak we also reveal a self-contempt, a disgust with ourselves and our humanity (see Nietzsche 1967a:67-69, 121-125; 1982:83-85, 143; 1989:149-150).

*Pity is not altruistic, but egoistic* Nietzsche is also highly suspicious of the claim that the morality of pity is altruistic. In the final instance, pity is always egoistic. The pitier's deed of pity is an attempt to get rid of his own pain. In pitying another, he feels more powerful and 'virtuous' than that person. The pitier's act of benevolence may also serve to assure him that he has defences lined up against the world's assaults. Because it is based on the fear he has for his own life, pity is egoistic (Nietzsche 1967a:19; 1982:83-85, 91-92). In this view, even the most generous and apparently unselfish person is, in the final analysis, an egoist, since he feels stronger, more virtuous and assured of procuring a place in heaven for himself. Nietzsche does not shun egoism as such, but the self-deception of those who believe and proclaim themselves to be altruistic.

Although for the most part Western culture has not openly embraced Nietzsche's extreme views on suffering and compassion, we find similar attitudes in contemporary liberal societies. A recent study in the USA has shown that 45 percent of all adults engage in voluntary work, helping others for at least five hours a week, but 54 percent believe that people generally bring suffering upon themselves and that charity is only a temporary 'Band Aid'. The vast majority believe that people have to find solutions for their troubles themselves, and that it is important not to get involved in the problems of others. One has to take care of oneself first and only if one has time and energy left, help others. The plethora of voluntary organisations aimed at relieving the suffering of the poor and needy has had the effect of placing limits on charitable feelings. By assigning clear roles to be fulfilled by different individuals and organisations it has protected people from being made unbearably miserable by the suffering they see (Morrison 1988).

## An Aristotelian Account of Compassion

In the remainder of this chapter I will develop an account of compassion which is based largely on Aristotle's analysis of the term in *Rhetoric* (II. viii).[4] In response to the Kantian objection I shall argue that although compassion does have an irreducible and undeniable affective or emotional dimension, it also has a definitive cognitive element. Compassion is not only an impulsive force, but involves thought or belief, an empathetic understanding of the other's situation. I shall contrast this view of compassion with accounts given by thinkers such as Adam Smith and Arthur Schopenhauer, both of whom place undue weight on the emotive element of compassion, thus falling prone to the denunciation of compassion as an irrational force which is likely to lead to a failure to understand and benefit the sufferer. The Nietzschean objection does hold, to a certain extent, with regard to the Augustinian view of suffering as punishment and compassion as the granting of consolation and forgiveness to those who deserve only blame. However, I shall indicate how these problems are largely avoided in the Irenaean tradition, which finds its roots in Aristotle's work.

Aristotle defines compassion or pity (*eleos*)[5] as 'a certain pain at an apparently destructive or painful evil happening to one who does not deserve it and which a

---

[4] Again, I am indebted to Nussbaum (1992, 1994 and 1996) for the analysis of Aristotle's account of compassion.

[5] In Aristotle's writings the Greek term *eleos* is generally translated as 'pity', which has roughly the same meaning as the term 'compassion' as used in contemporary writings. However, since the Victorian era onward, 'pity' has acquired nuances of condescension and superiority to the sufferer that it did not have before. As we shall see more clearly later, the way in which the compassionate person views the sufferer contrasts directly with the attitude characteristic of pity. Compassion involves a sense of shared humanity – a person's suffering is seen as the kind of thing that can happen to anyone, including oneself. In contrast, pity involves the belief that the sufferer has brought the suffering upon himself through misconduct or some other weakness in character. In order to avoid this connotation – which is particularly inappropriate in the context of health care – and for the sake of clarity and consistency, I shall translate the Greek term *eleos* as 'compassion', which for modern readers renders the meaning of this term more clearly than 'pity' does.

person might expect himself or one of his own to suffer' (*Rhetoric* II. viii). Compassion requires and rests on three beliefs:

1. the belief that the possibilities of the subject of compassion are similar to those of the sufferer;
2. the belief that the suffering is serious rather than trivial; and
3. the belief that the suffering was not caused primarily by the person's own culpable actions.

In what follows, I discuss these aspects of compassion in more detail.

*Similar Possibilities*

We feel compassion, according to Aristotle, whenever we are in the condition of remembering that similar misfortunes have happened to us or ours, or expecting them to happen in future. Neoptolemus finds it possible to identify with Philoctetes's plight because he has suffered similar misfortunes which, Philoctetes says, are 'the very counterpart of mine' (*Philoctetes* ll. 399-400). Philoctetes emphasises this aspect of the compassionate attitude when he says: 'You must have pity if you but think how all our mortal lives are set in danger and perplexity: One day to prosper, and the next – who knows?' (*Philoctetes* ll. 500-503). Compassion arises from an understanding of the other's plight and is made possible by the peculiarly human ability to identify with another, to see oneself in them. The compassionate person provides the sufferer with a way of overcoming the solitude of suffering, of sharing her feelings with someone who has experienced something similar. Rousseau (1909:203) argues that an awareness of one's own weakness and vulnerability to similar misfortunes is a necessary condition for compassion:

> In order to become sensible and compassionate the child must know that there are beings similar to himself, who suffer what he has suffered, who feel the sorrows which he has felt, and others of which he can form an idea as being able to feel them also. In fact, how shall we allow ourselves to be moved to pity if not by transporting us outside of ourselves and identifying ourselves with the suffering animal, by quitting, so to speak, our own being, in order to assume his? We suffer only as much as we judge he suffers; and it is not in us, but in him, that we suffer. Thus no one becomes sensible save when his imagination is aroused and begins to transport him outside of himself.

Rousseau's romantic view of compassion as a transportation of the self into the body of the other is problematic. Like Schopenhauer and Adam Smith, he suggests that the imaginative reconstruction of the condition of the sufferer involves an identity confusion in which the subject fails to distinguish his feelings and situation from the other person's. Schopenhauer gives the following account of compassion:

> [I]n *his* pain as such I directly feel, with suffering, *his* pain as I otherwise feel only my own, and on that account want his good directly, as I otherwise want only my own. This, however, requires that in a certain manner I should be *identified* with him, that is to

> say, that the entire *distinction* between me and that other person, which is the basis for my egoism, should be, at least to a certain extent, removed (translation and emphasis by Nussbaum 1996:34-35).

Smith describes the compassionate response as follows:

> [B]y the imagination we place ourselves in his situation, we conceive ourselves enduring all the same torments, we enter as it were into his body, and become in some measure the same person with him, and thence form some idea of his sensations.... His agonies, when they are thus brought home to ourselves, when we have thus adopted and made them our own, begins at last to affect us, and we then tremble and shudder at the thought of what he feels. For as to be in pain or distress of any kind excites the most excessive sorrow, so to conceive or to imagine that we are in it, excites some degree of the same emotion, in proportion to the vivacity or dullness of the conception (1976:9).

For these thinkers compassion involves a complete removal of the distinction between subject and object, a complete identification or 'becoming one' with the sufferer. Thus conceived, compassion does fall prone to the Kantian objection, namely that such identification with the other precludes a rational judgement concerning the nature, cause and seriousness of their suffering because it lacks the necessary distance between subject and object required for an objective judgement. Schopenhauer's account of compassion also falls prone to the Nietzschean objection that pity is fundamentally egoistic, since it is based on the fear one has for one's own life.

However, I believe that Kant and Nietzsche have been too quick in their rejection of compassion. In what follows, I develop an Aristotelian account of compassion that involves a dialectic between identification and distantiation, thus offering an intermediate position between the emotional and objective responses to another's suffering.

*Identification* An objective, distanced attitude is not sufficient for gaining an understanding of another's suffering. The distress of another will be an object of my concern only if I acknowledge some sort of community between myself and the other, to the extent that I am able, in my imagination, to see that suffering as a possibility for me, and to understand on the basis of my own experience what its meaning might be for the person who has it. Without this sense of commonness, 'I will react with sublime indifference or intellectual curiosity – like a Martian scientist, or a certain sort of god' (Nussbaum 1994:142). Such strangers cannot help being indifferent and unconcerned, since they have no idea at all what it means to be in pain or to be mortal. Whereas the cause and nature of physical pain can be explained through the scientific attitude, an understanding of suffering is made possible only by the inner, experiential sense of the importance of these matters for human beings.

It is helpful to examine Aristotle's analysis of *synesis* (understanding), which he defines as 'the critical quality answering to the imperative quality [of] practical wisdom' (*N. Ethics* VI. x). Aristotle opposes *synesis* to *episteme* (scientific knowledge), and characterises it as a variant of *phronesis* (practical wisdom). *Phronesis* is a form of reasoning that involves a distinctive type of mediation between the universal and the particular. It is not simply an application of universal rules to particular instances characteristic of science and deductivist ethical theories. *Phronesis* is a form of reasoning that yields a type of 'ethical know-how' in which both what is universal and what is particular are co-determined. For Aristotle, *synesis* and *phronesis* have the same subject matter. Neither involves scientific knowledge of things that are fixed and unchangeable. He distinguishes *phronesis* from *synesis* as follows: '[P]ractical wisdom issues commands, since its end is what ought to be done or not to be done; but understanding only judges' (*N. Ethics* VI. x). Where the subject of understanding is another person in his suffering, *synesis* (like *phronesis*) involves a mediation between the universal (the frailty or vulnerability of human beings in general) and the particular (the specific situation of the sufferer) in which both are co-determined. My understanding of human vulnerability enables me to understand the suffering of a specific person, which in turn improves my understanding of the human condition. This understanding can only be subjective; it is only through my being a person capable of suffering that I am able to understand the other's suffering. In his discussion of the hermeneutical importance of Aristotle's approach, Gadamer explains the term *synesis* as follows:

> It appears in the fact of concern, not about myself, but about the other person. Thus it is a mode of moral judgment.... The question here, then, is not of a general kind of knowledge, but of its specification at a particular moment. This knowledge also is not in any sense technical knowledge or the application of such.... The person with understanding does not know and judge as one who stands apart and unaffected; but rather, as one united by a specific bond with the other, he thinks with the other and undergoes the situation with him (cited in Bernstein 1986:100).

The belief that one has similar possibilities due to one's humanness is a necessary condition for compassion because it allows us to identify with the other. This identification is often made possible because the onlooker has had a similar experience. But it is quite possible to have compassion for someone, to imagine what that person is enduring, without ever having had a similar experience. Rousseau points out that one can be moved to compassion not only by witnessing the suffering of someone which is similar to one's own previous experiences, but also by forming an idea of a person's sufferings 'as being able to feel them also' (1909:203). The ability to *imaginatively* reconstruct the situation of another human being, without necessarily having been in the same kind of situation, is an indispensable characteristic of the compassionate person.

Compassion is closely connected to the belief that you yourself are vulnerable in similar ways. If you believe yourself to be self-sufficient, secure in your possession of the good life, you will suppose that what happens to others cannot possibly happen to you, that their misfortune could have been prevented by their own autonomous decisions and actions. This, according to Aristotle, will put you in a state of 'insolent pride' (*hubristikḗ diathesis*), in which the sufferings of others do not arouse compassion. On the other hand, if you believe that you are so badly off that nothing further could happen to you to make things worse, you will not be capable of compassion for others because you will be looking at their plight from the very bottom, from the point of view of one whose sufferings are complete (*Rhetoric* II. viii). Thus compassion requires fellow feeling, the judgement that your possibilities are similar to those of the suffering object. The atrocities carried out in South Africa during the *apartheid* era by people who otherwise adhered to the Christian belief that 'one should love one's neighbour as oneself', owed much to the belief that black people were essentially different from whites – in the words of H.F. Verwoerd, that 'they can never be anything but drawers of water and carriers of wood'. As a child of the *apartheid* era, watching 'them' labour from a distance, I was similarly guilty of forming a conception of blacks as somehow insensitive to pain, fatigue or revulsion. I was shocked when I first saw a black woman cry. In time I discovered that their apparent indifference in performing tedious forms of manual labour stems from necessity and fear, rather than insensitivity. Only then could I see them as human beings who suffer under an inhumane political system. Many of the attempts at changing the actions of whites are therefore directed towards changing their perception of 'non-whites' by making them aware of their similarities and drawing attention to the basic humanness shared by all.[6]

The importance of the virtue of compassion is shown in an illuminating way by John Deigh (1995) in his analysis of the psychopath. He defines the psychopath as a person who is able to grasp the social and moral values as they operate within his community, but who lacks any motivation to act accordingly: 'Though amoral, they appear nevertheless to be capable of reasoning, weighing evidence, estimating future consequences, understanding the norms of their society, anticipating the blame and condemnation that result from violation of those norms, and using these cognitive skills to make and carry out their plans' (1995:743). The lack of moral motivation cannot be ascribed to deficiencies in intelligence or rationality, but rather to a lack of empathy. Deigh convincingly argues that the absence of a motivation in psychopaths to act according to the societal norms is due to the fact that they lack the capacity to empathise with others. The psychopath shows no concern for the welfare of others, due to a failure to see others' purposes, though different from his own, as worthwhile. Deigh ascribes this deficiency in empathetic powers to stunted development or regression to an egocentric view. It stems from an inability to tolerate the clash of different perspectives with which one in whom the capacity for empathy has matured is presented. Thus empathy can be seen as a form of moral insight, allowing us to understand the other as a being worthy of respect.

---

6 See also Raul Hilberg's book, *The Destruction of the European Jews* (1985:274-293), in which he shows how the Nazi's portrayed Jews as non-human: either as beings of a remote animal kind, such as insects or vermin, or as inanimate objects, 'cargo' to be transported.

*Distantiation* Compassion, then, requires an empathetic identification with the other, an acknowledgement of the fact that one has possibilities and vulnerabilities similar to those of the sufferer. But it also requires an awareness and consideration of the other as different and separate from oneself. This identification does not involve thinking that one *is* the sufferer, or imagining one's own responses as *fused* in some mysterious way with those of the sufferer. Nietzsche is right that the reaction to another's suffering described by Schopenhauer precludes genuine altruism insofar as the subject focuses on himself, on his own suffering and fears. Smith's account of compassion, with its conception of ourselves as 'enduring all the same torments', causing us to 'tremble and shudder at the thought of what he feels' (Smith 1976:9) is similarly egoistic, insofar as one would be concerned with and attempt to alleviate the other's suffering only *because* it is a source of one's own suffering. By blurring the distinction between subject and object, such total identification precludes genuine compassion. However, Nietzsche's charge of egoism in no way threatens the Aristotelian account of compassion. Aristotle claims, for instance, that panic-stricken people do not feel compassion, because they are too taken up with what is happening to themselves (*Rhetoric* II. viii). If one's attitude is to be one of *altruism*, it is necessary to recognise the circumstances of the other as distinct from one's own, so that one is concerned with the well-being of the other as *other*, not merely as an extension of oneself. While it is true that compassion is made possible by an acknowledgement of the suffering person as one like me, one who counts as I count, this by no means implies that one is concerned mainly and primarily with oneself. As Nussbaum (1994:157) points out, in compassion one treats the other as one would wish in similar circumstances to be treated. This is very different from Nietzsche's suggestion that in pitying one uses the other as a means to one's own security or satisfaction.

Aristotle would also agree with Kant that Schopenhauer's account of compassion precludes rational judgement. Such 'losing of oneself' could well constitute an inability to assess the situation in a rational way. It is for this reason that Aristotle includes older people in his list of people who are likely to feel compassion, since they 'have practical wisdom and experience' (*Rhetoric* II. viii). A truly virtuous person does not only feel in certain ways, he also acts on the basis of a true and rational judgement. For Aristotle, being truly virtuous does not only entail having certain moral virtues, but also certain intellectual virtues, namely practical wisdom (*phronesis*), knowledge (*episteme*) and technical skills (*techne*).

To enable one to make an accurate estimation of the nature of the other's suffering, one should not merely equate one's own imagined reaction to a specific event with that of the other. As Nussbaum (1996:35) points out, the compassionate person has to remain aware of her separateness from the sufferer, because she needs to be aware of her own qualitative difference from the sufferer. To illustrate this point, consider the following situation:

> After numerous miscarriages and unsuccessful attempts to fall pregnant, Sarah finally falls pregnant but has to remain bedridden to enhance the chances of a successful pregnancy and birth. She thus suffers not so much as a result of physical pain or

> discomfort, but because of her concern or anxiety for the well-being of her unborn child. Chris, a staunch feminist who is dedicated to her career and who abhors the thought of having children herself, is alarmed by the very thought of being pregnant and the prospect of losing her freedom. She tries to comfort Sarah by assuring her that she will soon be able to return to work.

Clearly, Chris's attitude would not be welcomed by Sarah as one of true compassion, since it is based on a false belief concerning the cause of her friend's suffering and anxiety. She fails to respect the values, beliefs and life plan of her friend as different from her own by focusing instead on her own feelings about motherhood. To be able to feel genuine compassion we have to be aware that the sufferer's circumstances, values and beliefs differ from our own, so that what would count as being beneficial for a person in a specific predicament might differ significantly from what we would experience as beneficial when faced with a similar misfortune. Although we imaginatively project ourselves into the other's problem situation, in giving advice it is necessary to hold back from identification with the other person, retaining an awareness of the other as a person whose unique circumstances are different from our own.

Compassion, then, involves a dialectic between identification (focusing on similarities in past experiences and future possibilities) and distantiation (remaining aware of differences). If one's compassion were not to be merely an emotion, a 'feeling with' the other, but an understanding of the suffering of the other, one would have to remain aware of the circumstances, values, beliefs and life plan of the other as different from one's own.

The relationship between the subject and object of compassion, together with the notions of respect, altruism and benevolence will be discussed in more detail in the following paragraph, which concerns the second requirement of compassion highlighted by Aristotle.

### *The Seriousness of Suffering*

According to Aristotle, compassion is based on the belief or judgement that the suffering of the other is serious rather than trivial: 'All things are pitiable that are destructive, consisting of griefs and pains, and things that are ruinous, and whatever evils, having magnitude, are caused by chance' (*Rhetoric* II. viii). As we have seen, Nietzsche believes that pity is insulting to the dignity of the sufferer. According to him, pity makes the statement that the person's own efforts are not sufficient for flourishing. To pity is to insinuate that the person's loss of worldly goods is detrimental to his welfare. In certain respects, Nietzsche's argument is similar to that of Plato and the Stoics, who held that external goods are not really important. The good life required only intellectual virtue, the pursuit of truth as knowledge of the eternal, and the wise man did not concern himself with the fleetingness and contingency of worldly goods. According to this tradition, the most important thing in life is one's own reason and will, and one can achieve virtuous reason without the aid of external resources. The loss of external goods, such as friends, health and wealth, should not be considered occasion for suffering, since these things are only of minor importance. In this sense compassion involves a false belief, namely that something is important when it is not. Plato repeatedly emphasises that a change of fortune, such as Socrates's imminent death, is not an occasion for fear or lamentation, and hence, not for compassion. In the *Apology* (36b-38a) Socrates argues, for example, that such changes of fortune are trivial, since they happen only to the body, leaving the soul secure and self-sufficient. The false belief upon which compassion is based also brings with it an insult to the dignity of the sufferer: It implies that this person really needs and values worldly goods, whereas a virtuous and self-sufficient person does not depend on anything except his own reason.

The Aristotelian would react to the question whether the acknowledgement of need ever contributes to the good life (of either the pitied or the pitier) by firstly pointing out that the Stoic tradition's total disregard for the importance of worldly goods is unjustified. Aristotle's opinion of compassion as a virtue is based on the view, developed in the *Nicomachean Ethics* (particularly Books I, VII-IX), that the possession of a certain amount of external goods, in addition to intellectual and moral virtues, is necessary for the good life. The loss of such goods is therefore an occasion for compassion. In his *Rhetoric* (II. viii) Aristotle gives the following examples of conditions under which we should feel compassion: the death of a loved one, bodily injuries and afflictions, old age, diseases, lack of food, lack or scarcity of friends, deformity, weakness and mutilation. Whereas it is true that human beings value different things and have different conceptions of the good life, it is possible to identify certain things as necessary conditions for realising one's life plan, whatever this may be.

Secondly, the Aristotelian does recognise that an extreme reliance upon, and an over-valuation of, external goods are likely to distract people from leading a virtuous and flourishing life, and that intellectual and moral virtues are more important than these things. Compassion does not arise simply because someone is suffering, but because one judges his suffering to be serious. People may become deeply attached to things that on reflection we may think are either trivial or bad for them. Their suffering at the loss of these things may be real enough, even though the onlooker is not disposed to share in it. Nussbaum (1996:32) uses the following example to illustrate the fact that the sufferer's own judgement may be mistaken:

> Q, a Roman aristocrat, discovers that his shipment of peacocks' tongues from Africa has been interrupted. He weeps bitterly as a result of this, feeling that his dinner party that evening will be a total disaster. Seneca, his Stoic friend whom he implores to have pity on him, responds by laughing.

In feeling compassion for this man, one would fall prone to Nietzsche's objection that pity is an acknowledgement of weakness and insufficiency not only in the *pitied*, but also in the *pitier*, because it is based on an inappropriate valuation of worldly goods. One would also fall prone to the objection that pity is simply a case of 'emotional contagion', a loss of self which only increases the amount of misery in the world, without doing any good. In its simplest form, empathy does arise as a result of merely witnessing the pain of another as it is conveyed by her facial expression. By replicating the facial expressions of others we tend to 'catch' the emotions of others. Charles Darwin describes the reaction of his six-month-old infant son when the child's nurse pretended to cry:

> I saw that his face instantly assumed a melancholic expression, with the corners of his mouth strongly depressed; now this child could rarely have seen any other child crying, and I should doubt whether at so early an age he could have reasoned on the subject. Therefore it seems to me that an innate feeling must have told him that the pretended crying of his nurse expressed grief; and this through sympathy excited grief in him (cited in Gordon 1995:729).

This form of simulation or 'facial empathy' is a sympathetic response of a very primitive sort, since it is not *about* anything in particular. It does not focus on the event or loss that caused the facial expression. Human beings are able to recognise that the other is suffering and to empathise with him without there being any facial expression of pain or suffering, simply through communicating with him or by being aware of the negative event that he has experienced. This form of empathy is made possible by our awareness of the vulnerability of others to be damaged by certain events, losses and experiences; it therefore involves intellectual interpretation and not 'emotional contagion'. Compassion requires a normative judgement to the effect that the negative condition is relatively central to a person's life and well-being, describable as pain, misery, hardship, suffering, affliction, and the like. It involves the recognition that the situation matters deeply for the person in question and the judgement that the issue at question is indeed serious.

Finally, we can meet the objection that compassion is a disrespectful attitude by pointing out that the Aristotelian conception of compassion does not entail viewing the sufferer as weak or pathetic. In granting our compassion to another, we *acknowledge* that his sufferings indeed have importance, we agree that he has good reasons for suffering as he does. Indeed, by *not* feeling compassion for someone who suffers extreme misfortune, we are guilty of injuring his dignity. Philoctetes for instance says that he has sent many messages to his father to urge him to send an escort to take him home. This has not happened, which leads Philoctetes to believe that his father is either dead, 'or else my messengers, as well may be, made light of my affair' (*Philoctetes* ll. 497-499). The fact that he finally accepts that his father must be dead shows that he cannot believe that any of his messengers would be so callous as not to convey his message to his father. Smith writes (and here I do agree with him) that '[t]he cruellest insult... which can be offered to the unfortunate, is to appear to make light of their calamities. To seem not to be affected with the joy of our companions is but want of politeness; but not to wear a serious countenance when they tell us their afflictions, is real and gross inhumanity' (1976:15).

Compassion does not necessarily exclude or prevent respect for that person's dignity, since it includes an acknowledgement of the fact that he has good reason to suffer as he does. Once the importance of (a limited amount of) external goods and the legitimacy of the person's suffering as a result of a loss of these goods are recognised, no basis remains for the claim that the compassionate person disregards the dignity of the sufferer. This argument also supports the conclusion in the previous section, namely that compassion does not involve a complete identification with the other in which the subject loses himself or abandons his own perspective. Compassion requires that we *consider* the unique circumstances of the other in judging the seriousness of his suffering, not that we *adopt*, for the time being, his values, beliefs and experiences. By maintaining a certain distance from the sufferer the compassionate person is able to make a rational assessment of the importance of external goods. She is able to judge whether the loss of external goods is serious enough to warrant his compassionate concern, and hence is able to criticise those who attach inappropriate value to money, status or pleasure, such as the Roman aristocrat, who weeps because his shipment of peacocks' tongues is delayed. This does not, of course, imply that compassion always rests on a rational or true judgement of the seriousness of the suffering or the importance of external goods, but only that it does rest on *a* judgement – one that could be true or false. The tradition that favours compassion as a virtue is not prevented from judging that some appeals for compassion are illegitimate, and based on false evaluations.

An important question that arises with regard to the seriousness of suffering is the following: Does a person have to be aware of his negative condition to be the appropriate object of compassion? What if he does not experience his condition as negative because of an under-valuation of the importance or significance of his loss or deprivation? This question has been the subject of much debate. Blum (1980:508) argues that the object of compassion need not be aware of his condition for compassion to be the appropriate response, since he might be deceiving himself with regard to the existence or the seriousness of his suffering. This seems to imply that the subject should judge the seriousness of the object's suffering from his own perspective. Nussbaum agrees that suffering and deprivation often produce adaptive responses that deny the importance of the suffering. This is especially likely to happen when the deprivation is connected to oppression and hierarchy, and taught as proper through religious and cultural practices. She uses the example of women who live in rural villages in India to illustrate her point. These women are often severely undernourished and uneducated, but do not think their lot a bad one, since they have no idea what it is to feel healthy, and no idea of the benefits and pleasures of education. They believe that they are living a good and flourishing life, as women ought to. Nussbaum argues that since people's judgements about what is happening to them can go wrong in many ways, it is necessary for the subject not to rely only on the other's judgement of the seriousness of suffering. Pity takes the onlooker's point of view, informed by the best judgement the onlooker can make about what is really happening to the person being observed – taking the person's own wishes into account, but not always taking as the last word the judgement that the person is able to form: 'Implicit in pity itself is a conception of human flourishing, the best one the pitier is able to form' (1996:32-33).

The first objection that can be made to the views expressed by Blum and Nussbaum stems from the etymology of the word 'compassion'. As an *empathetic* emotion, compassion first of all involves a 'feeling with' or 'suffering with' another person, imagining what the other person is experiencing, given his beliefs, values and circumstances. It appears that it is clearly not possible for someone to 'suffer with' another in this way if the other is not suffering, or is unable to consider his condition as negative. Indeed, it is not clear whether one can at all say that someone is suffering if that person does not perceive his situation to be unfavourable. Suffering is, after all, a subjective experience and not an objective state. The view expressed by Blum and Nussbaum is contradictory: If the onlooker takes the perspective of the other, it would be logically impossible for him to 'suffer with' that person.

Secondly, failing to take the experiences of the other seriously is to fail to *respect* that person as a separate individual, as one whose experiences, values and beliefs differ from one's own. Ortony *et al.* (1988:95) offer the following example to illustrate this point:

> If Fred learns that the husband of his friend Mary was killed in a serious accident, Fred would ordinarily feel very sorry for Mary. But suppose Fred knew that Mary's husband habitually beat her, and that she no longer had any affection for him. In this case, we might expect him to feel less sorry for her because he would presume the event to be less undesirable for her. Indeed, it is conceivable that he would (rightly or wrongly) view such an event as being a desirable event for her, in which case he might even feel happy for her (appropriately or not, as the case may be).

Even though in most circumstances and for most people the death of a spouse would be seen as a tragic event (making compassion for those left behind an appropriate response), it is possible for a given individual in specific circumstances not to experience such an event as negative. For us to be truly respectful towards a person, we have to be sensitive to the individual's specific circumstances and her experience and interpretation of her situation. In other words, if compassion is not to prevent or preclude respect for the other, it is necessary for one's compassion to be appropriate, for one's judgement of the seriousness of the person's suffering to be based on that person's experience of her circumstances. The question is not how well or badly off the other person is according to some universal standard of 'human flourishing', as Nussbaum (1996:33) proclaims, but how *the other* is affected by the conditions or events, that is, in terms of her interests and values.

### *The Innocence of the Sufferer*

The third requirement of compassion, according to Aristotle, is the belief that the suffering which resulted from the loss or absence of external goods was not caused primarily by the person's own responsible actions. Compassion, Aristotle repeatedly insists, is closely tied to our sense of injustice since it sees its object as undeserving of the suffering (*Rhetoric* II. viii). This view of suffering is also reflected in Sophocles's play. Although legend has it that Philoctetes was bitten by a serpent as punishment for trespassing in a sacred precinct, Sophocles makes it clear that his suffering cannot rightfully be seen as 'punishment', since he was totally unaware of the fact that he was transgressing. Sophocles emphasises his innocence and goodness and thus the legitimacy of his appeal for compassion. Hence the chorus of soldiers says: 'This fate he endured, this wickedness, who had done no wrong by force or fraud to any on earth his whole life long, a lover of truth and gentleness' (*Philoctetes* ll. 683-689).

Aristotle's position in this regard can again be contrasted with that of Plato. For Plato, the only way to be seriously damaged by life is through one's own irrational choices, in which case the appropriate response is blame, not compassion. Plato insists that if a person's character is good, he cannot be harmed in any serious way – a view that leaves no room for compassion. If someone is suffering it is because he is guilty of irrational or evil conduct. Such a person deserves to suffer and thus cannot be the appropriate object of compassion, but only of blame.

Against this Aristotle argues that in order to feel compassion, we must believe in the goodness of at least some people; if you think nobody good, you will believe that everybody deserves evil fortune (*Rhetoric* II. viii). The issue of accountability and guilt is raised in an extremely vivid way by Helen Prejean in her book *Dead Man Walking* (1996). Prejean, a Catholic nun, describes her relationship with two death-row inmates. The reader is asked to judge whether the men awaiting execution deserve the nun's compassion, despite their atrocious crimes, and, on another level, whether the death penalty can ever be seen as proportionate to the crimes committed. The parents of one of the victims raise the question whether the nun's compassion is not best directed at them, who have suffered a terrible loss without in any way deserving it. While retaining an undiminished awareness of the horror of the two men's crimes, Prejean judges the punishment to be disproportionate to the crimes, and thus makes them the objects of her compassion. The basis of her compassion is the belief that no-one deserves to be killed by the state. It is made possible by her view of the murderers as fellow human beings and by her ability to identify with their plight. Prejean repeatedly asks herself whether, if raised under similar circumstances, she herself would not have turned out to be a criminal.

In requiring us to judge the innocence or guilt of the sufferer, compassion conveys respect. Insofar as we do feel compassion, it is either because we believe that the person is without blame for the loss or impediment, or because, though there is some fault, we believe that the suffering is not proportional to the fault (Nussbaum 1996:33). When a person's suffering does come about in a way for which he deserves some blame, the appeal to compassion must be accompanied by a claim that the sufferings exceed the amount of due punishment. If we believe that a person's suffering is the result of his own misconduct, we will blame and reproach him, rather than have compassion for him. In such cases the suffering is seen as just punishment that serves as a disincentive to repeat the offence.

We can now return to Nietzsche's objection that compassion is a form of disrespect towards the sufferer. His rejection of the 'religion of pity' is directed towards the Christian view of suffering as being connected to a sense of guilt and shame, with the implication that compassion inflicts a further insult to the dignity of the sufferer. Nietzsche's objection does hold with regard to the Augustinian tradition, which has followed Plato in many respects. However, it does not apply to the view of suffering and compassion contained in the Irenaean tradition, which has its roots in Aristotle's philosophy.

The Augustinian theodicy regards man as having been created by God in a finished state, as a finitely perfect being fulfilling the divine intention for our human level of existence, and then falling disastrously away from this perfect state.[7] St. Augustine (354-430 AD) accounts for evil in this world by arguing that although God created the world as good, things give rise to evil when that which is basically good is perverted and corrupted. Evil is a privation of that which is essentially good and is not God's responsibility – it can be accounted for as a *corruption* of what was designed by God in perfect order. Moral evil – the pain humans inflict upon each other – is sin, while amoral or natural evil, such as disease, floods, earthquakes and droughts, is God's punishment for the sins of mankind. In whichever way it is seen, pain is the collective responsibility of humans. Evil is either sin, or the punishment of sin. Since no one is without sin, everyone is guilty and as such deserves to be punished.

The Augustinian tradition emphasises the purifying or therapeutic properties of pain, which force the sufferer to reflect on the wrongs in his life and bring him to accept God's forgiveness. Because of the sufferer's guilt, he can only hope to solicit the pity of others. An illustration of the Augustinian approach to disease is given by Edmonds in her introduction to Tolstoy's work. She writes that 'The Death of Ivan Ilyich' is 'essentially a study in religious philosophy, written at a time when Tolstoy was concerned with the meaning and importance of life and death and human conduct. After his conversion Tolstoy condemned all his previous imaginative writings but the artist in him revolted and sometimes succeeded in persuading the moralist that art often preaches the more effective sermon' (1960:8). For Edmonds, the story serves the function of moving the reader to 'intense pity', and the main 'sermon' Tolstoy preaches is that prolonged physical pain has certain 'therapeutic properties'. It forces the sufferer to confess to his sins, and this enables him to die without fear of death and punishment. She cites the following passage to support her interpretation: '[W]hat hindered him [from dying] was his claim that his life had been good. That very justification of his life held him fast and prevented him from advancing, and caused him more agony than anything else' (Tolstoy 1960:159). Pain thus has a purifying effect since it forces the sufferer to accept responsibility for his sins. The implication of this view of suffering is that Gerassim's compassion cannot be appreciated fully. Following the example set by Jesus, Gerassim pities Ivan Ilyich despite his shameful state; offering the dying man the consolation he desires yet does not deserve.

---

[7] The term 'theodicy' derives from two Greek words meaning 'god' and 'justice'. A theodicy is an attempt to justify the goodness of God in spite of the presence of evil in the world. In the Judaeo-Christian tradition, it is an attempt to maintain two affirmations about God, namely that he is all-powerful (and *can* therefore prevent evil) *and* completely benevolent (and therefore would *want* to prevent evil).

The attempt to absolve God from responsibility for evil by placing all the blame for evil on the shoulders of mankind lies at the basis of the Nietzschean objection that compassion necessarily entails disrespect. In certain respects this objection is well-founded. In the first place, the view that God created the world as essentially good commits one to the notion of disease as having no independent reality and appearing instead as the absence of health, as the perversion or corruption of what was created as essentially good. The Bible contains numerous examples of the association of disease with dirtiness,[8] weakness[9] or a demonic presence.[10] Being ill is considered to be a state one should be ashamed of, serving as a symbol of one's sinfulness and shameful animal nature. In this view, human dignity derives from man's god-like qualities, from being made in the image of God (Genesis 9:6). Man has special standing because of his likeness to God, a likeness grounded in the capacities of reason, freedom, judgement and moral concern. This view of human dignity leads Kass to the conclusion that the notion of 'dying with dignity' is an oxymoron:

> [I]nsofar as we seek better health and longer life, insofar as we turn to doctors to help us get better, we necessarily and voluntarily compromise our dignity: being a patient rather than an agent is, humanly speaking, undignified. All people, especially the old, willingly, if unknowingly, accept a whole stable of indignities simply by seeking medical assistance (1990:39).

Secondly, the view that suffering is a punishment for the sins of mankind commits one to the view that no one deserves forgiveness or compassion. Although pain and suffering should bring only shame and guilt, God grants us his forgiveness as an undeserved favour, and Jesus bestows upon us his compassion despite our guilt. In the Christian tradition compassion became associated with forgiveness granted to the sufferer as the passive, pathetic and undeserving receiver of the mercy of one who is infinitely superior to him.[11]

This leads us to a third problem inherent in the Augustinian view of natural evil as God's punishment of our collective or individual sins, namely that compassion does not require a judgement of the sufferer as being undeserving of suffering. Indeed, the Christian is asked not to judge others, so that he will not be judged (see Matthew 7:1-6 and Luke 6:37-42). The recognition of human equality rests only on the collective sinfulness and guilt of human beings – the reason we should not judge others is because we ourselves are just as guilty as they are. Suffering, as well as

---

[8] In Matthew 8:1-4 a man with a 'dreaded skin disease' asks Jesus to 'make [him] clean'.

[9] See Matthew 9:35-38, where Jesus heals people with every kind of disease and sickness: 'As he saw the crowds, his heart was filled with pity for them, because they were worried and helpless, like sheep without a shepherd'.

[10] See Matthew 8:16-17, where Jesus 'drove out the evil spirits with a word and healed all who were sick'.

[11] In Matthew 9:1-7 a paralysed man is brought to Jesus, who says to him: 'Your sins are forgiven.... Get up, pick up your bed, and go home!', upon which the man got up and went home.

compassion among human beings, is a symbol of man's shared responsibility for the original sin. Hence Buytendijk argues that we can only understand the meaning and purpose of pain if we view it as a just and reasonable punishment for original sin. He cites the words of St. Thomas Aquinas to substantiate his argument: 'The flesh, conceived in sin, is forced to suffer pain, not only by principles of nature but by reason of necessity imposed by the guilt of sin.' According to Buytendijk, a sufferer can only discover the sense underlying the senselessness of pain if he shares in the solidarity of man in nature and sin. This acceptance of pain as punishment ultimately brings him to strive towards a 'more perfect and happy state', which is found only in heaven and can only be attained by his humble acceptance of God's forgiveness: 'The purpose of pain lies in its bringing man to himself in the midst of his affliction so that he shares in the distress of the whole community, in their fate and their longing for release' (1961:161-164).

It is exactly the promotion of compassion as a form of self-sacrifice that has led many Westerners to reject it in favour of the liberal philosophy of independence and self-fulfilment. For example, although 42 percent of Americans say 'I want to give myself for the benefit of others', when the sentence is rephrased – 'I want to sacrifice myself for the benefit of others' – only 15 percent are ready to do so (Morrison 1988). Quite understandably, most people do not want to be martyrs, or live like monks or nuns, and neither do they wish to be the objects of pity.

It is not difficult to see how Nietzsche could view the Augustinian attitude towards suffering and compassion as a denial of the joy of life and of the strength of the individual, and that he would advocate instead that the individual should resist the desire to become an object of pity and should strive to preserve his independence. The Nietzschean might point out that Ivan Ilyich, by accepting Gerassim's compassion, chooses the 'religion of comfort', captured in the pathetic picture of the sick man with his feet on Gerassim's shoulders. This silly position can only offer false comfort and diminish his suffering to mere physical discomfort. Ivan Ilyich grows as a person only when he accepts responsibility for his own life, when he reflects upon his life and acknowledges the awful truth, thus rejecting the religion of comfort. Initially, Ivan Ilyich's efforts are directed towards understanding the cause of his illness and finding a cure so that he could be rid of his meaningless suffering. As the illness progresses he contemplates the meaningfulness of his relationship with his family, friends and colleagues. Ultimately, he comes to contemplate both his faith in God and the meaning of his life, when he finally realises that 'it's not a question of appendix or kidney but of life and... death' (Tolstoy 1960:135). When he discovers the truth about his life, when he admits to himself that his life has been wrong, he experiences an exalted moment of freedom from pain and from fear of death before he dies:

> In place of death there was light.
> 'So that's what it is!' he suddenly exclaimed aloud. 'What joy!' (1960:160-161).

However, a complete rejection of the compassion and benevolence of others is not the only way in which we could maintain our self-respect and dignity in the face of pain. The negative implications of the Augustinian view are largely avoided in the Irenaean view of suffering and compassion. Following St. Irenaeus, John Hick rejects the Augustinian theory that the evil we find in nature is the result of man's sin and thus represents just punishment for his own wrongdoing. The theodicy problem, according to Hick, consists in the fact that 'instead of serving a constructive purpose pain and misery seem to be distributed in random and meaningless ways, with the result that suffering is often undeserved and falls upon men in amounts exceeding anything that could be rationally intended' (1966:369).[12] In viewing man as still in the process of 'soul making', Hick makes the implicit value-judgement that one who has attained goodness by meeting and eventually mastering temptations, and by rightly making responsible choices in concrete situations, is good in a richer and more valuable sense than would be one created *ab initio* in a state of innocence or virtue. In response to the question of why God allows innocent people to suffer, he asks us to imagine a world that contained no unjust and undeserved misery. Suffering would either be justly deserved punishment or it would serve a constructive purpose of moral training. In such a world, Hick argues,

> human misery would not evoke deep personal sympathy or call forth organized relief and sacrificial help and service. For it is presupposed in these compassionate reactions both that the suffering is not deserved and that it is *bad* for the sufferer. We do not acknowledge a moral call to sacrificial measures to save a criminal from receiving his just punishment or a patient from receiving the painful treatment that is to cure him. But men and women often act in true compassion and massive generosity and self-giving in the face of unmerited suffering (Hick 1966:370, emphasis in original).

It is the recognition that the suffering experienced by humans is often undeserved that allows one to feel compassion for them. For our purposes it is not necessary to discuss Hick's theodicy in any detail, apart from noting that he shares with Aristotle the view that human beings are largely responsible for becoming virtuous people. However, humans are not *completely* responsible for their well-being, since there are important features of human life that nobody fully controls, with the result that it is possible for a good person to suffer serious and undeserved harm. One cannot always avoid disease and injury through one's rational or virtuous actions.

The Aristotelian (unlike the Augustinian) does not view human beings as equals in sin and guilt. Because human beings are largely responsible for their own welfare and happiness they often deserve to suffer (or enjoy) the consequences of their actions. Yet human beings are equal in at least one respect, namely that they are mortal and thus subject to grave misfortune through no fault of their own. Being rich, powerful, wise or virtuous does not remove one from the ranks of humanity. When confronted with a suffering person it is necessary to judge whether

[12] We need not concern ourselves with the question whether Hick's theodicy succeeds in overcoming the problem of evil. For our purposes it is more important to focus on the implications of his theodicy for the meaning and significance of suffering and compassion.

he or she deserves misfortune. In feeling compassion one conveys to another one's belief in his innocence, and thus one's respect for him.

Suffering is not a *defect* in a perfectly created world. For Hick it is a necessary part of our development or growth as moral persons. Witnessing the undeserved suffering of others forms a significant part of our moral development, so that the sufferer is not simply viewed as a weak and passive receiver of compassion:

> It seems, then, that in a world that is to be the scene of compassionate love and self-giving for others, suffering must fall upon mankind with something of the haphazardness and inequity that we now experience. It must be apparently unmerited, pointless, and incapable of being morally rationalized. For it is precisely this feature of our common human lot that creates sympathy between man and man and evokes unselfish kindness and goodwill which are among the highest values of personal life. No undeserved need would mean no uncalculating outpouring to meet that need (Hick 1966:371).

While one need not agree with Hick that the suffering of human beings pays testimony to God's goodness in offering us a means of moral self-development or 'soul making', his view of suffering as undeserved has the positive implication that compassion is not associated with forgiveness. The patient need not be considered purely a pathetic recipient of the gifts others bestow upon him, but may bring to others the knowledge of what human fragility and finitude involves. This applies particularly to the dying patient who finds himself in a situation which is a very real possibility for every person. The attempt to understand and to get involved in the dying of another is an opportunity to help one to come to terms with the inevitability of one's own death. According to Lansberg, the compelling certainty of our mortality is, amongst other experiences, the result of the experience of the 'death of a fellow creature':

> The consciousness of the necessity of death is awakened only through participation, only through the personal love by which this experience is completely imbued. We have constituted an 'us' with the dying person. And it is in this 'us', it is through the specific power of this new and utterly personal being that we are led toward the living awareness of our own having to die.... My community with that person seems to be broken off; but this community in some degree was I myself, I feel death in the heart of my own existence (cited in Choron 1963:18).

The sufferer may also serve as a model of virtue, helping others to understand and cope with their own suffering. The change in Neoptolemus's attitude can be attributed largely to his witnessing Philoctetes's courage and moral goodness. Neoptolemus is initially convinced by Odysseus to play along in attempting to trick Philoctetes through a false show of compassion. He justifies his actions by saying that he has no choice but to 'obey my masters for duty's sake and for my own' (*Philoctetes* ll. 926-927). However, after communicating with Philoctetes and reflecting more on the matter, he is confronted with the dilemma – either to remain loyal to the unscrupulous Odysseus and carry out his orders to forcefully remove Philoctetes from the island, or to stand up for justice, here symbolised by the bow in the hands of the rightful owner. His choosing the latter option despite the risk to himself is evidence of his moral growth, which is only made possible through his contact with Philoctetes.[13]

## Conclusion

Through no fault of his own, Ivan Ilyich becomes the victim of a terrible disease, isolating him from his family and colleagues who are unable to identify with his plight. Instead, they view his illness as an inconvenience and they secretly hope for a quick demise, not for the sake of the dying man, but for the sake of what they could gain through his death. Although one would expect Ivan Ilyich's close family members and friends to be more capable of feeling compassion for him, Gerassim is the only one who finds it possible to identify with him. Gerassim stands in for the imaginative activity of the reader, for whom the story is a similar exercise of compassion.

Gerassim's compassion, like that of the chorus, does not entail disrespect. For instance, when Ivan Ilyich apologetically says that caring for a dying man has to be very disagreeable, Gerassim answers: 'Oh, why, sir, what's a little trouble? It's a case of illness with you sir' (Tolstoy 1960:141). When Ivan Ilyich wants to send Gerassim away so that the boy may get some rest, Gerassim answers: '"We shall all of us die, so what's a little trouble?" meaning by this that he did not mind the extra work because he was doing it for a dying man and hoped someone would do the same for him when his time came' (Tolstoy 1960:143). With his simple honesty, Gerassim conveys his belief in the seriousness of Ivan Ilyich's affliction and in the fact that he is not morally accountable for his misfortune. While Ivan Ilyich wonders why God is punishing him, Gerassim shows that it is not a question of guilt or punishment at all. Instead, he views Ivan Ilyich's dependency as due to the vulnerability to misfortune shared by all human beings. In this way Gerassim conveys his respect for his master, something which is strikingly absent in the attitude of all the other characters. While Ivan Ilyich suffers from a terrifying solitude, unable to discuss his condition and impending death with his family, friends and physicians, he regains his self-respect through Gerassim's understanding of his plight. Indeed, it is the lack of compassion shown by the other characters that conveys disrespect. For instance, while his physician is examining Ivan Ilyich, his wife describes how he made Gerassim hold his legs up. In response, 'the doctor

---

[13] Thus far, I have focused on the question of individual responsibility with regard to the sufferer's liability for the situation he finds himself in, arguing that compassion rests on the recognition of the sufferer's innocence. The objection raised by Plato and Nietzsche, namely that compassion necessarily entails disrespect, pertains not only to the sufferer's liability in bringing about misfortune, but also with regard to his responsibility for overcoming suffering on his own. According to these writers, compassion denigrates the sufferer's own efforts by implying that they are insufficient for flourishing and that the sufferer needs the help of others to overcome hardship. I shall examine this objection in Chapter Five, where I deal with the problem of individual self-determination and autonomy.

smiled with a bland condescension that said: "What can we do? These sick people, you know, do sometimes get such foolish fancies, but we must forgive them"' (1960:148). In contrast, Gerassim's attitude is not one of condescension or pity since he realises that *there is nothing his master needs to be forgiven for*.

Neither does Gerassim's compassion rest on false beliefs or irrational feelings. It is precisely his honesty in face of the terrifying truth that makes it possible for him to be compassionate. Again, this is in stark contrast with the deceit that surrounds the dying man:

> The awful, terrible act of his dying was, he saw, reduced by those about him to the level of a fortuitous, disagreeable and rather indecent incident (much in the same way as people behave with someone who goes into a drawing-room smelling unpleasantly).... Gerassim alone told no lies; everything showed that he alone understood the facts of the case, and did not find it necessary to disguise them (Tolstoy 1960:143).

For Ivan Ilyich, then, his acceptance of the compassion and dedication of Gerassim becomes his only means of comfort. Gerassim, through his understanding of the dying man's fears and needs and his acceptance of the inevitability of death, helps Ivan Ilyich to overcome his sense of shame and degradation.

An important point that arises from the discussion of the empathetic element of compassion is that it involves a sense of shared humanity and respect for others. It entails the recognition that there are deleterious events that may befall people through no fault of their own, simply because they are human. The compassionate person regards the sufferer as a fellow human being, whose suffering can be seen as the kind of thing that can happen to anyone who is mortal and human. In this way compassion promotes the experience of human equality, despite the existence and awareness of social inequalities. It also makes us aware of the injustices or undeserved misfortunes suffered by people. It is for these reasons that compassion should be praised as a virtue in itself; that is, apart from its value in giving rise to beneficent actions. Rousseau illustrates the moral value of the ability to identify with others, of being able to see others as beings that are subject to pain and suffering and thus share with oneself a common human vulnerability:

> Do not accustom your pupil to look down from the summit of his glory on the afflictions of the unfortunate and the toils of the wretched; and never hope to teach him to pity them if he considers them as strangers to himself. Make him clearly understand that the lot of these unfortunates may be his own, that all their misfortunes lie before him, and that a thousand unforeseen and inevitable events may at any moment plunge him into them. Teach him to count neither upon birth, not upon health, nor upon riches; show him all the vicissitudes of health... (Rousseau 1907:204).

The fact that compassion rests on a number of beliefs (namely, that the person is suffering, that the suffering is serious and that it is undeserved) shows that compassion has a definite cognitive basis. The relevant beliefs are not only a necessary condition for compassion, but also a constituent part of this emotion. Aristotle argues that emotions are not identified and distinguished by some special way they feel, but instead by the character of the beliefs involved. The cognitive component of compassion can be found in the fact that compassion involves an imaginative reconstruction of the sufferer's condition, one that may be true or mistaken.

Compassion is not only reconcilable with rationality, it also allows a more comprehensive understanding of the sufferer's condition than does a purely objective or scientific view. We have seen that suffering involves more than an emotional reaction to physical pain. It involves an interpretation of the significance of pain for one's continued existence. Similarly, empathising with another's suffering constitutes more than an emotional reaction. A person's pain may be explained in rational, scientific terms. For us to understand his *suffering*, however, requires more than a distanced, objective and scientific approach.

For the physician as medical scientist, the patient's experience and perspective of disease have no bearing on his assessment of its seriousness. A rational assessment requires an objective, distanced attitude. Different diseases and injuries are branded as more or less serious independent of the patients who suffer them. Therefore, in the attempt to reach the ideal of rationality, a purely medical-scientific attitude excludes a central aspect of a patient's condition from consideration, thus failing to form a complete understanding of a patient's plight. The compassionate attitude, I believe, forms a valuable corrective to this limited perspective on medical afflictions.

Finally, an important point that arises from this discussion is that compassion does not require total selflessness, as it does in the Christian tradition. For Aristotle, being a virtuous person is an intricate and necessary part of one's own happiness. By attempting to understand the suffering of the other one gains more insight into the mortal condition of human beings, thereby affirming, rather than denying, one's own dignity as a person.

# Chapter Four

# Benevolence and Beneficence

## Introduction

In the previous chapter I examined the empathetic element of the virtue of compassion as a corrective to the Cartesian-Newtonian paradigm of explaining disease. Benevolence – the desire to alleviate another's suffering or to benefit him or her – forms the second component of compassion and stems from the empathetic understanding of the victim's suffering. Medical practice has developed as a response to human dependency in the face of disease and injury, and thus is rooted in the virtue of benevolence. However, in much the same way that medical science operates within the confines of an outdated paradigm of disease which rejects the need and relevance of empathy as a virtue, in the sphere of medical ethics we find a rejection of the virtue of benevolence in favour of the principle of beneficence. Contemporary medical ethics takes as its foundation the rules and principles developed by nineteenth century philosophers and ethicists, in particular Kant and J.S. Mill. To fully appreciate the problems and challenges in current medical practice it is necessary to trace the deontological and utilitarian roots of the principles of medical ethics. After critically discussing the principle of beneficence as it operates within medical practice, I develop a teleological notion of 'responsible benevolence' as a means to overcome some of the shortcomings of principle-based ethics. I shall focus particularly on the role of compassion in motivating benevolence and will reconsider, in light of this, the appropriate goals of medical practice. First however, I discuss the second feature of suffering which typically results from serious disease or injury, namely the patient's helplessness in the face of pain and his consequent dependence on the help of others.

## The Second Feature of Suffering: The Helpless Patient

Henri Bergson writes that, '[i]n all pain, even in the most transient, the living being is momentarily helpless in the grip of a power which is deleterious to his vital integrity' (cited in Sauerbruch and Wenke 1963:116). Pain teaches us how unfree, transitory and helpless we really are, and how life is essentially capable of becoming an enemy to itself. The feeling of helplessness and abandonment is perhaps the greatest pathos of chronic pain. Despite the formidable advances in the management of pain, suffering caused by sickness and death still remains characterised by a single idea – the frailty of all that is human. Pain is not simply a disagreeable sensation. For the Western person who typically places much emphasis on the value of individual self-determination and independence, pain is experienced as a restriction of his freedom, as an impediment to activity and hence as a loss of independence and self-sufficiency.

The vulnerability of good people to reversals of fortune forms a central theme of tragedy. Tolstoy's Ivan Ilyich shares with Philoctetes the feeling of helplessness, dependence and weakness brought about by his physical condition. Both experience a tragic reversal of fortune in which they are prevented from acting nobly, losing control over their actions and bodily functions. It is therefore not so much physical pain as it is the restrictions brought about by illness and the consequent dependence upon others that constitute a major part of suffering. References to Philoctetes's helplessness, weakness and dependence are abundant in Sophocles's play. One description Philoctetes gives of his hopeless condition reads as follows: 'Not one to befriend me or lend me a helping hand in the trouble that racked me. Whichever way I looked, there was nothing, nothing beside me but misery, and that in abundance' (*Philoctetes* ll. 279-282).

The restrictions characteristically brought about by disease or injury are not limited to bodily movement or actions. Disease may also bring about a restriction of one's ability to think rationally and independently. For instance, after sending the chorus away Philoctetes immediately begs them to return, saying, 'I don't know what I am saying. Pain drowns my senses' (*Philoctetes* ll. 1192-1193). Pain makes the sufferer aware of his cognitive limitations since the ordinary person cannot explain the cause of pain. Although one may be aware of the exact location of pain, the typical patient lacks the medical knowledge to answer the questions concerning the nature and origin of the physical disharmony that produces the sensation of pain. He also lacks the medical knowledge and expertise to be able to overcome illness on his own. As the severity of pain increases, the ability to verbalise or explain experiences typically decreases, so that he may eventually manage little more than a moan or scream (see Scarry 1985).

The act of seeking help depends on our awareness and acceptance of our dependence on others, both to understand pain and to manage it. Pain reminds us of the fact that we are not totally self-sufficient, that there are times when we need the help of others to regain our health. In this regard pain serves to distinguish the human condition from that of the animal. While it is true that pain renders the sick or injured animal easy prey for its predator by forcing it into passiveness, this need not commit us to the pessimistic view that the only function of pain is to destroy or to assist in the annihilation of the organism. Through the capacity of human beings to sympathise with those they perceive to be in pain, they are inclined to be helpful. The ability to recognise that the other is in pain has given rise to numerous techniques to reverse or slow down the disease process, to alleviate pain and to render other forms of assistance. In this way pain may also draw our attention to the strength found in human community.

## The Benevolent Response

A close relationship exists between the empathetic and benevolent components of compassion. The concern for the other's welfare, together with the desire to alleviate his suffering, an understanding of which is made possible by empathy, characteristically leads to acts of benevolence. Benevolence can be defined as an active disposition moving us to bring about the welfare and to reduce the suffering of others. In addition to identifying with the sufferer, the compassionate person is inclined to act beneficently, to be helpful or merciful. Compassion is a morally-desirable character trait because it motivates the person to act beneficently.

On the face of it, the virtue of benevolence and the principle of beneficence seem to require exactly the same things: to benefit the patient, to prevent harm coming to him, and to remove or remedy it when it does. But as we shall see more clearly in the following sections, there are important differences between benevolence as a virtue and beneficence as a principle. With regard to *character*, deontological and virtue-based ethics both focus on the agent's intentions or motivation. However, deontological theories make their evaluation of character on the basis of a person's adherence to principles or duties, in other words, on whether he or she performs a given action because it is required by duty. Virtue is definable in terms of favourable attitudes towards duty. By contrast, virtue-based theories evaluate character on the basis of the person's dispositions or inclination. Virtue is not defined in terms of performing obligatory acts. The primary object of moral evaluation is not the intentional act or its actual consequences, but the agent's character. In this regard contemporary medical ethics has followed deontological theories. Benevolence is recognised as a *principle* or duty, rather than as a *disposition* or virtue. When there is a conflict between what their inclination or intuition disposes them to do and a contractual or professional duty, health-care workers are required to act according to the latter.

As far as judging *action* is concerned, virtue-based theories and utilitarian theories are both concerned with consequences. But whereas utilitarian theories judge a rule or action on the basis of its contribution to maximising happiness or utility, virtue-based theories focus on the goal or *telos* of life – living well and achieving excellence. Critics of virtue ethics have found the notion of 'living well' too vague to guide actions. The right action is seen as that which a virtuous person would do if he could, but what would a virtuous person do? Contemporary medical ethics has followed the rule-utilitarian tradition by formulating the duty to benefit others in terms of universal rules and concrete strategies geared towards attaining specific ends.

Some ethicists have argued that deontological and virtue-based theories should not be seen as rivals, but as two complementary aspects of the same morality.[1] Virtues are not originative or primary but rather derive from principles. Each principle has a corresponding virtue. The virtue of benevolence derives from the principle of beneficence, honesty derives from the duty to tell the truth, and so

[1] See Beauchamp and Childress (1994:66-69) and Frankena (1988:305-310).

forth. In this view, the virtues are motivationally indispensable – they provide the dispositions that generate right (i.e., principled) action. As Frankena writes: '[P]rinciples without traits are impotent and traits without principles are blind' (1988:307). In order to evaluate these positions on the role and primacy of the virtues it is necessary to examine the objections to the virtue of benevolence in more detail.

## Two Objections to Benevolence

The first question that will concern us here pertains to the morally-appropriate *motivational basis* for benevolence. Kant's objection to virtue ethics is that benevolence has to be motivated by a sense of duty, rather than sentiments or virtues such as compassion. There has been widespread disagreement about the question of whether benevolence must be rooted in virtues such as compassion or in an adherence to a principle or duty for it to be a morally-desirable character trait. The dominating tendency in Western moral philosophy – one which has also shown its face in medical ethics and practice – has been to place an almost exclusive emphasis on beneficence as a principle, while downplaying or rejecting the value of compassion in bringing about benevolence. This preference, I shall argue, is the unfortunate result of the Kantian attack on 'inclination' and the failure to distinguish two distinct positions, namely an ethic based on virtues and one based on emotions.

A second objection to compassion as a *benevolent concern* for the welfare of others comes from utilitarian theorists, namely that it is not sufficient for producing acts that are truly beneficent. Some would argue that it is exactly the compassionate person's emotional involvement that prevents him from acting beneficently. Health-care professionals can only succeed in benefiting patients if they are motivated by a sense of duty and possess the necessary medical knowledge and technical skills. There is no need for compassion or benevolence; indeed, these character traits can only be a hindrance. The second question to be answered here concerns the relationship between character and action, more specifically, whether an act should be judged on the basis of the agent's intended results or on the basis of the actual results.

In this regard it is helpful to note the difference between the concepts 'benevolence' and 'beneficence'. 'Benevolence' refers to the disposition or inclination to act beneficently, to seek to do or promote good and not evil, whether this aspiration is realised in practice or not. Benevolence is a matter of intention, not of outcome. By contrast, an act is beneficent if it actually produces good and not evil; beneficence is thus a matter of outcome, not of intention. For a person to be benevolent as well as beneficent, he must endeavour as well as succeed, but to be benevolent he must only endeavour (Frankena 1987:2). Because people do not always succeed in acting beneficently, despite their good intentions, the virtue of benevolence is said to have only limited value. If what is important in the moral life is to actually benefit others, some argue, the intention to benefit is not enough.

'Benevolence', says Frankena, 'means *willing* and genuinely *trying* to do or bring about good and not evil; but even a person who is benevolent in this sense may by inadvertence, bad luck, ignorance, or weakness fail to do or promote good, or even bring about evil' (1987:2, emphasis in original). Greek tragedy offers many examples to substantiate the claim that good intentions are not sufficient for the moral life. Neoptolemus and the chorus of soldiers are unable to help Philoctetes, despite their obvious feelings of compassion. Indeed, as is characteristic of Greek tragedy, it takes the divine intervention of Heracles to bring about a reversal of Philoctetes's fortune. The lesson of Greek tragedy seems to be that the only function of compassionate characters is to bring about feelings of pity and fear in the audience. They are powerless to help those in need.

In the following sections I discuss three ethical theories that have played an important role in the development of the principle of beneficence as it figures in modern medical practice. This will allow us to counter the above-mentioned objections in the subsequent account of the virtue of benevolence.

## Moral Motivation: From Virtue to Principle

### *Hume's Sympathy*

David Hume develops his theory of moral sentiments in *A Treatise of Human Nature* (first published in 1739) and *An Enquiry Concerning the Principles of Morals* (first published in 1751). He gives a naturalistic account of morality by emphasising the value of the emotions in bringing about the good of others. The fundamental drive of benevolence is emotional; it derives from the *feeling* that we care for the good of the other, a *concern* with his plight and a shared *desire* for the alleviation of his suffering.

Central to Hume's ethical theory is the concept of 'sympathy', which has to be distinguished from the virtue of compassion. We saw in the previous chapter that compassion is a disposition that involves not only emotion, but also reason and moral judgement. By contrast, Hume understands 'sympathy' to be the human capacity to be moved or affected by the happiness and sufferings of others – being pleased when others prosper, and distressed when others suffer. Sympathy is not itself a virtue but an emotion. It forms the source of moral approval that allows us to regard human dispositions as either vices or virtues.

Morality, in Hume's view, is based on the human capacity to have feelings of approval and disapproval. We approve of something and call it good because it produces a kind of pleasure in us, while we disapprove of and call something bad if it produces in us a kind of pain. Moral qualities do not exist in objects or actions. Instead, they are sentiments that other human beings produce in us. Moral judgements are primarily judgements about virtues and vices exhibited by others. Hume believes that when we praise any action, we regard only the motives that produced that action. The external performance has no merit – virtuous actions derive their merit from virtuous motives alone.

Hume's central claim is that the moral praise or blame we ascribe to people derives from an attitude or feeling of sympathy. The fact that we *feel* sympathy towards others explains why we judge as we do. Moral approval and disapproval does not derive from reason. Benevolence is a valued quality, indeed, the paradigm of natural virtue, because its exercise promotes the happiness or well-being of others. Through sympathy we take pleasure in the happiness of others, and are led to admire the quality which promotes it. Benevolence is a basic human disposition that stems from and is made possible by a feeling of sympathy, rather than a sense of duty. To understand the role of reason and emotion in Hume's ethics,[2] it is necessary to refer to the distinction he makes between natural and artificial virtues and vices. Natural virtues are inborn, either as actual character traits, or as propensities to develop them, while artificial virtues are habits cultivated to help society flourish. His main claim concerning the respective roles of feeling and reason is expressed in the following passage:

> Human nature being compos'd of two principle parts, which are requisite in all its actions, the affections and understanding; 'tis certain that the blind motions of the former, without the direction of the latter, incapacitate man for society (Hume 1960:493).

In this passage Hume makes both a positive and a negative claim about the role of reason. The negative claim de-emphasises the role of reason in moral decision-making by drawing attention to its lack of motivational force: '[R]eason alone can never produce any action or give rise to volition' (Hume 1960:413). He understands particular moral judgements as expressions of feeling, for it is the passions and not reason that motivate us to action. At the same time, however, he recognises that we invoke general rules when making moral judgements. He attempts to explain this by showing their utility in helping us to attain those ends that the passions set before us. The positive claim, then, is that reason directs feelings by acting as a corrective of feelings. Reason enables us to recognise the appropriate objects toward which feelings ought to be directed and to find efficient means of enjoying or avoiding these objects:

> [N]ature provides a remedy in the judgement and understanding, for what is irregular and incommodious in the affections.... This can be done after no other manner, than by a convention enter'd into by all members of the society to bestow stability on the possession of those external goods, and leave every one in the peaceful enjoyment of what he may acquire by his fortune and industry. By this means... the passions are restrained in their partial and contradictory motions (Hume 1960:489).

Whereas sympathy induces us to take account of the happiness and suffering of others, general standards or customs correct the operation of sympathy, so that we

---

[2] Hume uses the term 'reason' in a comprehensive sense to refer to our capacity to judge truth and falsity, that is, to obtain any kind of knowledge, whether from pure thought or from experience.

attach the same moral importance to the happiness or suffering of anyone. This prevents partiality and ensures that our actions actually contribute to the welfare of others.

Hume sees benevolence as an emotion-based disposition to care about the welfare of others. Its moral value derives from the fact that it gives rise to pleasure and reduces pain. To help ensure that these positive results are attained, it should be guided by critical and rational reflection, since it is through reason that we discover the consequences of various human qualities and actions. Despite the fact that Hume gives a much more prominent place to benevolence in his list of virtues than does Aristotle or Plato, he shares with the Greek thinkers the assumption that moral judgements are primarily judgements about character. We morally praise people for exhibiting virtues, and blame them if they exhibit vices. However, as far as the problem of moral knowledge is concerned, he disagrees with both Plato and Aristotle. For Plato moral knowledge is a purely intellectual acquaintance with abstract universal forms. In contrast, Aristotle holds that moral knowledge is to be derived from an empirical study of the facts of human existence. Hume denies that moral knowledge derives from reason at all, and considers it to be based within the sphere of sentiment and intuition. Despite the striking differences between Hume and Aristotle, the ethics of virtue suffered a severe but unfair blow with Kant's criticism of Hume, from which it never fully recovered. In what follows I examine the most important features of the argument Kant offers in favour of the view that benevolence has to be motivated by a sense of duty, rather than inclination.

### *Kant's Duty*

Kant has been the main opponent of sentiment, such as compassion, being considered a morally-desirable character trait. While granting that compassion has an undeniable motivational element, he argues that benevolence has to be rooted in the good will to be of any moral value. One has to perform benevolent acts, not because one is inclined that way by instinct or passion, or because such acts have favourable consequences, but simply through an acknowledgement of the fact that it is one's duty.

Kant begins his *Fundamental Principles of the Metaphysic of Morals* (first published in 1785) with the assertion that nothing can be called good without qualification except a good will. The value of the good will is entirely separable from the value of the results it brings about (1988:17). This claim derives its plausibility from the widely held idea that moral judgements of people focus primarily on their intentions – people are not morally blamed if, through no fault of their own, their good intentions lead to unfortunate results. Kant does not argue, at this point, that consequences are entirely irrelevant in moral assessment. We cannot characterise the agent's intention without reference to what the agent intends to accomplish. The contrast, therefore, is between the *intended* and the *actual* consequences. In Kant's view, the former are the objects of moral praise or blame.

Kant then introduces the central concept of duty which, 'in estimating the value of our actions always takes the first place, and constitutes the condition of all the rest' (Kant 1988:21). As Kant uses it the term 'duty' refers to the good will, as opposed to inclination. Actions have moral worth only if they are performed through duty and hence are governed by reason. To illustrate the difference between acting from duty and acting from inclination, Kant uses the example of the duty to maintain one's life. He says that most people have a direct inclination to maintain their lives, but their doing so is not necessarily morally praiseworthy. The care most people take to preserve their lives has no intrinsic worth since, although they act *as duty requires*, they do not act *because duty requires*. It is only when we find ourselves in a situation of utter hopelessness and have lost all enjoyment of life *but choose nevertheless to conquer our desire to die*, that our life-preserving actions have true moral worth.

In the same way Kant argues that the 'sympathetically constituted' minds of people who find pleasure in performing beneficent acts, who spread happiness and take delight in the satisfaction of others, have no true moral worth, even if they do not act from a motive such as vanity or self-interest. Not only are the actions of such people not praiseworthy, Kant seems also to regard them as positively blameworthy, for they allow their decisions to be governed by passion. In *The Metaphysical Principles of Virtue* (par. 34) he follows the Stoics in holding that this kind of benevolence is called 'softheartedness' and should not occur at all among human beings. If someone allows himself to be infected by another's pain, Kant argues, then two people suffer. In this way pity only increases the evils of the world.[3] He concludes that when we get rid of pity, that 'insulting kind of benevolence, expressing the sort of benevolence one has for an unworthy person', we will be able to think of the needs of others with 'an active and rational benevolence' (Kant 1964:121-122). Benevolence that issues from inclination does not include any rational ethical belief, and thus does not involve any distinctively moral motivation. Natural human inclinations can have no moral value unless they are primarily motivated by a concern for duty which, in turn, is based in reason. Kant's argument suggests that it is disrespectful to react to the suffering of others in an emotional manner, for as rational beings they deserve to be treated rationally, and not passionately.

Kant also suggests that inclination is not a reliable guide or motivation for acting benevolently, since the passions cannot be commanded:

> For love, as an affection, cannot be commanded, but beneficence for duty's sake may; even though we are not impelled to it by any inclination – nay, are even repelled by a natural and unconquerable aversion. This is *practical* love, and not *pathological* – a love which is seated in the will, and not in the propensions of sense – in principles of action and not of tender sympathy; and it is this love alone which can be commanded (Kant 1988:24, emphasis in original).

---

[3] Kant's argument in this passage shows an interesting resemblance to that of Nietzsche in *Daybreak* (1982:85-86).

In stating the second proposition of morality, Kant claims that the goodness of the good will is totally independent of the results at which it is directed. Although he previously held that the good will is independent of the *actual consequences* of the action, he now makes a stronger claim, namely that duty is to be contrasted with all specific purposes or intended consequences. An action done from duty derives its moral worth from the maxim by which it is determined. It does not depend on the realisation of the object of the action or even on the intended consequences, but merely 'on the *principle of volition* by which the action has taken place, without regard to any object of desire' (Kant 1988:24-25, emphasis in original). Kant seeks to detach duty from any idea of utility. The fulfilment of duty becomes an abstract moral requirement, and not something required for the effective functioning of social institutions. In other words, duty is to be performed entirely for its own sake, not in order to promote human happiness or fulfilment. Of course, Kant does not doubt that all men desire happiness and that the individual's moral perfection, crowned by the happiness that it merits, is the highest good conceivable. However, he believes that any moral precept designed to secure our happiness would be an expression of a rule holding only conditionally. And, as we shall see, all moral expressions that are genuine have an unconditional categorical character.[4]

But if duty is abstracted from all specific purposes, there appears to be no way of determining what this duty consists of. Kant addresses this problem by introducing the third proposition of morality: 'Duty is the necessity of acting from respect for the law' (1988:25). Since all considerations of inclination and result are excluded, duty must be defined not in terms of its content, but as a purely formal requirement – acting from respect for the universal moral law. Kant believes that a principle cannot be truly moral if it is tied to a particular content. The idea of duty involves acting on principle, that is, following a universal principle and not simply reacting to the immediate and particular situation. The moral law, in turn, is the expression of pure reason. Kant sees man as a divided being, composed of rational and emotional elements. The moral law is legislated by man as a rational being. It is simply an expression of our own free will. But since humans are also subject to act from inclination or passion, morality is something we have to obey, even when our inclinations would suggest otherwise.

If the principle of is a purely formal principle, how, then, are we to determine what the moral law commands? Kant claims that the moral law, although entirely formal, is not entirely empty. The supreme principle of morality is the principle of universalisability or the 'categorical imperative',[5] which states that 'I am never to act otherwise than so *that I could also will that my maxim should become a*

[4] See MacIntyre (1990:43-47) for a critical discussion of this point.

[5] Kant distinguishes between 'hypothetical' and 'categorical' imperatives, of which only the former are imperatives contingent upon some further end or goal. Hypothetical imperatives are of the form 'If end *x* is desired, then perform act *y*', while categorical imperatives are of the form 'Do act *y*'. An example of the former is 'If you want to pass finals, then study hard', while an example of the latter might be 'Tell the truth'.

*universal law*' (Kant 1988:27, emphasis in original). The fundamental justification for a maxim is its rationality, which requires that our practical maxims must be universalisable in the sense of being consistent, impersonal and impartial. Universalisability as *consistency* requires that one's reason for performing a certain action in certain circumstances must be a reason for one to perform *the same* action again in relevantly similar circumstances. Universalisability as *impersonality* requires that one's reason for performing a certain action in certain circumstances must be a reason for *anyone* to perform the same action again in relevantly similar circumstances. Universalisability as *impartiality* requires that one's reasons must give equal weight to everyone's desires and interests, including one's own.

One of the examples Kant uses to illustrate this principle is that of making a deceitful promise. When one is in distress and has to decide whether to make a promise that one has no intention of keeping, one should ask: 'Should I be content that my maxim (to extricate myself from difficulty by a false promise) should hold good as a universal law, for myself as well as for others?' Kant answers that one clearly cannot will this consistently, since with such a law there would be no promises at all. This maxim, as soon as it is made a universal law, would necessarily destroy itself. By making deceitful promises one would also be treating the other person as a means to one's own ends (Kant 1988:27-28, 50, 58-59).

Another example Kant uses is the obligation to help those who 'have to contend with great wretchedness'. Kant asks whether the prospering onlooker can consistently will that the maxim 'whenever anyone is flourishing and others are in distress, he will give nothing to charity' become a universal law. He argues that such a maxim would contradict itself, since many cases might occur in which one would need the love and sympathy of others yet, having willed the above maxim to become a universal law, would be deprived of all hope of the aid one desires (Kant 1988:51-52, 59). The implicit conclusion here – that one has a duty of benevolence – is problematical. Can one universalise the maxim, 'Whenever anyone is flourishing and others are in distress, he will give *something* to charity'? There seems to be no logical contradiction in the universalisation of this maxim, but anyone who tries to consistently act upon such a maxim would soon cease to flourish. Perhaps, then, one should change the maxim to read 'when anyone is flourishing and others are in distress, he will *sometimes* give something to charity'.

Kant's distinction between perfect and imperfect duties might help us to understand his position. Kant says that the duty of benevolence is an imperfect obligation towards others, which he defines as 'those which cannot be enforced'. By contrast, the duty to refrain from making false promises is an example of a perfect obligation towards others, since it allows no exceptions. Unfortunately Kant does not clarify the distinction between perfect and imperfect duties, and merely remarks in a footnote that he reserves an examination of the division of duties for a future metaphysic of morals (1988:49-50n). One possible interpretation of the categorical imperative is that the distinction between perfect and imperfect duties does not coincide with the distinction between obligatory and impermissible acts, but with the distinction between *permissible* and *impermissible* actions. On this reading, committing suicide would always be wrong or impermissible. Helping others, as an imperfect duty, would be *permissible*, rather than *obligatory* (see Norman 1986:104-105). But this interpretation is simply not consistent with what Kant says. He explicitly claims that refusing to help others in need is not universalisable, and it does seem to follow from this that helping others is *obligatory*, rather than just permissible.

Another interpretation of this distinction is given by Feldman (1988:266). Having an imperfect duty to perform a certain action makes it obligatory that one *sometimes* perform an action of that kind when the opportunity arises, while having a perfect duty requires one to *always* perform that kind of action when opportunity arises. This seems to be in line with Kant's description of imperfect duties, such as helping others and developing one's talents, as *contingent* or *meritorious* duties (Kant 1988:59). In contrast, the duty of non-maleficence or, as Kant refers to it, the duty not to intentionally withdraw from the happiness of others, can be seen as a perfect obligation. This interpretation seems plausible since it does make sense to say that negative duties, such as not committing suicide or not making false promises are of a kind that may be regarded as having no exceptions. The same can hardly be said of positive duties such as helping others or developing one's talents. But if this is Kant's position, it is inconsistent with the basic tenets of his ethics. Kant argues that duties are derived from reason alone. However, the implausibility of a perfect obligation to help others derives from its practical impossibility, and not from its logical inconsistency. One can imagine a society where the vast majority of its members are so affluent that it is possible for them to help all those in need. The duty of benevolence can, without logical inconsistency, be seen as a perfect duty. In most societies, however, it is simply not possible for affluent people to help all the needy people they encounter. Yet Kant repeatedly insists that moral knowledge is not to be 'borrowed from experience' but only comes through the exercise of pure reason.

It is also unclear how an imperfect or contingent obligation can be described as *universal*. Whilst Kant gives a central role to the principle of universalisability, which implies that maxims found to be universalisable allow no exceptions, he here admits that some duties do not have to be performed without exception. To this Kant might want to reply that while the maxim 'always help those in need' is not universalisable, the maxim 'sometimes help those in need' is. But this only leads us to a third difficulty: It is unclear how the duty to sometimes help others can withstand the tests of *impartiality* and *impersonality*. Given the (experiential) fact that man's ability to benefit others is limited, we have to discriminate between possible candidates for our benevolent acts. To have an imperfect duty to perform a certain action requires that one *sometimes* perform an action of that kind when the opportunity arises. By contrast perfect duties require one to always do that kind of action when the opportunity arises. The question we now need to consider is 'How are we to decide when this "sometimes" should be?' This surely cannot be decided through the use of pure reason alone. Yet, we are not to act according to our feelings or inclinations (the requirement of rationality), to favour friends and family (the requirement of impartiality), or to benefit those whom we know would one day return the favour (the requirement of impersonality).

The Kantian position is also extremely problematic with regard to the morally-appropriate motivation for benevolence. The first question that can be asked is whether benevolence is a duty at all. Why should one adopt benevolence as a principle? Kant identifies with the Stoic view that it is inappropriate to respond with distress to the present distress of another:

> It was a sublime way of representing the wise man, as the Stoic conceived him, when he let the wise one say: I wish I had a friend, not that he might give me help in poverty, sickness, captivity, and so on, but in order that I might stand by him and save a human being. But for all that, the same wise man, when his friend is not to be saved, says to himself: What's it to me? i.e., he rejected commiseration (1964:121-122).

It is unclear what sense Kant can make of the *need* for benevolence if one considers that he holds the dignity of reason to be complete in itself. As Nussbaum states: 'If people can exercise their most important capacities without material support, this very much diminishes the urgency of that support' (1996:46). It is also unclear what one's motive would be for helping someone in need, if not compassion. Kant tries to salvage the motivational foundations of benevolence by insisting that, since active benevolence is a duty, it is also a duty to seek out circumstances in which one will witness poverty, illness and deprivation, and in which one will not be able to avoid the pain of pity: 'For this feeling, though painful, nevertheless is one of the impulses placed in us by nature for effecting what the representation of duty might not accomplish by itself' (Kant 1964:122). With this statement Kant contradicts his earlier position. He makes a concession to the value of compassion, described as a 'painful feeling' and an 'impulse', in bringing about benevolent acts. He also acknowledges that a good will may not be sufficient, despite his belief that the good will, having failed to bring about any good results, will 'like a jewel... still shine by its own light, as a thing which has its own value in itself' (Kant 1988:18-19).

To clarify Kant's conception of virtue and its role in moral decision-making it might be helpful to refer to his distinction between 'the susceptibility for mutual feelings of enjoyment or pain' (sensitive humanity), and 'the capacity and will to share another's feelings' (practical humanity). The first is a simple case of feeling or sharing another's feelings. Since it is 'pathological' or 'sentimental' it is not a *moral* virtue. For benevolence to be a moral quality it should be inspired by duty, by an acknowledgement of 'the necessity of acting from pure respect for the practical law' (Kant 1988:28). The second, 'practical humanity', is rooted in the rational will and gives rise to an active kind of benevolence. It is this kind of benevolence that we have a duty to seek out. It is at this point that Kant's own rigid distinction between reason and emotion begins to fall apart. Is 'practical humanity' a rational or an affective force? On the one hand he admits that 'practical humanity' is a 'painful feeling', and as we have seen, he holds that the emotions cannot be commanded by reason. Yet he also considers it our duty to seek out this painful feeling, which implies that we can, after all, direct our feelings. Kant finds it impossible to develop his theory of benevolence as a morally-desirable character trait or duty without referring to the fact that human beings are *affected* by the sufferings and happiness of others.[6]

Like most of his predecessors, Kant treats the emotions as unintelligent parts of our animal nature. If compassion and benevolence were instincts or inclinations in this sense, they would indeed lack moral value since there is no conscious or rational moral choice involved. There is some plausibility in the idea that if an action is done simply because one enjoys it, it has no moral worth, since it does not involve any effort or will. But this is not the case with virtues such as compassion, benevolence and friendship. One may treat someone with kindness and compassion without necessarily feeling any love or affection for the person. One can act and feel toward strangers in ways that are fully characteristic of benevolence and compassion. What *is* common to both benevolence and love is that they involve a direct concern for the good of another person who is, for the agent, another self, and it is this concern that is morally relevant.

The requirement of impartiality excludes friendship as the appropriate basis for treating people in certain ways. But should our actions and behaviour towards our friends be dictated purely by a sense of duty? Is not the very fact that we enjoy serving our friends an essential part of friendship, paying testimony to the moral character and purity of our concern and regard for them? It is his concern with keeping emotion and reason neatly apart that lies at the basis of Kant's failure to appreciate friendship. His rejection of compassion as a morally-appropriate motivational force similarly stems from his failure to analyse or even recognise the cognitive basis of such sentiments. Kant's position is directly opposed to that of Hume. Whereas Hume held that the passions have to be guided by reason to enable them to reach their goal of benefiting others, Kant rejects the moral value of the emotions – benevolent inclination deserves praise and encouragement, but not esteem. Yet Kant and Hume share the assumption that morality is *either* the work of reason *or* it is the work of the passions. This initial assumption, as well as his own apparently conclusive arguments that it cannot be the work of reason, drives Hume to the conclusion that morality must be understood in terms of, explained and justified with reference to, the place of the passions and desires in human life. Conversely, Kant founds morality on reason because his arguments have excluded the possibility of founding it on the passions (MacIntyre 1990:49). The influence of Kant's philosophy on medical ethics also meant a rejection of the Aristotelian tradition, even though his criticism of the Humean position does nothing to

---

[6] This reveals another shortcoming of Kant's position, namely that he cannot justify the principle of benevolence without appealing to consequentialist considerations. Consistent and universal malevolence would be just as rational as consistent benevolence. The reason why we cannot will this to become a universal maxim is because of the adverse consequences an acceptance of a maxim of malevolence would have. The need for benevolence therefore cannot be promoted or justified in purely rational terms by referring to one's moral duty. I discuss this objection in more detail in the next section.

discredit the Aristotelian view of compassion. Aristotle's compassion, unlike Hume's sympathy, is not merely an emotion or instinct but involves and, indeed, requires both rational and moral judgement. With regard to the appropriate motivation for benevolence, our choice is between three distinct positions: the Kantian view that benevolence has to be motivated by duty, the maxims of which are discovered by reason; the Humean position which grounds benevolence in the emotion or sentiment of sympathy; and the Aristotelian position that bases benevolence in the virtue of compassion.

For Aristotle, virtues such as friendship do involve affection, but neither singly nor primarily. He defines friendship in terms of a common allegiance to and a common pursuit of certain goods. Friendship is not merely an irrational sentiment, a case of 'liking someone' because of his polite manners, beautiful face or pleasant composure. Friendship, in its ideal form, requires or presupposes a moral judgement of the person's character, respect for that person as an equal, as well as at least a certain level of identification with his goals, life style and interests.[7] Generosity towards one's friends is not motivated simply by feelings, but by one's *regard* for them.

Before developing a teleological or Aristotelian conception of benevolence it is necessary to focus on the utilitarian objection to Kantianism, namely that it is not sufficiently concerned with the consequences of an act in evaluating its moral value. This forms the second level of the debate concerning benevolence, namely whether our focus in evaluating acts should be on their results (beneficence) or the intentions underlying the act (benevolence). As we shall see, Mill's argument played a significant role in the replacement of the virtue of benevolence with the principle of beneficence.

## Consequences: From Benevolence to Beneficence

### *Mill's Utilitarianism*

Kant focuses on intention in judging actions rather than the actual consequences of the action. Utilitarians, by contrast, believe that intentions are not relevant in judging the moral acceptability of actions and take as the primary object of moral judgement the good or bad consequences of the action. In his well-known essay 'Utilitarianism', first published in 1861, J.S. Mill distances himself from the Kantian position, placing at the centre of his moral theory the very things which Kant wanted to exclude: the assessment of actions in terms of their consequences, their contribution to human happiness, and the prevention or removal of suffering. He did, however, retain certain aspects of Kant's theory of morality. Like Kant, Mill rejects those theories of morality that consider our judgements of right and

---

[7] For a critical discussion of the Kantian and utilitarian positions on friendship and impartiality, see Jeske (1997:51-72). For Aristotle's own analysis of friendship, see his *Nicomachean Ethics* (books VII and VIII).

wrong to be informed by a sense or instinct. According to Mill the only rational approach to morality is to believe that our moral faculty 'supplies us only with the general principles of moral judgements; it is a branch of our reason, not of our sensitive faculty; and must be looked to for the abstract doctrines of morality, not for perception of it in the concrete' (Mill 1987:273-274). Rational moral theorists agree that the morality of an individual action is not a question of direct perception, but of the application of a law to an individual case. However, they disagree on the source from which moral laws derive their authority. Some thinkers hold that the principles of morals are evident *a priori,* while others believe that moral knowledge is gained through observation and experience. In Mill's view, both these traditions fail to reduce the different principles to one first principle or common ground of obligation. His own goal is to develop such a fundamental principle of morality.

Although Mill appreciates Kant's attempt to lay down a universal first principle as the origin and ground of moral obligation, he claims that Kant cannot consistently defend certain rules and principles through the use of pure reason (or *a priori* knowledge claims) without reverting to *a posteriori* knowledge claims concerning the consequences of such principles and rules. He writes:

> [W]hen he begins to deduce from this precept [i.e., the categorical imperative] any of the actual duties of morality he fails, almost grotesquely, to show that there would be any contradiction, any logical (not to say physical) impossibility, in the adoption by all rational beings of the most outrageously immoral rules of conduct. All he shows is that the *consequences* of their universal adoption would be such as no one would choose to incur (Mill 1987:275, emphasis in original).

Mill explains that it is a mistake to speak only of actions done from the motive of duty, and in direct obedience to principle. One has a duty to act in certain ways *because* of the benefit that it brings. Following Bentham, then, Mill develops the principle of utility as the foundation of morals. Bentham's principle of utility, namely that an individual's actions are always motivated by their desire for pleasure and the avoidance of pain, has been rejected as advocating selfishness, since it focuses only on the results for the agent, and base, since it sees the good life in an Epicurean fashion as one of pleasure. Mill aspires to incorporate the insights that Bentham lacked in what is still a utilitarian framework. Mill's famous statement of the principle of utility reads as follows:

> [A]ctions are right in proportion as they tend to promote happiness, wrong as they tend to produce the reverse of happiness. By happiness is intended pleasure, and the absence of pain; by unhappiness, pain, and the privation of pleasure.... [P]leasure, and freedom from pain, are the only things desirable as ends; and... all desirable things... are desirable either for the pleasure inherent in themselves, or as means to the promotion of pleasure and the prevention of pain (Mill 1987:278).

Mill supports Bentham's departure from the dominant tradition in Western thought in his view that the capacity to suffer, rather than rationality, is the necessary and sufficient condition for moral standing. The principle of utility gains its universality from the fact that 'the ultimate end, with reference to and for the sake of which all other things are desirable (whether we are considering our own good or that of other people), is an existence exempt as far as possible from pain, and as rich as possible in enjoyments' (Mill 1987:283). But he puts a more altruistic slant on the doctrine of utility than does Bentham by emphasising the nobility of disinterested devotion to moral *duty*, and in this regard he follows Kant. Instead of merely attending to one's own happiness, one's actions should aim at the general happiness, regardless of whether this will increase one's own happiness. But in contrast to Kant he argues that happiness is the only thing desirable in itself. It is not sufficient only to have good intentions or a good will – we also have to benefit others. Whereas for Kant we have a duty to be *benevolent*, Mill's views imply that we have a duty to be *beneficent*. The principles of beneficence and non-maleficence are therefore central duties in the utilitarian framework. Mill shares with Kant the concern with universal principles and duties, but gives a different justification for this commitment. Whereas for Kant, the principle of universalisability is a formal principle discovered by pure reason, Mill defends a set of universal duties on the basis of the consequences they have for the general welfare of most people.

Mill's theory is an example of *rule*-utilitarianism, rather than *act*-utilitarianism, although this was not a distinction made in his time.[8] He suggests that we use utilitarian principles to establish rules of conduct. What justifies our adherence to these rules is their contribution to human welfare, even though he admits that the application of these rules may, in certain instances, have less than desirable consequences. Mill's concern with universal values is evident in the argument he develops to counter the possible objection that utilitarianism, in being concerned with pleasure or happiness as the sole and ultimate value, is a 'doctrine worthy of swine' (1987:278). There is a question concerning whether there is any way, besides instinct or passion, to prefer one pleasure above another. In response, Mill claims that there is a qualitative difference between pleasures. The so-called 'higher pleasures' are those that suit our nature as human beings and utilise or promote our capacity for intelligent activity. Despite his admission that there is a plurality of pleasures, and that different people have different preferences, he views a certain mode of pleasure as the morally-appropriate aim of our actions. Rather than leave the individual to decide which pleasures to strive towards in particular circumstances, he feels that we can, in principle, give an account of

---

[8] The rule-utilitarian considers the consequences of adopting rules, asking: 'What good or bad consequences will result from this kind of action in this type of circumstances?' A specific action is right if it conforms to a justified rule. The rule is not expendable in a particular context, even if following the rule in that context does not maximise utility. In contrast, the act-utilitarian bypasses the level of rules and justifies actions by appealing directly to the principle of utility, asking: 'What good or bad consequences will result from this action in this circumstance?' Moral rules are viewed as useful in guiding human actions, but also as expendable if they do not promote utility in a particular context.

pleasures that are universally desirable or valuable (even though they are not valued or desired by all). The morally-appropriate aims of our actions cannot be determined through the use of pure reason, but only through knowledge gained by those who have experienced both higher and lower modes of pleasure: '[T]he judgement of those who are qualified by knowledge of both, or, if they differ, that of the majority among them, must be admitted as final' (Mill 1987:282). No one experienced in both the higher and lower pleasures would prefer the latter.

In the third chapter of 'Utilitarianism' Mill introduces an important issue with regard to the principle of utility. He writes: 'What is its sanction? what are the motives to obey it? or more specifically, what is the source of its obligation? whence does it derive its binding force?' (Mill 1987:298). This is an important feature of his argument, but one that is often ignored or neglected by his critics and commentators.[9] This neglect is all the more striking when one considers the title of the chapter: 'Of the ultimate sanction of the principle of utility.'

Mill says that the principle of utility has all the sanctions that belong to any other system of morals. He first mentions certain 'external sanctions', such as fear of social disapproval and of God's punishment. These sanctions need not concern us here, and Mill himself does not discuss them in any detail. He devotes more attention to the 'internal sanction of duty', which he describes as a 'powerful natural sentiment'. He believes that this sanction will constitute the strength of the utilitarian morality if the general happiness comes to be recognised as the ethical standard. If perfected, this sentiment will ensure that the person would never think of or desire any beneficial condition for himself, unless it is also to the benefit of the other parties affected:

> So long as they are co-operating, their ends are identified with those of others; there is at least a temporary feeling that the interests of others are their own interests. Not only does all strengthening of social ties, and all healthy growth of society, give to each individual a stronger personal interest in practically consulting the welfare of others; it also leads him to identify his *feelings* more and more with their good, or at least with an ever greater degree of practical consideration for it. He comes, as though instinctively, to be conscious of himself as a being who *of course* pays regard to others. The good of others becomes to him a thing naturally and necessarily to be attended to, like any of the physical conditions of our existence. Now, whatever amount of this feeling a person has, he is urged by the strongest motives both of interest and of sympathy to demonstrate it, and to the utmost of his power encourage it in others (Mill 1987:304-305, emphasis in original).

Mill never gives a name to this sentiment; he simply refers to it as 'the social feelings of mankind; the desire to be in unity with our fellow creatures' (1987:303). This sentiment shows remarkable similarities to the Aristotelian account of compassion: a form of identification with our fellow human beings, an

---

[9] For example, Norman (1986:125) briefly mentions the four sanctions of the principle of utility, and Borchert and Stewart (1986:190-195) and Hamlyn (1988:275-280) totally ignore the issue in their detailed discussions of the basic tenets of Mill's utilitarianism.

unselfish concern for their welfare and a consequent motivation to benefit them. Mill appears to be baffled by the complexity of this sentiment, referring to it variously as a 'feeling' or 'desire', a 'conviction' as well as a 'force'. He thus defies the rigid distinction between reason and emotion. Mill is eager to point out that this sentiment is not merely an irrational force that distracts us from fulfilling our duties. He describes it as 'a powerful internal binding force' and in those who have it, 'it does not present itself to their minds as a superstition of education, or a law despotically imposed by the power of society, but as an attribute which it would not be well for them to be without' (1987:306). His difficulty in defining and clearly describing this sentiment reflects the fact that compassion is a complex mixture of emotional, cognitive and motivational elements. Mill could not fully appreciate this complexity since he still works within a dualistic framework according to which morality must be either the work of reason, or the work of emotion. Mill's struggle with the reason-passion dichotomy runs throughout his philosophy and his personal life. In his *Autobiography* he describes how, for six months, he was in a near-suicidal state of depression after being convinced that the exclusive cultivation of his analytical abilities had destroyed in him all capacity for emotion. The breakthrough came after he realised that his very depression was testimony to the fact that he is an emotional being: '[T]he oppression of the thought that all feeling was dead within me, was gone. I was no longer hopeless: I was not a stock or a stone' (Mill 1924:99). He was unable to make a similar breakthrough in his philosophical essays, at times considering the role of the emotions in moral decision-making, but ultimately coming out in favour of reason.

Like Kant, Mill finds it impossible to develop a theory of morality without referring to compassion as a motivation for benevolence. The role Mill affords to this sentiment as well as his implicit attack on the reason/passion dichotomy has been largely ignored by his followers and critics alike, who have tended to focus on his view of justice and the principle of utility. Utilitarianism has been adopted as a strategy of decision-making in everyday practice and policy-making that involves a dispassionate calculation of utility. The effect of the vastly over-simplified version of utilitarianism on medical practice has been significant.

## The Principle of Beneficence in Medical Ethics

Richard Taylor writes that:

> If I were ever to find, as luckily I never have, a man who assured me that he really *believed* Kant's metaphysical morals, and that he modelled his own conduct and his relations with others after those principles, then my incredulity and distrust of him as a human being could not be greater than if he told me he regularly drowned children just to see them squirm (1970:xii, emphasis in original).

Both Kant and Mill have, of course, received more than their fair share of criticism from fellow philosophers. I do not aim to provide a comprehensive critique of their theoretical positions but to examine some of the shortcomings of principle-based approaches within the field of medicine.

Contemporary medical ethics has been influenced by both deontological and utilitarian approaches. These two approaches are only mutually exclusive if one takes seriously the claim by adherents to both types of theory to have discovered the single foundational principle of ethics. Within a pluralistic moral framework, such as the 'four-principles approach' developed by Beauchamp and Childress (1994), it is possible to combine insights or aspects of both theories by separating two spheres of moral judgement. The first concerns the *character* of the agent, which can be described as either good or bad, and the second concerns the *act* itself, which can be described as right or wrong. This distinction makes possible the view that, although benevolence as motivation is relevant for judging character, an action should be judged on the basis of its consequences, i.e., as beneficial or harmful.[10]

### *Character*

Medical law and ethics have followed Kant in evaluating character on the basis of the person's adherence to principles or duties. The notion of 'negligence' has been developed in medical law to determine whether a health worker who has harmed a patient through his behaviour has done so because of a lack of motivation and effort in fulfilling his duties towards patients.

Hume's approach to judging character (i.e., focusing on emotions displayed by the agent) has been rejected, and with that, the Aristotelian position (i.e., evaluating character on the basis of the person's virtuousness or viciousness). The difference between these two positions is not always appreciated. In their discussions of the issues surrounding the motivation for benevolence contemporary ethicists have tended to present the conflict in a Kantian fashion, namely as one between reason (or duty) and passion, not recognising that virtue ethics represents a third and middle position between these two extremes. Frankena follows Kant in distinguishing between a love of neighbour that resides in the will ('practical love') and one that resides in inclination, the propensity of sense or in tender sympathy ('pathological love') (see Kant 1988:24). Frankena explains the difference in the following way: If one embraces benevolence as a *principle*, then one believes firmly and steadily that oneself and others should be benevolent or that it is good or desirable to be benevolent. Duty-ethicists point out that a disposition or trait is not a moral virtue unless it is in some essential way tied to a sense of duty. By contrast, adopting or displaying benevolence as a *disposition* does not entail believing this; one may just have a natural or motivational tendency

[10] Rachels argues, for instance, that the traditional relation between act and intention is mistaken: '[T]he intention is not relevant to deciding whether the *act* is right or wrong, but instead it is relevant to assessing the character of the person who does the act, which is very different.... A pure character cannot make a wrong act right; neither can an impure heart make a right act wrong' (1989:63-64).

to beneficence without believing that this is good, without making any value judgements about it at all, moral or non-moral. If one's benevolence commences from compassion, it would be regarded as an example of having benevolence as a disposition. Frankena claims that, for the most part, those who subscribe to an ethic of virtue hold that moral virtues are or should be *pathological* in Kant's sense. Benevolence cannot be *morally* good or virtuous unless it is tied to some *moral* principle or other, such as the principle of beneficence. Frankena concludes that a person cannot be morally good or have a moral virtue unless he or she acts under the aegis of some moral judgement, and perhaps only if he or she acts under that of moral duty (1987:1-2, 7-9).

I agree with Frankena that a person's intention or motive cannot be described as morally good if it is not accompanied by a moral judgement or if it is merely an emotional response. A disposition must be tied to a value judgement that a certain act is virtuous or that a given goal is worth striving for. Unfortunately, it is true that most supporters of virtue ethics have held that a disposition may be a moral virtue even if it is not accompanied by a sense of duty at all. But there is no reason why our choice should be between reason and emotion, or between duty and inclination. It is only under Kantian influence that contemporary virtue-ethicists have tended to present their position as favouring emotion above reason as the morally-appropriate motive for acting in certain ways. As I have argued previously, compassion and other virtues are not merely 'pathological' dispositions, they contain or are based on certain moral and intellectual judgements. The recognition of compassion as an appropriate motivation for acting morally therefore involves a transcendence of the reason-emotion dichotomy.

### *Action*

With regard to judging actions it is obvious that, *contra* Kant, medical practice is very much concerned with the results of treatment. Being appropriately motivated, accepting benevolence as one's duty, is simply not sufficient for producing acts that are truly beneficent. It is for this reason that, apart from adopting certain moral principles or duties, medical professionals are expected to have a certain level of competence (medical knowledge and technical skills) to ensure that they are not only willing, but also capable of benefiting patients.

In this regard, the ethics of virtue has once again been rejected. As a teleological theory, it is, of course, concerned with the consequences of actions. The virtues are often praised for the beneficent acts they give rise to. For example, Gennaro says that 'bad-intentioned people are, as a matter of psychological fact, more inclined to act rashly, irresponsibly, and (yes) wrongly.... Character matters because those who lack it are more likely to act immorally; it is not merely some causally irrelevant, additional fact about a person' (1996:220). In the medical field, however, it is often felt that no need exists for emphasising the virtues, since medical knowledge and technical skills allow physicians to benefit patients. The fact that they have the duty to act in certain ways is seen as ensuring that they do not act rashly or irresponsibly and thereby harm their patients. Indeed, medical professionals are encouraged not to become 'emotionally involved' with their patients since this would cloud their judgement, which has to be rational and objective at all times.

The virtues have also been rejected as being too vague with regard to the goals of actions. Hence it is often objected that a virtue-based theory, when confronted with the question of which actions should be performed, can only reply: 'Perform those actions that an exemplary moral agent would perform' (Beauchamp and Childress 1994:69). According to this line of reasoning, an ethic based on the obligation to benefit or not to harm others, and which also gives clear content to the notions of 'harm' and 'benefit', is more effective in promoting the well-being of patients than one based on the virtue of compassion.

The utilitarian aspect of the four-principles approach emphasises the principles of non-maleficence and beneficence, together with the principle of utility. The principle of non-maleficence is a negative duty – it states that one is never to harm a patient. Although this principle is often taken to be a perfect duty, this is untenable, since it is sometimes necessary to inflict a minor harm on someone in order to attain a major benefit. The principle of beneficence, on the other hand, asserts a positive obligation on the part of the medical professional to help patients further their important and legitimate interests. Because there are limits to what medical professionals can accomplish this can only be an imperfect duty. In addition to these two principles, the principle of utility plays an important part in medical decision-making. This principle requires the physician to weigh and balance possible benefits against possible harms for the specific individual in question. Because the moral life typically does not provide the opportunity to produce benefits or eliminate harms without creating risks or incurring costs, the principle of utility is an essential extension of the principle of beneficence. For example, where a major benefit can be produced by causing a minor harm, the requirement to benefit is overriding. It should be noted that the notion of utility as used by Beauchamp and Childress is not identical to the classical utilitarian concept thereof, which is an absolute and overriding principle. One of the key problems with classical utilitarianism is its disregard for individuals, insofar as it condones or even requires harming an individual or minority party to maximise overall happiness. In contrast, the principle of utility as employed by Beauchamp and Childress is one of a number of *prima facie* principles, and is limited to balancing benefits, costs and risks involved for a specific patient instead of determining the overall balancing of obligations (Beauchamp and Childress 1994:260, 263).[11]

The principle of beneficence in medical practice also moves away from utilitarian (and Christian) morality by requiring only *specific*, rather than *general*

---

[11] This approach is based on that of W.D. Ross in *The Right and the Good* (1930). Ross rejects the Kantian view that duties are universal and absolute, while arguing in favour of the view that they are *prima facie*, so that they may prevail on some occasions but overridden by another duty on other occasions.

beneficence. Specific beneficence is directed at specific parties, such as one's children, friends and family, whereas general beneficence is directed beyond these special relationships to all persons. The utilitarian morality has been criticised as being too demanding since it requires us to act impartially in order to promote the interests of persons beyond our limited sphere of relationships and influence. Beauchamp and Childress remark that it is 'overly romantic and impractical' to require us to have the same impartial obligation to strangers as we have to our own families (1994:264). This objection need not concern us here, since it is clear that medical personnel, at least in their capacity as health-care workers, do not have a positive and impartial obligation to benefit all people. Their obligation to benefit extends only to their patients. What is of interest here, however, is the nature of the 'special relationship' between doctors and patients. Those who advocate specific, rather than general beneficence, use as examples the special relationship between friends and family – people with whom one is intimately acquainted. It is the very intimacy of one's relationship with them that generates one's responsibilities towards such people. By contrast, doctors have a specific obligation towards their patients – people who are usually not their friends, family or acquaintances but most often total strangers. The significance of this, as we shall see, is that it often obscures the content of the terms 'harms' and 'benefits'. Whereas one is likely to know what one's friends or relatives would perceive and experience as beneficial or harmful, this becomes more difficult to determine if the other person is a complete stranger.

It is for this reason that Beauchamp and Childress point out that the general principles of beneficence and non-maleficence have to be more closely specified in terms of a set of rules. They follow in the tradition of Richard Cabot by specifying the goals of medicine in terms of purely physical harms and benefits (1994:193). The content of the terms 'harm' and 'benefit' is determined with reference to generally-accepted preferences, such as fertility to infertility, acute but brief pain to chronic pain, and life to death.[12]

Contemporary medical ethics has supplemented the Kantian principle of universalisability with utilitarian considerations by defining duties or principles in terms of ends or goals. In deciding whether a specific rule or maxim, such as 'One should provide terminal patients with assistance in dying if they so request', should

---

[12] Autonomists might want to reply that they do not hold any such general rules concerning the content of the concepts 'benefit' and 'harm', and instead believe that the good of a patient is that which the patient views as beneficial. I shall discuss this position in more detail in the next chapter. Suffice it to say at this stage that the implication of such a position would be that a conflict between the principles of beneficence and autonomy could never arise, since a patient's autonomous decision concerning what would benefit him would necessarily concur with what would actually benefit him. For instance, if a patient felt that amputating a perfectly healthy limb would be to his benefit, the physician should respect this decision *because such surgery would benefit him*. This is a position that not even the most radical autonomist would accept. The dilemma facing the physician is not whether to accept the patient's view of benefits or his own, but whether to respect the patient's decision, despite the fact that this would entail harming him.

become a universal law, the question to be asked is not 'Does it become self-contradictory?', but 'Would its universalisation lead to undesirable consequences?' or 'Would it tend to produce more suffering or less happiness than some alternative action?'. This appears to be the strategy that is most often followed in medical law in formulating legislation on controversial issues such as euthanasia, physician-assisted suicide, surrogate motherhood and abortion. However, while it might be true that a certain type of action, when universalised, would have certain consequences, it does not follow that an individual action of this kind would have such consequences. In other words, by adhering to general rules of beneficence and non-maleficence one might end up harming (or failing to benefit) specific individuals. In what follows I argue that this method of giving content to the rules of beneficence and non-maleficence lies at the basis of the dissatisfaction with a paternalistic ethic in contemporary Western societies.

## The Problems with Contemporary Medical Paternalism

The paternalist justifies making decisions on behalf of patients by referring to his medical knowledge and technical skills, the superiority of which is more striking today than ever before. Modern medicine is characterised by a technological sophistication pertaining to diagnosis, prognosis and modes of treatment previously unheard of. Whereas the physician of past eras made his diagnosis mainly through listening to the patient's complaints, the modern physician has at his disposal remote computerised machinery which offers a far more accurate scientific explanation of the patient's disease. Modern means of diagnosis and prognosis have enabled the physician to give an objective, scientific explanation of disease. The physician is also better able to predict the course of disease, if left untreated, and the dangers and benefits attached to different modes of treatment. These developments in modern medicine form part of the impressive progress of science during the nineteenth and twentieth centuries and the predictive powers of scientific explanations. Through their belief in the objectivity of scientific method, medical scientists have sought to gain access to knowledge about diseases which is impersonal, value free and universally valid. Whereas one might, with a certain level of legitimacy, claim that considerations of value should be excluded from procedures of diagnosing illness, there are two areas in which subjective judgements cannot be excluded from medical decision-making. The first concerns the way in which the individual patient is affected by disease (the suffering of the person), and the second concerns the goals of medical treatment.

### *Disease and Suffering*

Since disease is viewed in purely mechanistic terms as a physiological disorder, physicians focus their attention on restoring this disharmony. The principle of beneficence states that it is the duty of a physician to benefit patients. The term 'benefit' is understood as restoring health or, where this is not possible, relieving pain and alleviating physical discomfort. In the scientific view of medical disorders the choice of a mode of treatment is informed solely by a calculation, based on diagnostic and prognostic information, of *medical* risks and benefits, and the effectiveness of treatment is similarly calculated in terms of medical goals.

When it comes to restoring health and managing physical pain one can hardly underestimate the value of scientific explanations of physiological disorders. But while proving to be very effective in curing diseases, physicians' increasing reliance on medical technology and scientific explanations often results in a failure to alleviate suffering. The exclusive focus on relieving physical pain and discomfort is a failure to realise that, in the words of John Hick:

> [T]he greater part of human misery transcends physical pain. What makes an illness, for example, an experience of suffering is very often not pain as such but other elements in the situation: fear of permanent disability or of death; anxiety about one's family, or finances, or career; the frustration of one's plans; or the humiliation of helplessness and of dependence upon others (1966:356).

In this way a physician who focuses on the duty to relieve physical pain may fail to alleviate his patient's suffering. It is often assumed that the suffering of a patient is caused solely by physical pain, and that the management of pain will put an end to suffering. A physician who holds this view will be unable to care for the needs of a specific patient whose suffering is partly due to fear of death, grief, the frustration of goals and the like, which will not necessarily disappear when treated as pain. It is for this reason that the physician needs not only scientific knowledge of diseases, but also needs to cultivate the virtue of compassion.

The lack of compassion can, in part, be attributed to the shift in emphasis in modern medicine from history taking and communication with the patient to technologically-sophisticated diagnostic equipment. Together with increased patient loads and specialisation, this factor has contributed to less time spent with the patient, with a concomitant neglect of dialogue between physician and patient. In the editorial of a paediatric journal Prof. P.M. Leary expresses his alarm at hearing a colleague announce that he saved valuable time in his private practice by carrying out full physical examinations as mothers gave him their children's history. Leary points out that the value of history taking can be measured in both medical and humane terms. Communication firstly plays a role in facilitating correct diagnosis of the patient's medical problems. Listening to a patient's complaints informs the competent physician when deciding among the myriad of diagnostic tests available. Secondly, he says, relaxed interaction between parent and physician is 'wonderfully assuring and serves as an effective insurance against tearful or even violent opposition when the time comes for the shedding of clothes and the indignities of physical examination'. Leary also mentions the fact that communication gives the physician an opportunity to observe the body language of both parent and child and form impressions of bonding, child rearing skills, domestic interactions and general quality of life (1997:2).

By entering into a conversation with the patient, the physician may gain insight into the individual's life style, beliefs and values, his experience of illness and suffering, and may thus come to understand what it means for the individual to live with disease. In short, a compassionate understanding of a person's illness should, ideally speaking, accompany or supplement scientific knowledge of a patient's disease. General laws cannot explain the individual patient's unique experience, and a commitment to science disregards the fact that suffering comprises more than just physical pain. Spiro, in arguing for the importance of empathy in medical science, makes this point as follows:

> Training in continuing care will be of little value without doctors who know something of the life of the people whom they serve.... Science looks towards the general, but physicians deal with the particular. The individual is lost among our statistics and archetypes.... The problems of living – existential, socio-economic, and emotional – that account for 80 percent of visits to physicians' offices represent complaints that are unlikely to be switched on or off by an aberrant gene (Spiro 1993:12-13).

In multicultural societies such as South Africa, where a vast diversity of patients from different cultural, religious and socio-economic backgrounds converge, a compassionate understanding of the patient's situation is extremely important. The following case, which came up for discussion at a Bioethics seminar at the University of Cape Town's Medical School, illustrates this point well. The case was presented by a white doctor who worked in a clinic in Khayalitsha (a black township in Cape Town).

> An unemployed, single mother visited the clinic on several occasions with her severely-undernourished infant. Although there were no medical indications prohibiting breast-feeding, the mother refused to do so. Under pressure not to expend scarce resources unnecessarily, the doctor and a nurse attempted to explain to the young mother that there are many benefits to breast-feeding and that there is a significant risk of disease and infection with formula-feeding, particularly given the lack of adequate sanitation in the township. Their attempts failed to convince the mother.

The doctor was unable to understand the conflict between the mother's obvious concern for her child and her refusal to breast-feed, and seemed somewhat irritated at her stubbornness and stupidity. A social worker that attended the seminar shed some light on the mystery by pointing out that her refusal to breast-feed was probably due to the fact that she was a sex worker. Although there were no medical indications prohibiting breast-feeding, such an occupation does prohibit breast-feeding and may be the only means in which the woman can support herself and her children. The doctor's failure in this case was clearly not due to her lack of medical expertise but to an inadequate understanding of the mother's plight.

In contrast to the physician who relies solely on medical science to come to an explanation of the patient's condition, the compassionate physician attempts to understand her patient's suffering through an empathetic dialogue. By taking the patient's values seriously, the physician regards the patient as a being worthy of respect, as one whose suffering matters, and as one whose experience is unique, not to be explained fully with reference to medical facts and statistics. The compassionate physician realises that the well-being of an individual does not only depend on the satisfaction of his physical or medical needs, but also on the satisfaction of psychological and personal needs, all of which can be considered as *basic* needs. Unless a person's psychological needs are satisfied he could be seriously hindered in regard to almost any goal he wishes to attain. The same is true about personal needs and interests, such as religious beliefs, career aspirations and family obligations, which may be of overriding importance to the individual. Major curtailment of personal and psychological needs could qualify for consideration as serious harm and may outweigh physical harm in importance.

The first sphere in which judgements of value cannot be excluded in one's treatment of a patient is, then, the way in which disease affects the patient. The nature and seriousness of a patient's suffering is not necessarily proportionate to the nature and seriousness of his disease. As a means of understanding a patient's suffering, the scientific method is simply not adequate. The modern physician might want to respond that the primary duty or task of the physician as *medical* expert is to benefit patients by curing illness and relieving suffering due to physical ailments, and that it is the task of psychologists and psychiatrists, family and friends to fulfil their psychological or emotional needs. I agree that relatives and friends have an important role to play in this regard, and that they should not view the patient's predicament as a purely medical problem to be dealt with by medical professionals. In an age of technological miracles, people too often underestimate the importance of love and compassion at the bedside of a sick friend or relative, and through their own embarrassment or discomfort distance themselves from the patient. Yet this does not mean that physicians need not understand and respond to the patient's emotional suffering or that compassion is superfluous in the clinical encounter. A compassionate understanding is integral to the healing process. This is something that even advocates of the need for compassion in modern hospitals sometimes fail to appreciate. For instance, in his introduction to a compilation of papers on empathy in medicine, Spiro summarises its value as follows: '*Disease*, which is what diagnostic equipment displays, needs science for cure, whereas *illness*, the patient's suffering, needs the physician for care' (Spiro *et al.* 1993:2, emphasis in original). Empathy, as seen by most of the contributors to this volume, seems to be a strategy directed towards relieving a person's psychological and emotional suffering, whereas medicine is used to relieve their physical ailments. This does seem to suggest that communication and empathy are luxuries that the doctor may choose to bestow upon the patient if he has sufficient time to do so after fulfilling his primary duty, which is to cure disease and relieve physical pain. However, the medical treatment of physical pain and the compassionate treatment of psychological or existential suffering cannot be separated in this way. By combining empathy with scientific explanation, the physician does not take care of the patient's emotional needs only. In what follows, I argue that the value of compassion goes further than this – an empathic understanding ultimately enables the physician to realise the goals of medicine.

*The Goals of Medical Treatment*

The second sphere in which judgements of value are required pertains to the goals of medical treatment. A physician may harm (or fail to benefit) patients by focusing only on medical values in weighing harms and benefits, and by assuming that his hierarchy of values is supreme. For example, in the treatment of a thyroid tumour a choice has to be made between radiation therapy, surgery, and chemotherapy (or a combination of these). Each mode of treatment has its own potential risks and expected benefits. On purely medical grounds, there may be little value in favouring one mode of treatment over another, but the specific patient's values, life plan and beliefs may greatly influence the decision. A young woman who still desires to have children might consider the increased risks, pain and discomfort of surgery to be lesser evils, medically speaking, than the risk of infertility following radiation therapy. A physician who fails to consider the perspective of the individual patient, favouring some form of treatment based on his own judgements and preferences of medical risks and benefits, could be guilty of harming or failing to benefit a *specific* patient, although the same procedure and outcome might not be perceived as a harm, all things considered, by another patient. In fact, some patients might even see infertility as a benefit. In choosing among different modes of treatment, and in weighing up the risks and benefits relating to each, the physician should attempt to understand the values, life style and goals of each patient to be able to benefit the patient in terms of these. The value of compassionate dialogue does not only extend to emotional or psychological benefits, but may allow physician and patient to reach consensus on both the means and goals of medical treatment.

The following, not atypical, case further demonstrates the interconnectedness of medical, existential and psychological harms and benefits:

> Ms. Anderson was a 72-year old woman living on her own in relative poverty when she was found by public officials to have suffered frostbite of both feet, complicated by burns from her wood fire. Reports from several concerned parties led police to go to her home on three previous occasions; on the third visit, they entered and forcibly transported her to hospital. After one week of treatment, physicians urged amputation of both feet, now gangrenous, as a necessary life-saving measure. But Ms. Anderson could not be persuaded to consent to this surgery. She maintained that her feet were black because of soot or dirt and did not believe her physicians about the seriousness of the infection. She believed that her feet will heal without surgery, and refused to even consider the possibility that amputation is necessary to save her life.[13]

The physicians in this case were equally adamant in their belief that amputation was the only reasonable choice, refusing even to consider that the patient could be right. They made their analysis of harms and benefits exclusively in medical

---

[13] Adapted from *Department of Human Services v. Northern*, 563 S.W. 2d 167 (Tn. App. 1978), cert. denied, U.S. (1978). See Abernethy (1984:53-58) for a detailed discussion of the way in which physicians and judges handled this case.

terms, giving rise to a clear decision – not to amputate and so to risk death, or going ahead with the amputation to ensure survival. The result of this calculation of utility clearly points to the necessity of amputation. However, if one views the patient's particular circumstances – that she was unmarried, had no children or other relatives to take care of her, and lived in poverty – one might come to understand how the prospect of amputation and a consequent loss of independence would cause tremendous anxiety for this particular patient. To return to her home without her legs could be a fate worse than death.[14] If the doctors were serious about their desire to help this woman, then they ought to have discussed with her the options and opportunities open to her after the surgery. Such a discussion would, I believe, have enabled medical professionals to gain an understanding of what would be most beneficial (or the least harmful) for the patient given her specific circumstances. Instead, the subsequent discussion and court case focused on the question of whether Ms. Anderson was competent to refuse treatment, leading to a detailed examination of her mental and emotional state. Ms. Anderson died of pneumonia before a decision could be reached.

Another example of the conflict of values and beliefs that commonly arise between doctor and patient is that of the patient who refuses certain medical procedures for religious reasons. Jehovah's Witnesses believe that the biblical admonition to 'abstain from blood' applies to blood transfusions, and that such a procedure can never be justified, not even to save life. Here the conflict between doctor and patient is due to the physician's interpretation of the term 'benefit' as referring to physical benefits, while the patient also includes the loss of everlasting life in his calculation of costs and benefits. The physician who administers blood in the name of the principle of beneficence would not simply be guilty of violating the patient's right to refuse treatment or of injuring his dignity, but of seriously *harming* the patient. In focusing on universal standards of what the human good (clinically speaking) entails, and by relying solely on his medical knowledge and skills to attain these goods for his patient, the paternalist disregards the particular circumstances, values and beliefs of an individual patient. This could lead to a failure to conform to the very principle he uses to justify his actions, namely beneficence.

The above examples demonstrate that existential and psychological harms and benefits cannot be fully divorced from physical harms and benefits. Not only does the patient's physical condition have a direct influence on her emotional well-being, but her values and beliefs could determine whether medical treatment will benefit or harm her. To fully benefit patients, medical professionals should attempt both to reach a scientific explanation of a patient's medical condition,

---

14 This woman's situation is much like that of Philoctetes who, after his bow has been stolen from him, faces the choice between remaining on the island to face a slow and painful death, and returning with his traitors, thus giving up his independence, integrity and dignity. While losing one's weapon (or legs) might in most circumstances be seen as a much lesser harm than the risk of death, this is clearly not the case with either of these tragic figures.

basing their cost-benefit analysis on medical values, and to gain an empathetic understanding of a patient's condition.

Paternalistic actions often lead to grave harm for individuals considered as *persons*. There are usually alternative procedures to treat the same disease or illness, each with its own risks and expected outcome. The patient's experience, values, priorities and life plan need to be taken into consideration when selecting treatment. Together with the growing awareness and acknowledgement of a diversity of values, a growth and diversification of treatment possibilities is taking place in liberal societies. This renders it necessary for the choice of modes of treatment not to be based solely on the *physician's* assessment of *medical* risks and benefits. Since the terms 'benefit' and 'harm' have no universally-valid denotations but consist of a plurality of goals valued differently by different individuals, insight into the values, circumstances and beliefs of the person one wishes to benefit is crucial. I would certainly not want to suggest that all, or even most physicians lack such insight in their personal capacity as human beings. The more fundamental problem facing modern medical practice is that the prevailing system of values does not allow physicians to act according to their understanding of the individual patient's circumstances. Hence in private conversations with medical professionals I often hear them talk of what they did 'officially' and 'unofficially', for instance: 'Officially the child died because she was brought to the hospital too late after the drowning accident for me to be able to save her life. Unofficially, I let the child die after it became clear that she has sustained serious brain damage'. By excluding the virtues of compassion and benevolence from medical practice it has also given up much of what is significantly *human* about the enterprise. This objectification does not only pertain to the patient but extends also to the modern-day physician, who has become an expert in science and technology but has lost his insight into his patients as persons or – what is perhaps more common – is prohibited from using his discretion by certain set rules and policies.

The shortcomings of the principle of beneficence can be attributed to an over-emphasis of scientific knowledge (*episteme*) and technical skills (*techne*). The third intellectual virtue emphasised by Aristotle, *phronesis*, has characteristically been neglected or ignored by the scientific, instrumental rationality. As Flyvbjerg writes, we have become a 'civilization of means without ends' (1993:12). *Episteme* and *techne* are crucial for allowing one to attain set goals, but the virtue of *phronesis* enables one to have insight in to the good of man or the proper end of human life. Aristotle is concerned with *phronesis* as a core virtue that directs man towards the highest goal of his being, the good life, by forming the necessary condition for the possession of all the other virtues. My present project differs significantly from Aristotle's with regard to both aim and scope. I will not be concerned with the good human life or man's supreme destiny as such, but simply with the appropriate role and contribution of medicine and health-care professionals in making it possible for people to realise their conception of the good life. I will not attempt to advance some version of Aristotle's metaphysical biology. I agree with the liberal view that we cannot specify a single goal or function of human life, but I do think that certain conditions can be identified as necessary for being able to realise almost any conception of the good life. In what follows, I develop an account of benevolence as a disposition to do good to others.

## A Teleological Account of Benevolence

In Sophocles's tragedy the chorus of soldiers and Neoptolemus can do very little to help Philoctetes, despite their compassion. It seems that Greek tragedy is aimed simply at arousing the emotions of fear and pity in the audience, and then to reach a catharsis through employing the *deus ex machina* strategy. Hence it may appear that compassion is an agreeable sentiment or character trait, but of little motivational and ethical value. Aristotle does not explore the motivational function of compassion and its value in bringing about beneficent acts in his own discussions of tragedy. This apparent inability of virtue ethics to provide answers to the questions of doing is strengthened by contemporary advocates of virtue ethics such as Elizabeth Anscombe, Philippa Foot and Leslie Stephens, who emphasise character rather than action as the primary object of moral evaluation. Virtue ethics is put forward as an ethics of *being* rather than an ethics of *doing*. Stephens captures the spirit of contemporary virtue-based approaches in the following passage:

> [M]orality is internal. The moral law... has to be expressed in the form 'be this', not in the form 'do this'.... The true moral law says 'hate not', instead of 'kill not'.... The only mode of stating the moral law must be as a rule of character' (cited in Pojman 1988:289).

I shall be concerned with three objections to the virtues, namely (1) that they are simply modes of feeling, containing no cognitive element; (2) that they concern only *being*, and not *doing*; and (3) that they do not produce desirable ends.

### *Character and Passion*

I argued previously that the virtue of compassion contains both emotive and cognitive elements and will not repeat these arguments. This analysis of compassion is completely in line with what Aristotle claims about the virtues in general. In the *Nicomachean Ethics* Aristotle defines moral virtue as a state of character, rather than as a passion such as appetite, anger, fear and joy. The virtues are modes of choice that *dispose* rather than *move* us to act in certain ways, and the object of choice is the result of previous deliberation, rather than immediate desire. Yet the virtues are accompanied by emotions insofar as a virtuous person delights in doing the right thing. In Aristotle's view, Neoptolemus shows himself to be a better man than Odysseus 'because he is pained at telling a lie' (*N. Ethics* VII. ii), because he feels bad about acting viciously. Conversely, pleasure in doing virtuous acts is a sign that the virtuous disposition has been acquired. The pleasure felt in acting virtuously is not, however, a case of simple enjoyment of the consequences of one's action. It is, instead, a feeling of self-satisfaction that comes from the knowledge that one did not simply act under duress, or as the law or society demands, but from one's own free will and because one judged it the right thing to do. Aristotle writes that we should be educated 'both to delight in and to be pained by the things that we ought' (*N. Ethics* II. iii). It is sometimes difficult or unpleasant to act virtuously since it requires more effort, may lead to our own material disadvantage, or could disappoint social expectations. Yet at the same time we delight in acting virtuously because we have done what is noble.

In this regard one should note that Sophocles's tragedy is not merely an exposition of the irrational changes of sentiment displayed by the character of Neoptolemus. The play is essentially a lesson in morality. Neoptolemus has to choose between being an accomplice to the unscrupulous Odysseus, and standing up for justice. This choice is made difficult by the fact that the morally weak character, Odysseus, is also powerful and influential whereas Philoctetes, while morally good, completely lacks power and physical strength. Initially, Odysseus succeeds in convincing Neoptolemus to accept the selfish morality that it is acceptable to lie to and wrong another if your own 'success and safety depends on it' (*Philoctetes* l. 107). But the Neoptolemus we meet later in the play sets out to undo the wrong that he has already done, despite the fact that disobeying his superior's orders will be to his own disadvantage. He hands the bow back to its rightful owner and even prevents Philoctetes from killing Odysseus, who has now become their mutual enemy. It is clear that during the course of the play Neoptolemus does not only undergo a change of feeling, but also grows in moral knowledge and insight. It is exactly through witnessing Philoctetes's suffering and allowing himself to identify with his plight that Neoptolemus comes to understand that Philoctetes's existence would be even more desperate and miserable without his bow, which is his only means of defending himself and of procuring food.

### *Character and Action*

In response to the familiar objection that the ethics of virtue is not sufficiently concerned with action, I shall argue that the characterisation of virtue ethics as an ethics of being, rather than an ethics of doing, has been mistaken. It is only under the influence of monistic theories of morality that contemporary virtue-ethicists tend to construe virtue ethics as taking character as the primary object of moral assessment, with judgements of actions and their consequences being derivative of these character judgements.

Aristotle repeatedly emphasises the link between character and action. The appropriate motivation for acting in certain ways is the virtues. Virtue, he writes, is a 'state of character concerned with choice' (*N. Ethics* II. vi), with the choice being between different modes of action. In the *Poetics* VI he similarly emphasises the close relationship between character and action. In thinking about tragedy and its contribution to the moral life, he tries to explain why one should view the plot or action as an element of central importance. He argues that tragedy is a representation, not of men, but of action and life, of happiness and unhappiness – and happiness and unhappiness are bound up with action. In other words, the purpose of living is an end that is a kind of activity, not a quality. While it is their characters that make people what they are, it is only through their actions that they are happy or otherwise. Tragedies are not performed in order to represent character. Character is involved for the sake of the action. Character should be included in a good tragedy because it reveals personal choice, 'the kinds of thing a man chooses or rejects'. But the incidents and the plot are the end aimed at in tragedy and as always, Aristotle says, the end is everything. Virtue forms the moral purpose of the agents and thus naturally gives rise to action.

His discussion of *eudaimonia* (the good life) in the *Nicomachean Ethics* further supports the view that action is not only the natural culmination of character, but also a necessary companion of character. *Eudaimonia* requires not simply a good character but, in addition, action in accordance with character. Simply being good in the sense of feeling compassion and other virtuous sentiments is not sufficient for *eudaimonia*. The link between character and action is so close that Aristotle doubts whether a person who performs no actions at all could correctly be said to have a certain sort of character (*N. Ethics* I. xiii). He argues that a person cannot be good if he is being tortured, because such circumstances impede activity. Aristotle remarks that people who insist that such a person is still *eudaimôn*, so long as he is good, 'are, whether they mean to or not, talking nonsense' (*N. Ethics* VII. xiii). If there are certain external impediments that prevent a person from acting, such as a failure to help distant flood victims, they cannot be described as being either virtuous or vicious. The choice for moral theorists is therefore not between an act- and character-based theory. Being involves doing, and neither can be identified as the essence or focus of moral judgement.

A person cannot be truly compassionate if he does not perform compassionate actions, and cannot be truly benevolent without being beneficent. If it is in a person's power to help someone and he fails to even attempt to do so, this says something about his character: that he did not feel compassion, and that he is not benevolent. According to Aristotle, action is not only *capable* of showing character, it is also the natural expression of character and the best evidence of it (*N. Ethics* III. ii). He claims that the mere display of character without action would fail to have relevance for *eudaimonia*. For example, it would be unclear when Neoptolemus makes the transition from putting up a show of compassion to really feeling compassion, if one had to judge his character on the basis of his words and demeanour. In Aristotle's view, it is only when Neoptolemus hands the bow back to Philoctetes, when his actions match his compassionate words, that he truly shows himself as a virtuous man. This could not be said of him before, since his actions revealed something about his character, namely that he still gave priority to his own selfish interests and that he lacked the courage to disobey his master's vicious orders. Character and action therefore form an indissoluble union.

*Character and Ends: Responsible Benevolence*

A second objection to compassion as a *benevolent concern* for the welfare of others is that it is not sufficient for producing acts that are truly beneficent. The question is therefore: Can a person of good intentions be praised if his well-intended acts fail to reach their goal?

One may grant that a person does have a moral virtue if he really tries to be beneficent, whether or not he has much or any success at actually being beneficent. But to be benevolent in its full or ideal form one must not merely be sincere in one's attempts to do good. One must also have, so far as it is in one's power, the other things needed for doing what, *qua* benevolent, one wants to do. There is, in other words, a moral obligation not to make certain intellectual mistakes. Following Frankena (1987) I shall refer to benevolence in its ideal form as 'responsible benevolence', that is, benevolence that involves the exercise of certain intellectual qualities. Apart from the moral virtues such as courage, truthfulness and compassion, Aristotle also emphasises the intellectual virtues, namely *episteme*, *techne* and *phronesis*. A person of good character possesses all of these virtues, and could be held morally accountable if he failed to produce the desired ends through lack of knowledge or skills.

Of course, it is not in all cases that we would hold someone accountable for failing to benefit another because of a lack of intellectual virtues. Aristotle says that 'we punish a man for his very ignorance, *if he is thought responsible for the ignorance*, as when penalties are doubled in the case of drunkenness' (*N. Ethics* III. v, emphasis added). It is only when a person can be expected to possess certain knowledge and skills that we hold him liable. For instance, a mother who does not know how to feed her child properly is morally blameworthy, since, except in extreme cases, we can legitimately expect her to acquire such knowledge. Her not having it shows a lack of concern for her child. As Aristotle puts it, she is 'ignorant through carelessness' and thus shows a lack of benevolence.[15] Responsible benevolence requires certain skills and knowledge and, as such, has a cognitive or rational element. Apart from *feeling* concerned about another's plight and *wishing* to do well, the virtuous person should know how to benefit others.

---

[15] This was the reasoning used by the court in *R v. Burney [1958] NZLR (CA)*, in which a conviction for manslaughter was upheld when parents of a young girl failed to get medical attention for their daughter who died after suffering from malnutrition, staphylococcal bronchial pneumonia, anaemia and chronic skin sepsis. The court held that ignorance that the child needed medical attention may in itself have been negligence and that such negligence could not be invoked as a 'lawful excuse' if that lack of knowledge was 'neglectful and inexcusable'. The decision in *R v Burney* was explained in the following way in *R v. Walker [1958] NZLR 810 (CA)*: '[I]t was not necessary, in order to constitute the offence under section 151 [i.e., the duty to provide the necessaries of life], that the omission to perform the duty should be wilful or intentional, but that it was sufficient if the conduct of the accused in omitting to perform the duty showed negligence of a sufficiently high degree to incur criminal responsibility' (cited in Collins 1992:193).

According to Frankena responsible benevolence involves the following intellectual qualities: (1) having a habit of thinking clearly and logically, plus having the factual and other knowledge that is relevant to one's decisions; and (2) having at least a considerable share of the ability and skill needed to carry out those decisions, that is, to do the good one wants to (1987:3). Medical education is geared precisely towards fostering responsible benevolence. Apart from being appropriately motivated, health-care professionals are also expected to have a certain amount of medical knowledge and technical skill to be able to succeed in their attempts to benefit patients. But is this sufficient? One should note that Frankena only includes the first two intellectual virtues in his analysis of responsible benevolence, namely *episteme* and *techne*. As we have seen before, a physician may still fail to benefit a patient despite his possession of the required knowledge and skills. A crucial requirement for doing 'the good one wants to do' is not only having mastered the relevant knowledge and technical skills, but also to know what this 'good' entails. It is in this regard that the third intellectual virtue, *phronesis*, is extremely important.

*Phronesis* is the ability to deliberate well about what sort of things lead to the good life, not only for oneself, but for human beings in general (*N. Ethics* VI. v). The emphasis on *phronesis* allows us to find an answer to the question concerning the limits to be placed on medical competence. Medical competence has generally been understood in terms of the possession of scientific knowledge and technical skills. The result of this is that physicians may fail to contribute to the good of patients by a very excess of medical competence. Instrumental and scientific reason operates within a hierarchical opposition between competence and incompetence, truth and error, success and failure, so that the notion of 'excessive competence' cannot be grasped in this context. But if competence is understood not only as scientific knowledge and technical skills but also as practical reason, it becomes clear how the very success of technical procedures can fail to benefit a patient, or how medical skills can be overused, or used inappropriately. Aristotle defines virtue as the mean between two corresponding vices or extremes, the excess and the defect, and practical wisdom is the virtue that allows its possessor to determine the mean in every particular situation. There are no fixed standards, no absolute (Platonic) ideal of competence. Instead, 'the agents themselves must in each case consider what is appropriate to the occasion' (*N. Ethics* II. ii). In his attempt to follow the mean as method, a person of practical wisdom develops habits of making choices that are both relative and proportional to the time and place, the individual, the available resources, etc. In the medical field, practical wisdom is the ability to apply scientific knowledge and technical skills in a way that is appropriate to the specific situation.

Aristotle's conception of *phronesis* provides an attractive alternative to the attempt by most modern ethical theories to emulate science through trying to specify universal principles and duties that can, in each and every specific situation, be applied deductively. Unlike deontological and utilitarian theories, virtue ethics does not lay down universal rules and principles that prescribe which actions one should perform. According to some critics, it is this feature that forms the basis of its inadequacies. Louden argues that, due to the very nature of the moral virtues, there is a very limited amount of advice on moral quandaries that one can reasonably expect from the virtue-oriented approach. For him, virtue ethics is structurally unable to say much of anything about the question 'What ought I to do?' (1997:201-216)

However, it should be clear by now that a virtue-based ethical theory is not confined merely to recognising a certain set of qualities as virtues and the corresponding set of defects as vices (based on a consideration of their contribution to the realisation of the common good of the community). It also identifies certain types of action as doing or producing harm of such an order that it destroys the bonds of community. Acts such as murder, theft and perjury render the doing or achieving of good impossible in some respect, at least some of the time. In an Aristotelian society the table of virtues will teach its citizens what kinds of action will gain them merit and honour, while a table of legal offences will teach them what kinds of action are regarded not simply as bad, but as intolerable. While an ethic of virtues does lay down general rules of conduct, these rules are not seen as either absolute or universal, but as guidelines. Because *phronesis* takes the good of man as its focus, it cannot strive towards the objectivity, universality and the certainty characteristic of scientific knowledge. *Phronesis* is concerned with the particular and the changeable and thus we should not expect precision or exactness from it.

In response to the objection that 'general rules' are still not specific enough to guide action, one is tempted to follow Mill when he writes, 'there is no difficulty in proving any ethical standard whatever to work ill, if we suppose universal idiocy to be conjoined with it' (1987:296). In some sense Mill's somewhat arrogant remark is particularly appropriate. Aristotle does view a certain kind of intelligence – practical wisdom – as a condition for being a good or virtuous person. Whereas for Kant and most modern thinkers one can be both good (by having a good will) and stupid, for Aristotle stupidity of a certain kind precludes goodness.[16] General rules serve only as guidelines for those who have not yet, through experience, acquired practical wisdom. Because of the polymorphous nature of the good and bad for man, and the infinite variety of moral contexts, particular problems will always arise that are not solved by the simple application of rules. According to Aristotle, it is impossible to construct general rules that will encompass all human situations. A virtuous person has to be able to judge and do the right thing at the right time and place, and in the right way. He has to be able to act *kata ton orthon logon*, that is, 'according to right reason' (*N. Ethics* VI. i).[17] Practical wisdom involves skills of perception and insight, a situation-specific

---

[16] See Aristotle (*N. Ethics* VI. xii), as well as MacIntyre's discussion of this point (1990:154-155).

[17] I use MacIntyre's translation, which conveys more accurately Aristotle's de-emphasis of rules than Ross's translation, which reads, 'in accordance with the right rule'. See MacIntyre (1990:152-153) for a more detailed discussion of this point.

'know-how'. These skills are only developed through recognising and acting on what is relevant in concrete moral contexts as they arise.

In the medical sphere the virtue of responsible benevolence includes insight into the best interests of the particular patient, and a consideration of his circumstances, values and beliefs. It is true that Aristotle does not offer a clear strategy for dealing with cases where conflict arises between different goals or, in the case of clinical decision-making, where there are conflicting views of the patient's best interests. He seems to assume that the virtues form a perfect unity, that people within a community share the same goals, and that views conflict simply as the result of flaws in character or unintelligent political decisions. I will deal with this problem in more detail in the following chapter. At this stage I only wish to note the following. The compassionate person judges the seriousness and nature of a person's suffering primarily in terms of that person's perspective and circumstances. In the same way, benevolence involves helping the person in terms of and in consideration of his particular values, beliefs and circumstances. Thus Neoptolemus's attempt to benefit Philoctetes follows directly from his compassionate understanding of the latter's plight. He realises that if Philoctetes were to return with the soldiers, he would lose his independence, integrity and self-respect, and thus discontinues his attempts at persuading him to do so. He helps Philoctetes in the only way he can, by returning his bow.

What then, in the Aristotelian view, are the proper ends of medicine? Being the son of a practising medical man, Aristotle regularly speaks of medical knowledge with high respect and often makes use of medical illustrations and similes throughout his writings. From these it is clear that he views the actions of physicians as directed towards restoring, maintaining or improving the health of a human being. Stated as such, there is nothing remarkable in this view, and it seems simply to express the dominant view of medicine held by the Greeks and most other societies throughout the ages. It is important to notice, however, that for Aristotle the aim of physicians is not health *as such*, but health *for something*. Aristotle's main interest is with the supreme destiny of man or the good life, towards which bodily health is a means and a necessary condition.

The next question to be considered is: 'To what extent should the physician become involved in the moral life and happiness of his patient?' In an attempt to answer this question, the Rev. Joseph Owens (1977:127-142) develops an Aristotelian account of the relationship between medicine and ethics. The premises of his argument are as follows:

1. The supreme goal of ethical life (and the source of true happiness) is the life of contemplation and theoretical speculation.
2. Bodily health is an integral constituent of a complete life span in which a person can fulfil his or her destiny in the sense of realising the goal of life. In other words, a complete life span is a requirement of the human happiness that constitutes the goal of Aristotelian ethics.
3. The end of medicine is health.

From these premises Owens concludes that 'medicine comes in global fashion under the direction of ethics, and is an aid in attaining the supreme goal for which ethics strives' or, stated otherwise, 'ethics requires that the practice of medicine be directed to and subordinated to the general human good'. The point Owens is making – that medicine should have as its goal enabling individuals to live a good life by improving or maintaining their health – seems obvious, but is often forgotten in technological medicine. The good life, rather than health, is the final or ultimate goal. The physician should ask what form of treatment (if any) would best enable the individual patient to flourish. Owens further points out that the medical art is similar to the virtue of *phronesis* in its focus on the individual patient. Medicine aims not at health as such, but at the health of a particular person. Just as one would not be a better physician having contemplated, in Platonic fashion, the idea of health itself, so no philosopher who inquires into specific ethical dilemmas will profit much from contemplating the supreme and universal good. There is no universal conception of the good life, as there is no single conception of health and disease.

Again, this seems to be a fairly obvious point, but one that is often forgotten by medical scientists. The following case, discussed at a Bioethics seminar at the University of Cape Town, illustrates this well:

> Prof. Steve Louw, a prominent South African physician, researched the prevalence of Alzheimer's disease among Africans in Langa, a group whose mental and physical health has been largely neglected in the *apartheid* era. He was surprised to find, during his preliminary research, that African people do not perceive 'dementia' as a disease at all. They thought of it as a normal deviation of growing old and related it to the causal influence of ancestors. The question was whether there was any point in continuing his research in this area.

It is unclear why the question of continuing the research should arise at all if it is obvious that it would not contribute to the welfare of the subjects of the study. African families generally tend to accept mental illness more readily and cope with it more successfully than other population groups, and do not need counselling and treatment to facilitate coping with the condition. The most plausible explanation for Louw's uncertainty is that he was torn between the scientific endeavour that aims to obtain knowledge for its own sake (assembling statistics as to the prevalence of a disease within a specific community) and his goal as a medical practitioner, which is to benefit individual patients and communities.

I therefore agree with Owens that medicine is a moral enterprise, if by this he means that health is a necessary, though not sufficient, condition for a good life. But Owens has more in mind when he says that the end of medicine is directed towards the fulfilment of the human good. He argues that the end of medicine is not only health, but also the betterment of patients' moral conduct through the improvement of their moral judgement. In other words, the end of medicine is also to make people better agents, acting ideally as he or she ought to act. This view of the goal of medicine is fraught with difficulties. As Spicker (1977:150) points out, it is *hubris* of the worst kind to advocate that medical practitioners ought to attempt to affect directly their patient's conduct, moral judgement and happiness through medical intervention, moral persuasion or education. But more importantly, as a Christian moralist Owens makes the assumption that there is a single valid conception of the good life towards which the wise doctor can and should steer his patient. This assumption cannot be attributed to Aristotle, who left the content of the good life largely open. There is no golden pathway to a heaven of any kind. Each individual is to pursue the good life for him- or herself. One person cannot take responsibility for the other's moral goodness or happiness. Owens makes the mistake of concluding from premises 2 (that health is a necessary condition for happiness) and 3 (that the end of medicine is health) that the physician should also assume direct responsibility for the happiness or moral goodness of the patient. He is led to this conclusion by the following argument: For Aristotle, man is a composite of body and soul. This composite is an essentially changeable nature, changeable through both moral persuasion and physiological alteration. And since body and soul cannot be separated, the task of the physician includes both physiological alteration and moral persuasion.

By restoring, maintaining or optimising health (i.e., by removing factors that may hinder patients from acting and choosing freely), physicians certainly play a role in making it possible for their patients to participate in the moral life. Aristotle says that 'no activity is perfect when it is impeded, and happiness is a perfect thing; this is why the happy man needs the goods of the body and external goods, i.e. those of fortune, viz. in order that he may not be impeded in these ways' (*N. Ethics* VII. xiii). Patients may unknowingly participate in behaviour that may negatively affect their health, and here physicians and other health-care workers have the duty to inform them of the relevant medical facts. But this is very different from the more specific point Owens also makes, that physicians should persuade patients to act morally, to 'follow their better moral judgement' (1977:137). A simple example can be used to illustrate this difference. A doctor becomes aware that his patient is participating in potentially dangerous sexual activities. Clearly, the appropriate response would not be appropriate for the physician to lecture his patient about the virtues of monogamy and the sinfulness of promiscuity, as Owens would have it. The duty of the physician is simply to inform the patient of means of protection against disease or unwanted pregnancy and so to prevent her ideals from being thwarted. The general goodness and happiness of the patient ought not and cannot be the object of the physician. It can only be the particular enterprise of the person herself.

### *The Good of the Benefactor: Beyond Egoism and Altruism*

In the previous chapter I argued that the Christian ideal of selflessness falls prone to the Nietzschean objection that pity is a form of self-denial and hence conflicts with virtues such as courage, pride and self-respect. In the same way benevolence, if conceived as a concern for the good of the other which necessitates a total disregard for one's own interests, cannot be called a virtue in the Aristotelian sense.

Western society tends to regard selflessness as a virtue that stands opposed to the vice of selfishness. However, if one applies Aristotle's doctrine of the mean, benevolence would be a mean with respect to (1) an exclusive concern for one's own well-being, and (2) an exclusive concern for the good of others. The Aristotelian would therefore regard both selfishness and selflessness as vices. Following the dominant Christian tradition, Wallace rejects this conclusion. He considers examples of cases where the benefactor helps others to his own disadvantage, and argues that an excessive concern for the good of others – and a consequent neglect of one's own interests – cannot be considered a vice. The conditions of benevolence are (1) a direct concern for the good of others, (2) giving up something that one has some reason to value and thus to keep, and (3) giving more than one is generally expected to give. When someone gives away so much of his time, energy and possessions that he is unable to meet his own needs and responsibilities, we would still consider him virtuous, since his behaviour has the most important characteristics and consequences of benevolence and serves to affirm the value of persons. We would call such generosity *excessive benevolence*, he argues, rather than a vice that is the opposite of the virtues that are forms of benevolence. This excess does not thwart the functions of benevolence, and thus benevolence is not, in Aristotle's sense, a mean between too much and too little concern for others. Wallace is suggesting that one can never be too generous. Indeed, he defines 'primary benevolence' as a direct concern for the good of others, while he uses the term 'secondary benevolence' to refer to cases where one's primary motive is to be a good person. This motive, he says, makes one's actions egoistic in the final instance (1978:139-158).

Accounts of benevolence that hold complete selflessness forward as the ideal have been widely criticised as being unrealistic and demanding more than what is humanly possible (see Kekes 1987:21-36). Indeed, popular opinion holds that we cannot oblige people to sacrifice themselves, to make martyrs out of themselves. People who do sacrifice themselves for others are, nevertheless, praised as performing supererogatory acts. However, I believe that such selflessness is not only an unrealistic and overly demanding ideal, but that it is not praiseworthy. This view can be supported with reference to Aristotle's discussion of the question of whether a man should love himself or others most (*N. Ethics* IX. viii). Aristotle notices that people criticise those who love themselves most, since they do everything for their own benefit. By contrast, those who sacrifice their own interests for the sake of another are considered good. As is currently the case, the popular view in Greek society seems to have been that altruism necessarily requires selflessness, while self-love necessarily entails greed or selfishness. Against this Aristotle argues that one should distinguish between a lover-of-self who assigns to himself a greater share of wealth, honours and bodily pleasures at the expense of others (selfishness), and the lover-of-self who is anxious always to act justly, temperately and virtuously with the aim of securing for himself 'the honourable course' (self-interest). While he condemns the first form of self-love, he argues that the person who is concerned with his own goodness or virtue is actually a greater lover of self than the selfish person, since he assigns to himself the things that are noblest and best. Such love of self is therefore more appropriately described as self-regard, self-respect or proper pride.

Ideal benevolence does not and should not require selflessness. Benevolence is not only directed towards the good of others, but also forms a necessary part of one's own good or happiness. Virtue cannot be divorced from self-interest. Our legitimate concern with ourselves includes a concern with the honour, respect and gratitude one can expect in return for one's virtuousness. It also includes a concern with one's own material welfare and needs. To help others to such an extent that one is unable to meet one's own needs and obligations, while undeniably a form of benevolence or generosity, does not constitute *responsible* benevolence. Such extreme generosity is due to errors in judgement or a failure to consider one's own future needs and responsibilities towards others. Unless one believes in a heavenly reward, making a martyr of oneself reveals a lack of self-respect.

Aristotle provides a detailed account of the virtue of liberality in administering one's wealth and possessions. The liberal person refrains from giving to anybody and everybody, so that he may have something to give to the right people, at the right time, and where it is done for a worthy cause. But the liberal person will also accept generosity from others, when it is appropriate. Being too generous with one's possessions is a vice (prodigality or extravagance), since it prevents one from fulfilling one's responsibilities towards others and towards oneself. Prodigality, he says, 'exceeds in giving and not in taking, and falls short in taking' (*N. Ethics* IV. i). When Aristotle writes that the good man 'is related to his friend as to himself (for his friend is another self)' (*N. Ethics* IX. iv), he does not mean, as Wallace suggests, that the good man should *substitute* his friend's interests for his own, or that he should be concerned more with the friend's happiness than with his own. Instead, for Aristotle 'the good man should be a lover of self (for he will both himself profit by doing noble acts, and will benefit his fellows)' (*N. Ethics* IX. viii). Hence in true Aristotelian spirit Jane Addams, a pioneer in modern social work and the first woman to receive the Nobel Peace Prize, said that one of the things that motivated her to become involved in community service was that it helped unfold her interests and capacities so as to create a richer self through relationships within a community (Martin 1994:317-319). Self-interest and altruism therefore combine in ways that are mutually supporting, rather than mutually exclusive.

## Conclusion

Medical practice has tended to view understanding and helping the patient as two separate activities, while at the same time holding a very restricted view of what it is to understand and benefit a patient. As far as *understanding* a patient's condition is concerned, medical practice has focused largely on gaining scientific knowledge about the patient's disease through the use of diagnostic equipment. In the sphere of *helping* the patient, a similar focus on purely rational and scientific means of treatment is found. The choice between various modes of treatment is made through a calculation of utility, by weighing and balancing *medical* risks, benefits and harms.

The paternalistic physician accepts as his primary responsibility or obligation the principle of beneficence. This duty serves as motivation to benefit patients, which he is able to do because of his medical expertise. The weakness of this position is the assumption that medical values are the only values that are relevant in deciding on a course of treatment, that they possess an absolute quality which overrides other (non-medical) values, and that in assessing the relative weight of medical harms and benefits the physician is in a better position to make the final choice. The patient's hierarchy of goods does not always coincide with that of the physician. In assuming that it does or that it should, the paternalist not only disregards or injures the dignity of the individual by rejecting her perspective, he may also be guilty of harming his patient.

The focus on technological means of diagnosis and treatment, together with the use of universal rules of beneficence and non-maleficence, has resulted in a neglect of compassion as a means of both understanding and alleviating the individual patient's suffering brought about by illness. For the compassionate person, helping a patient forms part of understanding his suffering. In response to the objection that the virtues, due to their emotional component, often prevent us from acting beneficently, I have argued that apart from its role in understanding suffering and conveying respect to the sufferer, compassion plays an important role not only in *motivating* us but also in *enabling* us to benefit others. Whereas the affective and altruistic dimension of compassion serves to motivate the onlooker to benefit the sufferer, the understanding gained through the empathetic identification with the sufferer allows the onlooker to truly benefit him. Compassionate benevolence, in its ideal form, is more intimately linked to beneficence than is usually granted.

While scientific knowledge and modern technology do form significant parts of understanding and helping a patient, the intellectual virtues of *episteme* and *techne* need to be accompanied by the virtue of *phronesis*, which pertains to the valued goals or *telos* one attempts to achieve through one's actions. It is through a lack of this virtue that the physician, despite his possession of medical knowledge and technical skills, may fail to benefit a patient. This failure is, I have argued, due to an undue emphasis on a scientific explanation of a patient's physical condition and the consequent attempt to benefit a patient in terms of purely medical values.

Aristotle's failure to recognise the close relationship between compassion and benevolence in tragedy therefore cannot be attributed to any internal inconsistency that would prohibit a compassionate person from acting benevolently, or from knowing what the right action would be. The passivity of the chorus in Sophocles's tragedy can be attributed simply to the contingent fact that there was little man could do in ancient times to reverse the bad fortune inflicted on him by the gods. Where such reversals did occasionally occur they could only be attributed to divine, rather than human, intervention. Hence the popularity of the *deus ex machina* as a strategy for allaying the tension in Greek tragedies: It is an admission of man's powerlessness to change the good or bad fortune bestowed upon him by the gods. In most cases, the best person could do was simply to *be* friendly, honest, faithful, wise, etc. Advances in the areas of knowledge and technology have, however, allowed us to influence or change the course of nature, making it possible for contemporary virtue-ethicists to explore the link between compassion and beneficence, or character and action. The lack of power of Neoptolemus and the chorus is merely a contingent fact and in no way stems from their compassion for Philoctetes.

In Chapter Five I re-examine the principle of patient autonomy, its philosophical roots and its shortcomings. I also develop an account of respectfulness as a virtue that enables one to act in ways that would contribute to the good of the patient.

# Chapter Five

# Autonomy and Respect

## Introduction

We are told that Philoctetes was banished to the island of Lemnos because his incurable wound aroused so much revulsion among his comrades and his tortured cries desecrated the silence in the camp. Then, ten years later, the leaders of the expedition return to the island in search of Philoctetes. They have learned that they cannot win the war without him and his magic bow. Knowing that Philoctetes would not willingly surrender the bow or return with those who have done him a great injustice, they plan to trick him into returning with them.

A contemporary moralist would say that the injustice done to Philoctetes involves a disrespect of his autonomy, of his right to know the truth and to determine his own future. The notions of individual freedom and autonomy have become so deeply ingrained in modern thought that few people ever ask the more fundamental question: 'Why is it wrong to violate someone's right to autonomy?' Why is it immoral to use lies and deception to convince Philoctetes to leave behind the desolate island and his subhuman existence?

Along utilitarian lines one may argue that by deceiving Philoctetes the soldiers take advantage of his vulnerability. Although they promise him that he can expect a good outcome if he returns with them, they do not really have his best interest at heart. They do not offer him the opportunity to make a free and informed decision about matters that will significantly impact upon his future well-being. Even if the soldiers were well-intentioned, their lack of respect for his wishes would still be immoral since they have no way of knowing what the true needs and interests of Philoctetes are. There is no single or universal conception of pleasure or happiness, pain or suffering. Disregarding the autonomous wishes of a mature person is wrong because it usually leads to undesirable consequences for that person. Respecting individual liberty is among the most important means of securing happiness.

Alternatively, one may take the Kantian or deontological view that lying, deception and appeals to emotion are forms of disrespecting Philoctetes's autonomy, and wrong simply by virtue of this. The consequences that would follow from such actions are irrelevant for deciding the morality of these acts. It is not altogether clear whether Philoctetes will benefit most from returning with the soldiers or from remaining on the island, yet it is clear that the soldiers' behaviour is both insulting and disrespectful. Philoctetes's decision to remain on the island without his bow should be respected regardless of the consequences. To respect someone's autonomy is to respect his dignity as a person, to acknowledge that he is a rational creature with ends of his own.

Roughly speaking, these two positions form the basis of the arguments used to justify the centrality of individual freedom and autonomy. In contemporary Western medicine, the concern with self-sufficiency takes the form of the principle of respect for patient autonomy. In this chapter I examine the philosophical roots of this principle in an attempt to discover the nature and origin of the difficulties experienced when applying it in medical practice. In what follows I discuss the third feature typical of human suffering, namely the loss of self-respect as a result of one's physical weakness and dependence on others. This will enable us to determine whether the recognition of patient autonomy is an appropriate response to suffering.

## The Third Feature of Suffering: The Disrespected Patient

It is commonly understood that self-respect involves recognising and valuing oneself as a being with dignity. The dominant Western conception of personhood grounds dignity in three things: equality, agency and individuality.

1. *Equality.* Although various accounts have been given in support of the notion of equality, the dominant tendency in Western philosophy has been, in one way or another, to ground the equality of all persons in rationality. In this view, what distinguishes human beings from other animals (as 'lower beings') is their capacity for rational decision-making. Arguing from within the Christian tradition, Kass makes the point that 'human life is to be respected more than animal life, because man is more than an animal; man is said to be God-like... [since] he shares in reason, freedom, judgement, and moral concern' (1990:37). He attributes the patient's loss of self-respect to the assault on rational capacities. Illness tends precisely to underline the patient's ignorance or lack of medical knowledge and further to impair his powers of rational moral deliberation.
2. *Agency.* Self-respect involves a proper appreciation of ourselves as responsible agents, but illness prohibits us from acting out our responsibilities towards ourselves as well as others, forcing us instead to recline into a degrading state of passivity and dependency. Hence Kass (1990:39) remarks: '[B]eing a patient rather than an agent is, humanly speaking, undignified.'
3. *Individuality.* Finally, illness undermines individuality. This includes striving to live according to a conception of life that gives expression to one's ideals and commitments, and is expressed in the pursuits and the projects that define and befit one as the particular person one is. The disappointment of personal standards and expectations held by any self-respecting person is thus

often regarded as a degrading form of self-betrayal and accompanied by a sense of shame.

Both Ivan Ilyich and Philoctetes are reduced to an ignoble state, unable to further their own goals or to act independently, losing their self-respect and even expecting others to despise them too. Ivan Ilyich suffers immense embarrassment and shame at his needing assistance in his 'evacuations'. We are told that 'this was a continual misery to him: misery from the uncleanliness, the unseemliness and the smell, and from knowing that another person had to assist him' (Tolstoy 1960:140). Philoctetes has the same apologetic attitude; he seems to expect others to be disgusted by his physical state. He refers to his condition as causing an 'intolerable offence'. When he reawakens from a pain-induced stupor, he is surprised to find Neoptolemus still by his side. He says: 'You are a true nobleman to endure it all so bravely, the cries, the foulness, which I have afflicted you with' (*Philoctetes* ll. 866-867).

In what follows I discuss the Platonic and Nietzschean view that the only way in which a sufferer can regain or maintain his self-respect is by bearing hardship on his own. Underlying this view is the belief that the benevolence of others merely accentuates or affirms the undignified and disrespectful state of the sufferer, and that he can only overcome suffering through recognising and affirming his self-sufficiency and independence as an autonomous being.

## The Self-Sufficient Sufferer

One of Plato's objections to compassion or pity, we have seen, is that it is an irrational sentiment. Against this I have argued that compassion is based on a number of beliefs or judgements (that the other's suffering is serious, rather than trivial; that it is undeserved and therefore cannot be seen as just punishment for wrongs committed; and that the suffering is due to our shared vulnerability to misfortune). With this, we have answered the Platonic objection that the emotion of compassion is inappropriate and irrational since it is based on false beliefs. But Plato's argument against compassion pertains not only to the irrationality of compassion as a response to tragedy, but also to the view that benevolence undermines the person's self-sufficiency. Compassion and benevolence make the sufferer less able to achieve a self-sufficient demeanour, and suffering itself is a weakness that reveals the unwarranted importance that the sufferer attaches to external goods in leading a good life. His dependence on material goods and other persons shows that he lacks self-sufficiency. In short, the Platonic objection to the virtues of compassion and benevolence is that concern for the other's welfare and attempts to benefit him insinuate that he lacks the ability to attain his goals without help. Hence Plato's Socrates says that 'a good man is pre-eminently capable of providing himself with a good life entirely from his own resources, and is absolutely the last person to need anyone' (*Republic* 387d). From this perspective Philoctetes displays heroic qualities when he survives on his own on the island for ten years. He loses his dignity when, upon arrival of the soldiers, he appeals to their pity and accepts their help. The appropriate response to tragedy is not compassion, but disgust at the sufferer's pathetic display of weakness and lack of self-command.

Nietzsche supports a similar view when he objects that compassion and benevolence reduce the sufferer's worth by implying that she lacks the self-sufficiency to further her own interests. Pity denigrates the sufferer's worth by insinuating that she is not self-sufficient. Nietzsche views the appeal for pity as a pathetic attempt by the weak to regain some sense of power and importance by inflicting pain on others (1986:38-39). Despite his renunciation of the Stoic attitude toward pain and his affirmation of the positive value of suffering, Nietzsche shares with the Stoics an admiration for the person who overcomes suffering on his own. The heroic person opposes those who 'flee into the conscience of the others and into the lovely temple of the religion of pity', who find their own way 'too hard and demanding and too remote from the love and gratitude of others' (Nietzsche 1974:269-270). Nietzsche's hero sees suffering as an opportunity for self-development.

Nietzsche's position on the value of maintaining one's self-sufficiency and independence, even in the face of extreme pain and suffering, has been widely criticised. For instance, Buytendijk grants that this doctrine of heroism was an honourable attempt to free European civilisation from a vulgar naturalism, a culture in which enjoyment and leisure were the only ideals sought after. Yet he warns that the ethical results of this attitude were disastrous, resulting in the 'cold climate of pessimism and pride' in which 'love and simplicity... wither away' (1961:149-150). Others have argued, and rightfully so, that the Nietzschean attempt to overcome suffering by heroic courage may not only serve to increase the patient's isolation and sense of abandonment, but can also lead to greater harm to the physical organism. The refusal to share one's suffering or to accept the help of others is not always a sign of courage, but of obstinate pride. As Ambrose Bierce puts it: 'If courage is manifest in endurance of profitless discomfort it is cowardice to warm oneself when cold, to cure oneself when ill, to drive away mosquitoes, to go in when it rains' (1993:234).

This attitude toward suffering is not restricted to eccentric philosophers. In liberal societies admission of dependency is often seen as a sign of inadequacy and as grounds for disrespect. In his discussion of the 'politics of pain' Sternbach describes chronic-pain patients as 'petitioners for aid', and suggests that they use their suffering to get attention from others. He cites the following statement, made by a patient suffering from benign chronic pain:

> When I was first hurt I used to get a lot of sympathy and pity from the nurses and volunteers in the hospital. I used to eat it up, and really enjoyed feeling sorry for myself. Then I got tired of the whole thing. I figured it wasn't getting me anywhere, so I got out of the hospital and took a job and started going to school at night (Sternbach 1974:11).

This portrait of a patient reinforces the association of dependence with weakness, inadequacy, pity and disrespect. A courageous patient would bear pain with dignity and would overcome suffering by regaining self-control and independence. Liberal culture equates independence and self-sufficiency with being worthy of the respect of others and oneself, while dependence goes hand in hand with pity and disrespect. Problems related to power, dependency and respect are found in numerous forms in contemporary medical practice. Skevington for instance found that patients tend to assume a subordinate position within the power structure when they enter the health-care system to seek help for the relief of their symptoms. This makes them vulnerable to exploitation – one person's ignorance is the other person's power. The presence of pain and the uncertainty that often accompanies terminal or chronic illness accentuates any existing power differential. Studies of help-seeking show that people are more likely to ask for help when they expect to have an opportunity to return it in a reciprocal relationship. When deciding whether to seek support people often take into account not only their own costs and rewards but also those of their potential helper. In studies where helpers' tasks required a high level of involvement it has been found that less help was sought, due to the perceived imbalance in the social relationship. This behaviour has been partly explained by the results of laboratory studies, in which people who asked for more help reported feeling less comfortable about asking and believed that their helper would view them as less competent as a consequence (Skevington 1995:189-191).

Few people voluntarily take the solitary and 'heroic' road by proudly and courageously attempting to endure or overcome illness through the use of reason and will-power alone. People typically acknowledge their dependence on medical professionals and other caregivers to overcome illness. Yet maintaining their dignity and self-respect seems to require that they accept the help of others *only on their own terms,* in this sense still 'taking one's own way', as Nietzsche proclaimed, and remaining an agent rather than merely a patient, as Kass would have it. The recognition of the principle of respect for patient autonomy is an attempt to restore some form or degree of self-respect by allowing the patient to have a decisive share in decisions about medical treatments. It is usually argued that, although the typical patient may be restricted from *acting* autonomously by virtue of illness or injury and may thus depend upon others for fulfilling some of his needs, this is no reason to disrespect his autonomy of *thought* and *will.* In this way, it is hoped, the patient can maintain his self-respect and the respect of others, despite his dependence upon them.

## The Principle of Autonomy in Medical Ethics

In textbooks on medical ethics the principle of patient autonomy is asserted and defended using a mixture of deontological and utilitarian arguments, without always recognising the vast differences between these positions. For example, after briefly discussing Kant's and Mill's arguments, Beauchamp and Childress maintain that 'these two profoundly different philosophies both provide support for the principle of respect for autonomy' (1994:125). Brazier (1991:40-43) combines Kantian and utilitarian reasons in support of obtaining informed consent:

1. to safeguard the patient's autonomy;
2. to manifest respect for persons;
3. to enhance the quality of care; and
4. to prevent abuses in medical practice and research.

The first two reasons concern respect for autonomy as an end in itself, while the second two concern the consequences of obtaining informed consent. Although it is usually possible to realise both of these ideals, conflicts may arise in which the question of why one needs to respect patient autonomy is extremely important. This failure to recognise that Kantian and consequentialist theories provide two vastly different conceptions and justifications for respecting individual autonomy lies at the basis of the difficulties experienced in reaching consensus on the application of the principles of autonomy and beneficence in medical practice. We can only begin to overcome these difficulties by clearly distinguishing these positions.

*Kantian Autonomy*

The Kantian does not justify the duty to respect patient autonomy with reference to the consequences for the individual or society. By respecting a patient's autonomy, by not treating someone as a means to an end, one acknowledges his or her dignity as a person. The recognition of patient autonomy constitutes a rejection of the view that patients are passive recipients or objects that undergo some action. It is an attempt to restore their sense of self-respect as rational and independent beings who have their own values and goals.

Kant provides a detailed analysis and justification for the principle of autonomy in the second section of his *Fundamental Principles of the Metaphysic of Morals,* where he claims to provide a metaphysical basis for the principle of universalisability. The second formulation of the Categorical Imperative highlights the idea that morality requires respect for persons as autonomous beings: '*So act as to treat humanity, whether in thine own person or in that of any other, in every case as an end withal, never as a means only*' (1988:58, emphasis in original). The dignity of human beings lies in their autonomy, in their capacity to be self-determining beings. Unlike animals, plants and objects, human beings are capable of deciding and acting autonomously, by which he understands that they are not determined by external causes but have a will of their own. If, as a rational being I believe that others should respect my autonomy, it follows from the principle of universalisability that I should also respect theirs. In other words, since one necessarily regards oneself as a rational being, as an end rather than merely a means, consistency requires that one accept that everyone else is justified in regarding themselves as rational beings who, because they are free, rational and autonomous agents, have ends of their own. If I am to act consistently, impartially and rationally, I should not treat human beings as mere means to my own ends.

Kant next invokes the idea of the will of every rational being as a universally legislative will, an idea which he also expresses in terms of the notion of 'autonomy of will' and opposes to the notion of 'heteronomy'. One is acting autonomously if one does so purely from duty, in other words, if one can will that one's action become a universal maxim. Whenever the will does not make its own law, it determines its actions from a heteronomous principle; if the will does not act from duty, then it must act from inclination or self-interest. One's dignity as an autonomous, rational being depends on one's irrational or emotional side obeying the universal law discerned through one's reason.[1]

What sense, then, can the Kantian make of the generally-accepted view that we have an obligation to help others? Kant illustrates the Categorical Imperative by applying it to the question of whether we have a duty to help people who are in distress. He describes a man who is flourishing yet contemplates giving nothing to charity, and asks whether we can universalise the maxim 'Whenever anyone is flourishing and others are in distress, he will give nothing to charity'. Kant argues that all men have a natural end in their own happiness. He admits that human life would continue even if no one contributed anything to the happiness of others, as long as they did not intentionally harm anyone, so that the above maxim could be a law of nature. But he does not believe that an agent can consistently will that maxim to become a universal law. He argues that a situation might arise in which the agent needed the love and sympathy of others. By a law arising from his own will, however, he would have robbed himself of all hope of their help. In other words, he will find himself in the contradictory situation where he both desires the help of others but has already willed that no one should give charitable aid to others. Therefore, he cannot consistently will that the maxim become a universal law.[2]

A number of critics have found Kant's reasoning to be defective, arguing that there is no logical inconsistency in universalising the maxim. I will not repeat this criticism here, but instead will explore a different problem regarding the obligation to benefit others. Kant maintains that treating people as beings who have ends requires that the agent be motivated by other people's ends as if they were his own.

---

1 Kant believes that the moral law cannot be defined by its content. Duties do not derive their moral force from the benefits or disadvantages that would follow from a certain action or policy. Their moral force derives instead from their universalisability, which is a purely formal principle. The principle of universalisability describes the form that moral obligation must take. Substantial moral rules can be worked out by asking in the case of any particular action 'What is the maxim I am following here?' and 'Can this maxim be universalised?'

2 His argument in a later section is equally unclear: '[T]his would only harmonize negatively not positively with *humanity as an end in itself*, if everyone does not also endeavour, as far as in him lies, to forward the end of others. For the ends of any subject which is an end in himself, ought as far as possible to be *my* ends also, if that conception is to have its *full* effect with me' (1988:59, emphasis in original).

This involves a concern for their interests, helping them to promote their happiness and to prevent their suffering. But how are we to determine what the interests of others are? In his *Metaphysical Principles of Virtue* Kant gives this reply:

> I can benefit no one (with the exception of minors and the mentally deranged) according to my own concept of happiness, but only according to the concepts of him whom I think of benefiting; I actually do not benefit him when I urge a gift (1964:118-119).

This passage raises various questions. Firstly, one may ask: 'What if the other's conception of happiness (or his view of what will benefit him) is so mistaken that acting according to his will would surely do him more harm than good?' Kant explicitly rejects paternalistic actions, saying that benefiting someone according to your own conception of happiness is to deprive that person of his freedom (1964:118). The principle of autonomy, or the duty to respect the dignity of a person, receives priority over the consequences for the individual concerned. But how are we to relate this to the view that paternalistic acts actually *do not benefit people* (as Kant claims in the passage quoted above)?

Kant's answer to this question would again be that the notion of treating others as ends (benefiting them in terms of their conception of happiness) is not justified with reference to the actual consequences. The requirement to respect people stems from something much more fundamental, an attitude not just towards their interests, but towards the *persons* themselves, 'not on account of any other practical motive or any future advantage, but from the idea of the *dignity* of a rational being' (1988:63, emphasis in original). In the kingdom of ends, Kant explains, everything has either value or dignity. Whatever has value is replaceable, whereas whatever is above all value, and therefore cannot be replaced, has dignity. As possessors of dignity, persons are the proper objects of the attitude of respect. To attempt to convince someone to perform according to certain principles or duties would be to disrespect him as a rational being. Kant argues that actions that have intrinsic worth are secure in the disposition of mind. For this reason,

> [they] need no recommendation from any subjective taste or sentiment, that they may be looked at with immediate favor and satisfaction... and nothing but reason can *impose* them on the will; not to *flatter* it into them, which, in the case of duties, would be a contradiction' (1988:64, emphasis in original).

The difficulties with Kant's position appear when we attempt to apply his reasoning to the following case: John discovers that his friend Nick is severely depressed and is contemplating suicide. Does John have an obligation to try to prevent Nick from committing suicide? And how should he go about doing so? One alternative for John would be to respect Nick's dignity as a person by providing him with a rational argument against suicide. He could point out, for instance, that by committing suicide Nick would be violating a perfect or absolute duty towards himself. Nick cannot consistently will that the maxim 'whenever continuing to live will bring anyone more pain than pleasure, he will commit suicide out of self-love' becomes a universal law of nature. But what if John's attempt at rational persuasion fails, as it almost certainly would? It seems to follow from Kant's argument that by appealing to Nick's emotions or, failing that, by forcefully restraining him, one would treat Nick with disrespect. If John succeeded in preventing Nick from suicide, Nick's maintaining his own life would be a case of acting in *conformity* with what duty prescribes, but not acting *from* duty or for the sake of duty alone. One cannot force upon someone the will to act from duty (see Kant 1988:33).

One might want to reply that, because the decision to commit suicide is not universalisable and hence not rational, Nick is clearly not an autonomous person. John need not respect his autonomy and would therefore be justified in forcefully interfering with Nick's plan to jump off the bridge. This raises the question as to *who* these persons are whose autonomy we should respect – all human beings, or only the rational ones among them? According to one interpretation of Kant's position, all human beings are to be respected as persons. In the *Fundamental Principles of the Metaphysic of Morals* he refers to the subjects of morality as 'persons', as 'rational beings' and as 'humanity'. It would seem that he believes that all human beings, regardless of their individual capacities, ought to have the same moral protection. Non-rational or 'heteronomous' beings – those we need not respect – would include all non-humans. The controlling idea seems to be that human *nature* is rational, and the extent to which one deserves to be regarded and respected as an end in itself is determined by the norm for the species, regardless of one's individual characteristics. According to this interpretation, it would be wrong to convince the suicidal person not to take his life by means other than rational argumentation, despite that person's lack of autonomy, since he is worthy of respect by virtue of being a member of the human race.

This interpretation does not fit well with the passage (cited above) from *Metaphysical Principles of Virtue* in which Kant excludes 'minors' and the 'mentally deranged' from those who have to be benefited according to their own conception of happiness. Why does he allow for paternalism in these cases? It would be inconsistent with Kant's argument to say that one would be justified not to act according to their conception of happiness in order *to protect them from harm.*[3] Neither could it be that these people *do not have a conception of happiness* or cannot convey it to others, since even a baby can convey to its mother that it would be happier if fed or cleaned. The only remaining alternative

[3] One might want to interpret Kant as saying that the principle of autonomy is (at least partly) designed to supplement the principle of benevolence insofar as it provides an answer to the question 'What does is mean to *benefit* someone?' But while the view that one should respect someone's views and perspectives *so that* one may be able to benefit him seems an attractive one, it is an incorrect interpretation of Kant's ethic. Kant repeatedly emphasises that the principle of autonomy is not to be justified on consequentialist bases.

seems to be that they are excluded *because they are not rational beings* or have no *rational* conception of happiness. Thus a second interpretation of Kant's position on the appropriate subject of respect would hold that one is justified in forcefully interfering in the suicidal person's plans, since he is not a rational being and hence is not worthy of respectful treatment.

A third interpretation of Kant's position is even more extreme with regard to the respect owed to irrational people. In a set of notes written in 1764, Kant confessed that he despised the ignorant masses at one time, but that Rousseau taught him to honour men, to recognise their worth, and to establish the rights of humanity (see Acton 1970:42). Yet by basing the rights of humanity and human dignity on rationality, Kant again finds it difficult to respect irrational people. At times he hardly seems able to hide his contempt for people whose conceptions of happiness do not meet his standards of rationality. He argues that it is one's *inclination* to strive after happiness, *reason* that allows one to determine whether a person (including oneself) is worthy of happiness, and sense of *duty* that forms the universal and sole condition of one's worthiness to be happy. He then says that a sluggard who desires soft pillows to while away his life in sweet idleness, and the drunkard who desires wine and other intoxicating spirits, *are not worthy of happiness*. It follows that one is not obliged to make these people happy if it is in one's power, not because wine would hardly contribute to the drunkard's well-being, but because people like him are not worthy of happiness (1964:148-150). According to this line of reasoning, the suicidal person is irrational and oblivious to duty, and hence not worthy of happiness or our concern.

Whereas the first interpretation of Kant's position on the treatment of irrational people sacrifices beneficence for respect, and the second allows for benevolence at the cost of respect, the third requires neither respect nor benevolence as a moral obligation. These are only some of the difficulties experienced when trying to apply Kant's abstract and universal principles to everyday situations where we encounter people with different conceptions of happiness and different levels of autonomy. In what follows, I discuss the shortcomings of the Kantian justification of the principle of respect for patient autonomy in the context of modern medical practice.

One of the most prominent supporters of the Kantian view that patient autonomy is the primary duty of a physician is Ranaan Gillon in his *Philosophical Medical Ethics* (1995). He argues that an ethic that confines itself to the promotion of ends inclines toward paternalism, since it requires one to promote the happiness and prevent the suffering of others even at the cost of imposing on them, if necessary, the means of their happiness. In the Kantian ethic the basic requirement is respect for the other person's pursuit of her own ends through her own free action, and one is required to help in the promotion of those ends only in ways that are compatible with that basic respect. By complying with the wishes of the patient the caregiver conveys respect, regardless of the consequences for the patient.

Gillon defines autonomy as the capacity to think, decide, and act (on the basis of such thought and decision) freely, independently and without let or hindrance.

He does recognise that the autonomous person does not exist in reality and that disease and disability tend to impair people's autonomy. Since autonomy is a matter of degree, and is never found in an absolute state, the question arises as to how much autonomy is 'sufficient' for a person to be respected as an autonomous agent. In response to this question Gillon warns against using a stricter criterion for competency than those set democratically, for example, in permitting a person to vote, to consent to sexual intercourse, or to get married. In contexts such as these we should make a *prima facie* assumption in favour of autonomy. The mere presence of intrinsic pressures such as stress, neurosis, and grief, although they may diminish a person's autonomy, do not justify overriding what is left. Among the cases where respect for autonomy is not the answer, Gillon mentions children, patients whose autonomy of thought is severely impaired by delusions or hallucinations, and patients whose volitional autonomy is grossly impaired by intrinsic or extrinsic factors. Following Kant, Gillon does allow certain exceptions to the duty to respect the wishes of the patient. These exceptions are not justified by the consequences that would follow if one were to respect the wishes of children and mentally-disabled people. Instead, overriding a person's wishes is justified if (and because) that person is not, in his present state, a sufficiently autonomous or rational being.

The first shortcoming of holding forward respect for autonomy as the ideal is that in accepting a *prima facie* assumption in favour of autonomy one is likely to overlook the extent to which the patient may be vulnerable and dependent. By focusing one's efforts on respecting the autonomous 'parts' of an individual, as Gillon seems to suggest, one does not pay sufficient attention to the fact that a patient's judgement may be significantly impaired and that she may need the assistance of others in making a decision. Thus Campbell points out that the converse to saying that autonomy is always a matter of degree (i.e., that there is no time *t* when individual *x* is wholly autonomous), is that in *every* situation the individual will have *some* dependence on others (1991:103). An obvious result of focusing on autonomy in abstraction from dependency is that it will often amount to a failure to benefit 'autonomous' patients who refuse treatment by virtue of fear, ignorance or the like, and not because the proposed treatment conflicts with their moral or religious beliefs.

To overcome the conflict between the principles of beneficence and autonomy Lasagna suggests that 'people ought to be allowed to make the wrong decision if they so desire' (1977:45). The problem with this view is that people simply do not desire to make wrong decisions. Their decisions may not conform to the physician's views, and might for this reason be seen as 'wrong' by the physician. But people generally want to make a decision that is in their best interest and accords with their moral views and religious beliefs. Simply being informed of the relevant facts may not be sufficient to enable them to make this decision. Thus the physician who relies solely on the consent of the patient before commencing with treatment would often fail to act according to the values and beliefs of a patient, by not realising or by ignoring the extent of the particular patient's dependency and her vulnerability to human weaknesses such as fear, trauma, and ignorance.

A second shortcoming becomes apparent when one considers that the implication of the priority given to the principle of patient autonomy is that patients who refuse to give consent for potentially beneficent treatment can only be medically benefited at the cost of either overriding their expressed wishes – which puts the physician in danger of litigation – or having them legally declared incompetent. According to Gillon the most plausible justification for overriding a patient's decisions is that 'such patients do not have sufficient autonomy of thought for their self-damaging decisions to require the respect due to autonomous agents' (1995:121). For instance, in the case of Ms. Anderson (cited in the previous chapter), her refusal to consider the necessity of amputation was used to base the court's opinion that she was incompetent to make a rational decision as to the amputation of her feet. This was despite the fact that she was described as 'an intelligent, lucid, communicative and articulate individual'. Being declared incompetent by a court is not, I believe, to be very respectful to an 'intelligent, lucid' individual, a finding that is nevertheless necessitated by the very approach that emphasises the individual's right to respect. The physician who adheres strongly to the principle of patient autonomy would only be able to act against or without the patient's consent (in an attempt to benefit that patient) at the cost of having him/her legally declared incompetent. Furthermore, if one considers that the court order will allow medical professionals to use physical force to subject the patient to surgery, the amount of respect shown to 'incompetent' patients becomes highly questionable. Although this kind of coercion need not be thought of as a violation of the patient's autonomy, which may already have been destroyed, it will still be experienced by the patient as painful and humiliating.

In short, then, the problem with the Kantian emphasis on the principle of autonomy is that it views autonomy as giving people respect, value and proper motivation, while irrationality and dependency are regarded as moral defects. According to Kant, a person's autonomy has to be respected because his dignity – indeed, his 'sublimity' – comes from being morally autonomous. The very attempt to distinguish between autonomous and non-autonomous patients implies disrespecting those who are judged to be non-autonomous. The amount of respect owed to an individual is based on a judgement of his rationality or level of intellectual autonomy. Thus the degree to which a patient's wishes, values and decisions are to be respected is determined by an evaluation of that person's ability to understand and rationally weigh up medical facts. The Kantian ethic has too-limited a conception of respect for persons.

### *Utilitarian Liberty*

Another justification for adopting the principle of respect for patient autonomy is that it serves to protect patients from harmful intrusion, and so contributes to efficiency in medical practice. Modern science and technology have not only increased the physician's ability to benefit patients, but also to harm them. As medical practice has become ever-more sophisticated the age-old fear that the patient would be exploited for the sake of medical research or personal enrichment has intensified. The principle of respect for patient autonomy constitutes one measure to protect the typically weak and ignorant patient from harm and exploitation. The duty to obtain informed consent is also justified by referring to the positive consequences for patients. Liberals often point out that individuals hold different values and different conceptions of the good, so that even a well-intentioned physician who fails to obtain informed consent may fail to benefit patients. Liberals have rejected the paternalist's argument that physicians should make decisions on behalf of their patients because their superior knowledge and insight render them more capable of knowing what the interests of their patients are. Physicians have expertise in the medical arena, but that is not always sufficient for determining what is necessary for the good or happiness of their patients.

J.S. Mill makes out a detailed argument for the supremacy of individual freedom in *On Liberty,* an essay first published in 1859. His statement of the principle of respect for autonomy reads as follows:

> [T]he sole end for which mankind are warranted, individually or collectively, in interfering with the liberty of action of any of their number is self-protection. That the only purpose for which power can be rightfully exercised over any member of a civilized community, against his will, is to prevent harm to others. His own good, either physical or moral, is not a sufficient warrant. He cannot rightfully be compelled to do or forbear because it will be better for him to do so, because it will make him happier, because, in the opinion of others, to do so would be wise or even right. These are good reasons for remonstrating with him, or reasoning with him, but not for compelling him or visiting him with any evil in case he do otherwise. To justify that, the conduct from which it is desired to deter him must be calculated to produce evil to someone else. The only part of the conduct of anyone for which he is amenable to society is that which concerns others. In the part which merely concerns himself, his independence is, of right, absolute. Over himself, over his own body and mind, the individual is sovereign (1985:68-69).

At first glance, Mill's position on the relationship between the principles of autonomy and beneficence does not differ significantly from that of Kant. Like Kant, Mill rejects paternalism. He argues that society may not interfere in individual autonomy for the sake of that person's welfare, which does seem to imply that liberty has precedence over both social utility and individual benefit. In her introduction to Mill's *On Liberty* Himmelfarb says that Mill's primary intention in this essay was to establish liberty, not to rest his case on utilitarian principles, so that, as for Kant autonomy is not a means to attain happiness, but an end in itself (1985:30).

The differences between Kant and Mill, specifically with regard to the relationship between individual autonomy and beneficence, are significant. What distinguishes Mill's position from that of Kant is that Mill bases duties towards oneself and towards others in the principle of utility rather than an abstract principle of rationality or universalisability. Himmelfarb overlooks the fact that Mill makes an important qualification *before* developing his argument in favour of individual freedom. In his introduction to *On Liberty* Mill states that 'this doctrine is meant to apply only to human beings in the maturity of their faculties. We are not speaking of children or young persons below the age which the law may fix as that of manhood or womanhood'. Mill's reason for excluding these people is not their irrationality or lack of autonomy as such, but their welfare: 'Those who are still in a state to require being taken care of by others must be protected against their own actions as well as against external injury'. For the same reason he says that despotism is a legitimate mode of government in dealing with uneducated people or 'barbarians', provided that the end is their improvement and that the means are justified by actually effecting that end. However, as soon as most members of a community have attained the capacity of being guided to their own improvement by their own reasoning and beliefs, forceful interference and penalties for non-compliance are no longer permissible as a means to their own good (Mill 1985:69). Mill therefore holds that mature people should be allowed total freedom (except where their actions harm others) because they are generally competent to make their own decisions and procure their own happiness:

> Each is the proper guardian of his own health, whether bodily *or* mental and spiritual. Mankind are greater gainers by suffering each other to live as seems good to themselves than by compelling each to live as seems good to the rest' (1985:72, emphasis in original).

Although he admits that people will sometimes make mistakes and harm themselves, Mill believes that respecting individual autonomy will, *as a rule,* contribute to the greater good of the greatest number. He remains constantly aware of the threat of disutility that lies in democracy, where people are politically free yet governed by the 'tyranny of the majority' or by 'the prevailing opinion and feeling'. People should be free to develop their individuality. He advocates 'different experiments of living', 'varieties of character' and 'different modes of life' – not for the sake of liberty as such, but for the sake of utility – and he claims that 'the free development of individuality is one of the leading essentials of well-being' (1985:120). Mill's position on liberty is therefore fully reconcilable with his rule-utilitarianism. Respecting individual freedom is a rule any civilised society should follow with regard to its mature citizens for the sake of the greatest happiness of the greatest number. Of course, Mill does not believe that mature persons will always make decisions that would further their best interest. Although intervention might be necessary to protect individuals from harming themselves in a particular situation, he believes that such intervention is not warranted because society as a whole would be better off if no exceptions were allowed to the rule of respecting individual liberty.

To appreciate the differences between Kant and Mill on the relationship between autonomy and beneficence it is useful to compare the implications of their thought on suicide. I discussed Kant's view on suicide in the previous section. The closest Mill comes to discussing the topic of suicide is when he considers to what extent we may justifiably restrict individual liberty for the sake of preventing an accident. He uses the example of a person who is about to cross a bridge that is known to be unsafe. Someone who notices this, but has no time to warn him of the danger, would be justified in grabbing him and turning him back. According to Mill, such forceful interference would not constitute an infringement of his liberty. Liberty consists in doing what one desires, and we can safely assume that the unsuspecting man does not desire to fall into the river. However, Mill continues, when there is only a possibility or suspicion that the bridge is unsafe, no one but the person himself can judge whether he has sufficient motive for incurring such a risk. He should be warned of the danger since that would allow him to make a free choice, but not forcibly prevented from exposing himself to it (Mill 1985:166). But what if someone does desire to fall into the river with the intent to die? What would Mill have said about intervention if the person approaching the bridge knew of the danger and was intent on self-destruction? Mill argues that we would all be better off if everyone increased his disinterested and unselfish attempts to promote the good of others. We should try to persuade the person to change his judgements or help him to strengthen his will. But in the final instance, he argues, it remains the prerogative of the mature person to act as he sees fit:

> Considerations to aid his judgement, exhortations to strengthen his will, may be offered to him, even obtruded on him, by others; but he himself is the final judge. All errors which he is likely to commit against advice and warning are far outweighed by the evil of allowing others to constrain him to what they deem his good' (Mill 1985:143).

Mill further argues that society has no right to interfere if a person only harms himself through his actions. So-called 'duties to ourselves' are not socially obligatory unless circumstances render them at the same time duties to others:

> The term duty to oneself, when it means anything more than prudence, means self-respect or self-development, and for none of these is anyone accountable to his fellow creatures, because for none of them is it for the good of mankind that he can be held accountable to them (Mill 1985:145).

Mill's account of individual freedom provides little scope for justifying intervention in suicide. Even if one is of the opinion that most people who embark on suicide do so irrationally, it follows from his view that once it is known that a prospective suicide is not a child or mentally ill, intervention should cease or should not be attempted.

Ironically, the only argument Mill offers that can be used as a reason to interfere in someone's suicide attempt is also useful as an argument in favour of suicide in certain circumstances. Mill argues that no person is an entirely isolated being, since it is impossible for a person to do anything seriously or permanently hurtful to himself without also harming others. If he squanders his money or property, he harms those who directly or indirectly derive support from it, thereby also reducing the general resources of the community. If his bodily or mental faculties deteriorate, he disqualifies himself from rendering the services he owes to his fellow creatures generally, and may also become a burden to them. For this reason the state or society has the duty to interfere for the sake of others (Mill 1985:146-147). In other words, although the best interest of a specific individual (the principle of beneficence) does not warrant interference in his liberty, the welfare of society (the principle of utility) does. This line of reasoning has some awkward results. It follows that, if a person is already a financial and emotional burden on others due to illness or incapacity, and is unable to contribute to the welfare of society, he should not be discouraged from committing suicide if he so desires. Society can only gain from his death. Indeed, the implication of the utilitarian view is that it would not only be morally permissible, but obligatory to actually persuade such a person to commit suicide, or even to actively kill him if this would contribute to the welfare of society as a whole.

We are now in a position to appreciate the shortcomings of a utilitarian approach to medical care, more specifically, why respect for patient autonomy often fails to further the welfare of patients. I shall focus on the South African situation since medical practice in that country clearly demonstrates the shortcomings of modelling medical science and practice on standards developed in Western liberal countries. Just as medical scientists in South Africa have attempted to maintain 'international standards' and have largely ignored traditional African medicine, South African medical law has incorporated into what is predominantly an African culture principles and standards that fit more comfortably in Western contexts. The principle of respect for patient autonomy, together with the duty to obtain informed consent, is a prime example.

The shift in decision-making authority from doctor to patient necessitates a standard of *competence* whereby an individual's capacity to form and communicate his conception of his best interest is judged. In contrast to the Kantian justification for patient autonomy, the emphasis is not on respecting individual self-determination as an end in itself, but as a means to ensure welfare. When setting the criterion for competence the question is not whether the patient is sufficiently autonomous for his autonomy to require respect, but whether he is capable of making a responsible decision with regard to his health.

On the question as to who is competent to participate in medical decision-making, the rule-utilitarian (in contrast to the act-utilitarian) does not judge every specific case on its own merits. This would require hospital personnel to decide whether a specific patient needs to be protected from his harmful actions or decisions by overriding his wishes. The danger of such a policy is that a patient would be considered competent if he agreed with the doctor's recommendation, but incompetent if his decision conflicted with that of the physician. This approach would only pay lip service to the principle of respect for patient autonomy. To avoid this objection a rule-utilitarian approach would have to establish very lenient standards of competency. Following Mill, for example, only children and mentally-handicapped persons would be considered incompetent and in need of protection against their own harmful decisions and actions. South African medical law sets equally lenient standards of competence. Strauss explains the approach as follows: 'In principle the motive upon which a refusal of medical treatment, or a specific form of treatment, is based, should be legally irrelevant. It does not matter whether it is upon religious grounds, out of fear, or out of a desire to die an early death' (1991:32). The only exceptions to the rule of respecting the patient's wishes that are recognised in South African medical law are emergency cases, minor children, patients who are in an unconscious or semiconscious state, intoxicated, under the influence of drugs or premedication, and traumatised or mentally-ill patients. Although it is granted that mature people will sometimes make decisions that would be detrimental to their own happiness, this does not warrant intrusion or interference since, on the whole, respecting the freedom of mature people is seen as leading to the greatest benefits for the greatest number.

The obvious problem with the utilitarian justification for the principle of respect for individual freedom is that mature people, particularly the ill, are simply not as rational and as competent as Mill believes they are. One of the complicating features of medical practice is that serious disease and injury tend to impair people's competence. Individual freedom or self-determination goes hand-in-hand with self-reliance as a central moral value. Yet patients are by definition not self-reliant – they seek the help of physicians precisely for this reason. A patient's reasoning may be impaired through lack of sufficient medical knowledge and insight or an inability to clarify his moral principles and values. This is especially true in a country such as South Africa, where the average patient has very little understanding of Western medicine. In a private conversation a general practitioner explained this as follows: 'Most African people do not have a scientific understanding of the cause, nature and treatment of physiological disorders. Many believe, for example, that AIDS can be cured or prevented by having sexual intercourse with a virgin, or do not understand why they should complete the full course of antibiotics even if they are feeling better.' Due to cultural differences that often exist between patient and professional, as well as the fact that the *apartheid* system has left the country with the legacy of a poorly-educated population, even intelligent and alert individuals may lack the ability to clearly articulate their beliefs and values or to make free and fully informed decisions about their treatment.

A patient's volitional autonomy (i.e., his autonomy of will or intention) may be impaired through fear, neurosis, anguish or stress. Cultural differences between doctor and patient may augment the extent to which a patient's autonomy is reduced through emotional and psychological suffering. The typical patient in South Africa is not only faced with the puzzle presented by his physical condition; he also must deal with a hospital environment which he may find foreign and alien. He is withdrawn from the familiar surroundings of home and family, which form a central part of identity and personhood in African traditions.

The dangers of strictly adhering to the rule 'Respect the wishes of competent patients' became clear to me during a conversation with a group of young doctors who had only recently graduated from medical school. As far as they were aware, the criterion for competence commonly used at their hospital is the mere presence of a decision by the patient. They all agreed that they would never treat an adult patient against her wishes, except if she were unconscious. When I confronted them with the possibility that a patient's refusal of life-saving treatment may be the result of shock, trauma, fear or ignorance, one doctor answered simply: 'One has to respect the autonomy of the patient. You can't take any chances.' It appeared that the reason he would not try to convince certain patients of the necessity of treatment was that he did not consider their lives to be worth living. He explained that most patients who use the public system lived in poverty, were uneducated and usually unemployed. One of his colleagues explained that there is no justification for going to such lengths to benefit patients because the hospital – and the country – is already over-crowded.

This attitude towards patients may be striking with regard to its underlying racism, and I would by no means suggest that it is representative of those medical personnel adhering to the patient-autonomy model. But it is important to note that, in the utilitarian scheme, there would be little reason to interfere if a person's refusal of life-saving treatment also happened to contribute to the benefit of society as a whole. In this way the principle of patient autonomy is used to disguise the (utilitarian) judgement that society would be better-off if certain patients died or were left untreated. What should be a further cause of alarm is that the legal system quite comfortably accommodates the attitude expressed by these doctors: If patients who are considered competent under medical law refuse potentially-beneficent treatment after being informed of the medical facts and options, they may be left to their own devices on the precept that their freedom is being respected. Their refusal thus absolves the physician from all responsibility for the consequences of the failure to treat.

Respecting individual freedom may increase social utility, but often at the cost of benefiting a specific individual. One should further note that the cases in which harm would result from respecting individual freedom within the domain of medicine are far more frequent than Mill would concede, since patients are necessarily vulnerable. The possible harm is also usually more serious than Mill could foresee. I strongly doubt whether one can describe someone's refusal to undergo surgery for a life-threatening condition as 'an experiment of living' or a 'different mode of life'.

Patients who refuse treatment due to either ignorance or fear are considered to be competent by South African legal standards. These standards are in line with those recognised in most countries where the principle of respect for patient autonomy is upheld. The most obvious problem comes from basing the standards of competence in the South African context on those recognised in developed Western countries, thus ignoring the extent to which the autonomy of the typical patient may be impaired. However, the difficulties experienced with the informed-consent model, although more marked, are by no means peculiar to the South African context. A number of studies conducted in the USA found that the idea of patient autonomy is still a distant ideal, and that the legal requirement of obtaining informed consent has not succeeded in protecting the interests and rights of vulnerable patients. Despite advances in palliative care, many patients still experience significant pain during the last days of their lives.[4]

## A Teleological Account of Respect

In the remainder of this chapter I argue that the problems inherent in the rule-utilitarian and Kantian justifications of the principle of respect for patient autonomy can be overcome by a broader interpretation of the concept of 'respect' as a virtue. I shall base the analysis of the virtue of respect on the arguments in Chapter Three concerning the compatibility of the notions of compassion and respect, and will draw from aspects of traditional African and Aristotelian virtue-ethics.

In developing an account of respect we need to avoid the pitfalls of the utilitarian and Kantian conceptions of individual freedom and autonomy. A major problem with the principle of respect for patient autonomy is that it is based on a recognition of human dignity as being founded in rationality. The patient-autonomy movement of the 1960s brought with it the conviction that patients are, or should be, equal partners with physicians in making decisions about their own treatment. This conviction of equality between doctor and patient is supported by and modelled upon Kant's notion of rational beings as forming a 'kingdom of ends'. The problem with this position is simply that the typical patient is not, and cannot be, an equal partner in clinical decision-making since he lacks the medical knowledge necessary to do so.

As a consequence, the problem of the power differential between doctor and patient remains unresolved. Ignoring or disregarding the unequal nature of a relationship merely serves to underscore the inequality. The emphasis on autonomy as an ideal, as well as the responsibility placed on the patient to make decisions, may only serve to aggravate the problem, since the autonomy of the typical patient, relative to that of the doctor, is necessarily reduced through lack of medical knowledge and the debilitating effects of illness. This problem cannot always be overcome simply by informing the patient of medical facts, since the information may only serve to accentuate the patient's lack of insight into medical matters.

We need a conception of respectfulness that does not derive from the notion that individuals are, or should be, *independent*. Western philosophers have tended to place much emphasis on independence and individual self-sufficiency. Liberal individualists such as Robert Nozick (1974) see the right to freedom from interference as the fundamental right from which all others are deduced. John Rawls (1971) is careful not to justify positive rights with reference to human welfare and dependence. The acknowledgement of positive rights is the outcome of a hypothetical contract between disembodied and rational participants. As we

---

[4] See, for example, the studies conducted by Lidz *et al.* (1982) and Lidz *et al.* (1984) on informed consent, as well as the study conducted by SUPPORT in 1995.

have seen, Nietzsche declares the lonely sufferer a hero. A number of communitarian and feminist critics of liberalism have rejected the ideal of individual autonomy and have argued that human beings are essentially related, dependent or communal beings. We need not repeat the communitarian objections to liberalism but need only note how an ethic that emphasises autonomy, self-sufficiency and independence as central moral values may serve to increase the suffering of patients, their feeling of helplessness, isolation and loss of self-respect. Illness, to a greater or lesser extent, deprives one of independence. In making independence the basis of respect, dependence becomes viewed and experienced as grounds for disrespect, and hence as moral inadequacy. (This may also explain why doctors are notorious for being 'bad patients' when they are 'reduced' to the ranks of patienthood.)

Some critics have argued that respect for persons who are autonomous (rational and free agents) may differ from respect for persons who are not autonomous. In the case of non-autonomous patients, the emphasis shifts from respecting the wishes of a patient to restoring or enhancing patient autonomy. In this view, one would be justified in overriding a patient's wishes when respecting his wishes would lead to a loss of, or injury to, his capacity to become a self-determining or autonomous individual. Acting against such a patient's wishes is not disrespectful, since one still respects his autonomy by viewing it as the goal of treatment.[5] This position has clear advantages over the Kantian one, since the duty to respect autonomy extends not only to those who are regarded as autonomous, but also to those who have the potential to become autonomous or regain their autonomy. However, the shortcoming of this approach is that the chronically dependent become an embarrassment to the dominant moral value of autonomy:

> Fragility and vulnerability, rather than being seen as appropriate parts of life from the cradle to the grave, become obstacles to be overcome by the self-sufficient man or woman. The *successful* patient is always the one who transcends the state of patienthood. Such a philosophy feeds on many modern myths about illness and about the power of medical science, and eventually leads to childish illusions about human capabilities and human survival (Campbell 1991:105-106, emphasis in original).

By viewing a patient's extreme and prolonged dependency as a defect or failure, as something that needs to be overcome if he is to regain his dignity, an ethic that emphasises autonomy as a central moral value may serve to increase the suffering of the chronically or terminally ill. This shortcoming is particularly serious in the context of euthanasia, since the dilemma of these patients is exactly that there is little or no hope of their physical health being restored or their recovery from a totally dependant state. We therefore need a conception of respect that relies neither on the patient's present autonomy nor on the possibility of regaining such autonomy.

---

[5] Pellegrino and Thomasma (1988) promote a form of autonomy-enhancing beneficence.

*The Bases of Respect*

In 'The Death of Ivan Ilyich' the difference between the virtue of respectfulness and respect for patient autonomy is clearly illustrated. Piotr, the footman, dutifully obeys the sick man's orders, always 'ready to do his bidding'. Yet Piotr does not in any way contribute to Ivan Ilyich's well-being or sense of dignity. Ivan Ilyich senses that the footman does not help him out of kindness or compassion, but purely from a sense of duty. After being asked by Piotr whether he wants his tea, Ivan Ilyich thinks to himself, 'He wants things done properly, and that requires the gentry to take tea in the morning'. When Piotr then asks whether he wants to move to the sofa, Ivan Ilyich interprets it as 'He wants to make the room tidy, and I'm in his way. I am dirt and disorder' (Tolstoy 1960:144). By contrast, Gerassim does not merely obey his master's commands or respect his wishes; his attitude is one of total acceptance of Ivan Ilyich as a person. For instance, he performs the 'disgusting task' of assisting the man with his 'evacuations' with a smile. We are told that 'Gerassim did everything easily, willingly, simply and with a good nature that touched Ivan Ilyich. Health, strength and vitality in other people were offensive to him, but Gerassim's strength and vitality did not fret but soothed him' (1960:142).

I agree with utilitarians that the moral status of human beings (and other animals) should not be made to rest on their rational nature, but on their capacity to suffer. We are not equal with regard to our capacity for rational thought, but with regard to our shared vulnerability to suffering. At the basis of compassion lies an identification with the sufferer as a fellow human being, a recognition that similar misfortunes may also befall one, insofar as one is human. In what follows, I relate the beliefs underlying compassion to the virtue of respect.

*Dependency* The recognition of equality with regard to the respect owed to others requires the recognition that dependency is a characteristic feature of human beings. The compassionate person recognises that people are not to be held fully responsible for their welfare, that there are grave misfortunes that may befall people simply because they are human beings. One may define dependency as being in relationship to others in a manner which makes them necessary for the fulfilment of some or all of our needs. Thus conceived, all humans are dependent, in some way or another, and for us to disrespect someone because of her dependency would be to disrespect humanity as a whole.

The compassionate physician respects the patient as a human being, one with a greater or lesser degree of dependence on medical care. Respect does not depend on whether the patient is judged to be (capable of) making rational decisions and acting freely – more often than not, a patient would not be autonomous in this restricted sense, due to illness, medication taken, or lack of medical knowledge. Hence Campbell writes: 'To be a creature is to be born of others, to know ourselves through them, to depend upon them and create dependency, to know the pain of losing them and finally to be the instance of that pain to others' (1984:96). Thus the patient's dependency is not valued negatively as a *lack of* autonomy or as *in*competence. Whereas the current political mood with its emphasis on individual self-determination tends to view dependency as moral inadequacy, the compassionate physician views suffering and dependency as the result of our shared human vulnerability to illness, disease and injury. In short, dependency is not a basis of disrespect, but a simple fact of human life.

*Innocence* The virtue of respectfulness may be based on the recognition that the suffering of the patient is undeserved and hence morally arbitrary. Neither autonomy nor dependency carries intrinsic moral value. As Campbell makes this point: 'The autonomous crook is still a crook and the autonomous parent could well be guilty of neglect' (1991:105). Respect for patients may be based on the recognition that a patient's dependency as a result of illness or injury is morally arbitrary. For the most part, the suffering we come across in the medical field is clearly undeserved. Even in cases where the illness was the result of the patient's own irresponsible behaviour – for example where a smoker contracts lung cancer, or an unfaithful husband AIDS – the suffering by far exceeds the level where we could consider it to be a just punishment for wrongs done by the sufferer.

The view of illness as punishment is reflected in the treatment of sick people in biblical times and throughout the Middle Ages. Leprosy was viewed by physicians and the public as a disease caused by moral corruption and often linked to illicit sexual intercourse. It is because of such beliefs that people who suffered from leprosy and even non-contagious skin diseases such as psoriasis and eczema were ostracised from society for centuries. Prior to a more scientific understanding, patients with malignant diseases were subjected to cruel prejudice. In the late nineteenth century cancer was often associated with venereal disease, with the result that cancer patients were barred from hospitals. In 1884 a certain Mr. and Mrs. Astor offered to completely finance a cancer ward for the Woman's Hospital of New York. Their offer was rejected, partially because hospital board members were frightened of having cancer patients in the same facility with other women.

Despite the fact that medical science has revealed the causes of disease as physiological, rather than metaphysical, the idea that disease is a form of deserved punishment seems to live on in modern thought. Boeyink distinguishes between 'deserved' and 'undeserved' pain, saying that if pain is accurately viewed as deserved, one can, in acceptance of this fact, develop a sense of responsibility for the disease or injury which causes that pain. This sense of responsibility can accept pain as following from one's own culpable actions and thereby furnish an explanation of the reason for the illness and its consequent pain. It is an answer, Boeyink concludes, to the question 'Why me?' (1974:90). The same way of thinking about disease is often used to furnish an answer to the question 'Why them?' We resist the idea that disease strikes randomly, and find comfort in the thought that the cause of a disease can be traced back to the person's life style or environment. In this way the concept of 'deserved pain' may serve to distance the onlooker from the sufferer.

Prejudice is particularly marked with regard to psychiatric illness. Peschel and Peschel claim to have observed many physicians who make the most brutally insensitive remarks about patients with certain kinds of neuro-biological disorders such as schizophrenia, anxiety disorder, and obsessive-compulsive disorder. Physicians may even joke about the idiosyncratic behaviour of such patients, despite the fact that their 'behaviours' are the behavioural *symptoms* caused by their aberrant neuro-anatomy or neuro-chemistry (1993:115). Such a lack of empathy can be attributed to a false belief about the nature and cause of 'psychiatric' disorders, as opposed to 'physical' disorders. The prejudice towards 'mental' patients seems to rest on the belief that while people cannot fully be held responsible for physical ailments, a strong and intelligent person should be able to control his emotions and behaviour by exercising his power of rational faculty.

*Seriousness* The compassionate person recognises the extent of our dependence on external goods, including health and medical care, and our coinciding dependency on each other in attaining or retaining these goods. The sufferer becomes an object of our compassion because we realise the importance and value certain goods have for him, in terms of his values, beliefs and needs. Compassion is based on a judgement to the effect that the suffering of a person warrants our concern. While it is true that people are by nature dependent upon each other, this does not imply that we cannot decide when demands made upon us for dependent relationships are appropriate and justified. The subject chooses to bestow compassion on the sufferer because he judges the sufferer's loss as one that is significant rather than trivial. Recognition of interdependence does not exclude respecting someone as a separate individual who is free to hold certain beliefs, values and life plans. The compassionate person shows his respect by imagining what the other person is experiencing, given her unique circumstances, and by trying to offer advice or engage in actions that would alleviate her suffering.

### *The Telos of Respect*

Recognition of the seriousness of a patient's suffering, the legitimacy of his dependency on others and the morally arbitrary nature of his condition form the bases of the virtue of respectfulness. But the notion of treating someone with respect is still one without any clear content. Does respecting someone require treating him according to his wishes (whether or not one thinks his decision is right), or does it require treating him in a way that would further his interests (according to some objective measure of 'best interest')?

As we have seen, a deontological ethic focuses on respect for autonomy as an end in itself, while the utilitarian ethic views autonomy as a means to maximise utility. By contrast, a teleological account of the virtues does not entail viewing respect as either a means or an end. For Aristotle, the means cannot be adequately characterised without reference to the ends, and *vice versa*. The virtues are those qualities the possession of which will enable an individual to achieve a good life and the lack of which will frustrate his movement toward that end or *telos*. But the *telos* is not a final goal that can only be reached *after* a period of struggle. The goal of life is to be found in the living. What constitutes the good life for humans is a complete human life lived at its best. The exercise of the virtues is a necessary and central part of such a life, not a mere preparatory exercise to secure such a life (see MacIntyre 1990:148-149).

But what are the implications of this conception of the good life for the virtue of respect for patients? After all, the physician's primary concern is not his own good or happiness, but that of the patient. If a virtue is defined in terms of its contribution to a specific *telos*, we are again confronted with the question: 'According to whose conception of the patient's good should the physician act?'

For Aristotle, the *telos* of human life is to achieve happiness. On this basis MacIntyre (1990:150) argues that an Aristotelian theory of the virtues presupposes a distinction between what any particular individual at a particular time takes to be the good for him and what is really good for him as a person. This seems to imply that the physician would be justified in scrutinising and overriding, if he deems it necessary, the patient's decisions. But is it at all plausible to distinguish between true and mistaken conceptions of the good life? The standard liberal challenge to Aristotelian moral reflection is that the very notion of a single human goal evinces an ethical monism that does violence to modern experiences of pluralism, the diversity of goals and aspirations, and the reality of moral conflict. A monistic theory of morality would incline towards paternalism, and would fail to acknowledge and further the different goals and aspirations of different individuals. If the good life consists in freely cultivating the virtues and furthering one's goals, an institution that forced upon participants or clients a specific view of the good would rob them of the opportunity to live a good life.

But Aristotle's theory does not commit us to a specific, narrowly-conceived conception of the human good. His starting point in the *Nicomachean Ethics* is not the affirmation of moral consensus but the recognition of moral disagreement. He acknowledges the fact that different individuals and societies conceive differently the nature of the good. Of course, Plato's *Republic* begins with a similar recognition of the problem of ethical relativism in the face of the diversity of conceptions of the good life. Yet unlike Aristotle, Plato attempts to overcome the problem of relativism by isolating a single, universal and objective human goal. By contrast, Aristotle leaves the content of the good life largely open. It is for the person of practical wisdom to decide in each particular context which action would enable her to achieve a good life. The nature of the good life is not determined according to some universal conception of human happiness. Similarly, the basic conception of neo-Aristotelianism is that moral reason consists not in a set of moral principles that are apprehended and defined through procedures of detached rationality, but in the concrete embodiment of certain human capacities in a moral subject who knows those capacities to be constitutive of a consummately desirable life (Beiner 1992:149). The content of the human good is not to be grasped by pure reason alone, but arises to self-consciousness in the embodied praxis of a moral agent who makes good choices and is pleased by activities that confer worthy pleasures.

Thus conceived, the physician's role in the good of the other is to enhance certain capacities for living a good life. By helping in the restoration of their health, physicians and other health-care professionals enable patients to act freely in pursuit of the aims or goals defined by the patient themselves. They do this by healing the body or easing its discomforts, but they should also attempt to restore the factors that may impede the patient in making free and informed decisions about his health, such as lack of understanding, fear or emotional suffering. If the concern at hand is the good of the patient, it follows that decisions should be made with consideration of the unique circumstances of that particular person. The focus should be on benefiting the patient in terms of her values and beliefs. The duty to respect individual freedom and self-determination should not be viewed as a *negative* obligation or as a duty of *non-interference*, but as a *positive* responsibility necessitating a certain degree of *interaction* or *interference*.

In response to the charge that Aristotelianism is rooted in ethical monism and hence inclines towards paternalism, one should further point out that the Aristotelian does not attempt to impose a single conception of the good life by the fiat of reason. Yet at the same time he or she does not deny the existence of patterns of coherence and shared values. When Aristotle speaks of a single end shared by all human beings, he refers to the fact that all human beings share an interest in living well. We will necessarily have certain shared concerns and interests that affect our ability to live well. We may grant that contemporary societies are characterised by an absence of a single cultural tradition or a shared conception of what the human good involves. Yet we should not emphasise these differences at the expense of the things that make us similar to each other. We can identify certain capacities as being necessary (although not sufficient) conditions for living a good life, whatever its specific content. Among these requirements is health, which refers to certain capacities of an organism that allow it to engage in activities of different kinds. Medicine involves the needs and interests that we all share. All of us wish to avoid untimely death and unnecessary suffering, and we all wish to be cared for when we are in pain. Hauerwas remarks that 'medicine provides a powerful reminder... of our "nature" as bodily beings beset by illness and destined for death. Yet medicine also reminds us it is our "nature" to be a community that refuses to let suffering alienate us from one another' (1986:7). If a patient chooses a mode of treatment that would inhibit his capacity for freely engaging in certain activities, it is possible to say that he chooses wrongly. For instance, if someone chooses to suffer from a fully treatable condition we can say that she is mistaken, that she is inhibiting her capacities or limiting her potential. In this sense there may be a distinction between what any particular individual at a particular time takes to be the good for him and what is really good for him as a person.

The Aristotelian would also provide for the possibility that the patient's wishes are not authentic. The values and beliefs of a patient cannot always be gathered from the wishes she expresses concerning her treatment. Our hero Philoctetes repeatedly expresses the wish to die. At the height of the tragic tension the only choice left to him seems to be that between dying a prolonged and agonising death or putting a quick end to his hopeless situation. Yet by killing him, by respecting his autonomous decision, the chorus of soldiers would certainly not respect him as a person, since his own actions and attitude – his eagerness to return to his family, his persistent attempts to maintain his life and improve his fortune – show that his death wish cannot be considered as authentic or as an accurate reflection of his values. An important requirement for being virtuous is having certain intellectual skills, which includes the ability to act and decide on the basis of true and rational judgements. Much of the suffering experienced by patients is due not only to physical pain, but to anxiety and fear, a feeling of powerlessness, a sense of isolation or solitude, and an inability to understand the nature, cause and seriousness of their symptoms. But such reactions are not a sign of immaturity or stupidity. The most 'competent' patient may have difficulty in understanding complex and unfamiliar medical facts. If a patient's decision rests on false beliefs, is ill-informed or stems from emotions such as fear, the physician would not be contributing to his good if he were to act according to these wishes. Instead, the physician should use his medical knowledge and experience to facilitate such understanding and thus to alleviate emotional suffering. What the patient is told should not be determined with reference to some (legal) standard of what counts as informed consent, but should depend on the particular patient's abilities, needs, expectations, fears and wishes. It is exactly by taking the emotional and existential suffering of the patient seriously that the physician demonstrates respect for the patient.

Rather than viewing patient autonomy as the goal of treatment or as a requirement for having one's wishes respected, a respectful physician responds to the patient's present and future well-being, to his good in general. The question to be asked when deciding on treatment is not: 'What are the wishes of the patient?' or 'What mode of treatment will maximise the patient's autonomy?' but 'What would contribute to the well-being or happiness of the specific person?' The patient's well-being is here not only understood in terms of his physiological condition, but also in terms of his emotional and psychological health, which can be impeded by emotions such as fear or by lack of understanding. An important part of respecting a patient is to engage him in a compassionate *dialogue,* which has the twin aims of helping the patient to overcome emotional suffering and misunderstandings, and enabling the physician to gain an understanding of the values, beliefs and circumstances of the patient.

The recognition of human dependency does not preclude an appreciation of, and respect for, the other as a being who is free to hold certain beliefs and values. In this regard, the traditional African conception of freedom provides a more viable alternative to the dominant Western conception of individual liberty. Shutte (1993) develops an account of 'freedom in dependence' that is based on traditional African thought and closely resembles the Aristotelian view. At the basis of the African conception of freedom lies the view that 'a person depends on persons to be a person' (as expressed in the Xhosa proverb 'umuntu ngumuntu ngabantu'). Thomist philosophy and traditional African thought hold in common the conviction that, in order to develop as persons, we need to be empowered by others. Our capacity for free self-realisation requires a certain kind of influence provided by other persons. Individual freedom and community with others need not be seen as an opposition, as is the tendency in the Western liberal tradition. Instead of the misguided desire for total independence often found in contemporary European philosophy and culture, African thought does not view dependence as a moral defect. Instead, dependency forms the basis of one's personhood. Community defines the person as a person, not some isolated static quality of rationality, will or memory (Menkiti 1979:158). Personal identity is not defined in terms of some or other essence or natural property but in terms of relationships. Instead of the Cartesian maxim 'I think, therefore I am' African culture is based on the notion 'I participate, therefore I am' (Taylor 1963:41). The strength the individual finds through his dependence on others and their influence on him is not seen as a lack or defect, but as a universal and defining characteristic of human beings.

In the patient who refuses treatment due to fear or ignorance, we find a lack of integration between his cognitive, volitional and emotional life. To simply act according to the patient's wishes under the pretext of respecting his autonomy is to hamper such a person's ability to attain happiness. Therefore the task of medical professionals is not simply to carry out the wishes of the patient, but also to enter into conversation with that person, to seek to integrate the patient's cognitive, volitional and emotional life. To succeed in bringing this about, the professional needs the virtue of *phronesis* or discernment, which can be defined as 'sensitive insight involving acute judgement and understanding'. The person of discernment 'is disposed to identify what a circumstance calls for in the way of human responsiveness' (Beauchamp and Childress 1994:468). Vulnerable and dependent patients may, for instance, need a more sensitive approach, while other patients may prefer a clinical, factual approach. African people, who are known for their high estimation of family life, may need to discuss their illness with family members before deciding on treatment. It is exactly through gearing communication towards meeting the specific patient's needs that one respects her as a unique human being.

Freedom does not involve the capacity to think, decide, and act (on the basis of such thought and decision) independently or without external influence. The Western notion of the individual as an independent agent and decision-maker totally disregards the fact that people are essentially social beings and, as such, depend upon one another for their welfare. Leading a good life is not entirely up to the individual in question. We all need, to a greater or lesser extent, the influence of others to be able to reach our goals and fulfil our ideals. The virtues of respect, compassion and benevolence are based on the recognition that others depend on our help and influence for their well-being.

### *Consent versus Consensus*

The aim of medical treatment should be to enable the patient to lead a good life. This is only possible if the physician has clear insight into the beliefs, values and circumstances of the individual patient. But isn't one of the aims of the legal requirement of informed consent exactly to help the patient to overcome ignorance and fear by informing him or her of the relevant medical facts? In this section I shall argue that the legal requirement of obtaining informed consent does not guarantee that this will be the case. Instead, doctor and patient should enter into a dialogue aimed at reaching consensus on the ends of treatment, so that neither the physician (as in the paternalistic model), nor the patient (as in the autonomy model) is the primary decision-maker. The virtues of respect and benevolence can only be integrated through engaging in a compassionate dialogue with the patient, in which the physician seeks to understand the suffering, values, beliefs and circumstances of the patient.

Bearing in mind that physicians in most countries are legally obliged to obtain informed consent before any medical intervention, we seem to have a culture of lawlessness in many hospitals. A study of doctors' behaviour conducted at the University of Cape Town's Medical School found that a significant proportion of doctors claimed *not* to obtain informed consent for a variety of procedures (Henley *et al.* 1995:1273-1278). A series of sociological studies conducted in the USA had similar results. Qualitative methods were used to explore the reality of how informed consent actually operates in routine everyday treatment settings. It was found that the rational, linear model of informed consent as envisioned in law and bioethics does not exist (Lidz *et al.* 1982 and Lidz *et al.* 1984). While these studies refrain from commenting on their findings, Dr. Robert McGee (1976) openly expresses the feelings of many doctors in an article entitled 'To Hell With All Those Laws – Let's Be Good Doctors!' McGee argues that physicians have a moral right to ignore law and regulation when they believe these to be harmful to the medical interests and welfare of individual patients. The physician must run the risks of breaking the law, or being sued, or of doing that which is not sanctioned by statute if that is what is required to be a good physician. This includes ignoring informed-consent requirements or turning off respirators without court approval. 'Do what your conscience dictates', he pleads, 'follow your best medical judgement, and take your chances. If you don't you'll be doing your patients a disservice. There is no way to practise good medicine if you let yourself get mired in the wonderland of tangled law that legislators and lawyers have erected around us' (1976:92).

Not surprisingly, many ethicists strongly disapprove of the view that the physician's moral duties allow him a special licence to break the law.[6] A culture of lawlessness should indeed cause alarm, since health-care professionals too often coalesce to protect their own interests and cover up their mistakes. Yet what the critics fail to recognise is that this phenomenon is symptomatic of a more fundamental conflict that currently exists between medical law and practice. Absolute rules and prohibitions are not conducive to good medical practice, since the latter requires sensitivity for the particular and changing contexts of physician-patient encounters. It seems safe to say that the reason that doctors often fail to obtain informed consent as envisioned by law is not that they ignore the values and

---

[6] See, for example, the Round Table Discussion between Daniel Callahan, Robert Daly, Sissela Bok and others, reprinted in Spicker and Engelhardt (1977:223-245).

needs of individual patients. More often than not, they believe that better service can be rendered by taking a less strict approach to obtaining consent. The UCT study showed that the majority of doctors supported a patient-centred standard for determining the kind and amount of information to disclose:

> What patients are told depends on a combination of social, ethical and medical factors. These include the context and tradition of medical care, the attitudes, values and mutual expectations of the patients and health professionals, the duration of the doctor-patient relationship and the nature of a patient's condition and treatment (Henley *et al.* 1995:1273).

A 'patient-orientated standard' would not only require the doctor to control the amount and type of information revealed. It may also necessitate an appeal to the emotions of the patient or require physicians not to convey information that would unnecessarily upset sensitive patients. The UCT study's findings would only cause alarm if, like Kant, one believes that the attempt to convince someone to act according to duty through means other than reason, fails to respect the person as a rational agent. In this regard we should heed the words of Shutte:

> [E]ven the most radical and all-pervasive influence of other persons on me need not diminish my freedom of choice and action as long as this influence is strictly a personal one; it must be the effect of an attitude that is expressive of the genuine personal growth and fulfilment of the other person. Such an attitude of wise and loving affirmation of me, emanating from the other's clear-sighted and whole-hearted acceptance of themselves, actually enhances and promotes my freedom through a progressive integration of my cognitive, volitional and emotional life (1993:89).

Patients are often grateful to medical personnel or other persons for convincing them to undergo treatment. The moral acceptability of medical decision-making does not depend on the presence or absence of informed consent, but on whether or not the decision stems from a consideration of and insight into the needs, vulnerabilities and values of a particular patient. The UCT study suggests that physicians are sensitive to the particular context of their relationship with a patient, and that they recognise the highly individual nature of patients' informational requirements and expectations about the doctor-patient encounter:

> [T]here is convincing evidence that informed consent as envisioned by law does not exist in reality, even in highly developed countries, and that medical care is governed far more 'by the logic, logistics, and the ethos of medical practice than by the legal ideal of individual autonomy' (Henley *et al.* 1995:1277).

The informed-consent model has shortcomings for both 'competent' and 'incompetent' patients. First, the legal requirement of informed consent does not guarantee that the patient will receive the type or amount of information he requires, nor does it ensure that his suffering will receive the necessary attention. With regard to competent patients, the ultimate goal of informing a patient of medical facts often boils down to procuring a signature on a consent form. Conversation between doctor and patient may be limited to that which is required by law, instead of being directed by what the individual patient is able to understand and requires knowing. The result of this may be, for instance, that the more inquisitive may not receive the detailed information they require, while others may be bombarded with information they either do not understand or do not desire to have. The danger of inadequate or unsatisfactory communication between doctor and patient is even more pronounced with regard to patients who are found 'incompetent' but are still conscious and able to communicate. If it is decided that the patient is incompetent to give informed consent, communicating with the patient is no longer a legal requirement. But being incompetent to participate in medical decision-making does not necessarily imply that the patient's suffering cannot be alleviated through a compassionate discussion.

A second shortcoming of the informed-consent model is that the wishes expressed by the patient may not be authentic, in accordance with the values, beliefs and interests of the patient, even if the patient is considered competent to participate in clinical decision-making. The case of the Jehovah's Witness can again be used to illustrate this point. Some Witnesses affirm a doctrine of strict liability – the blood transfusion itself is seen as defiling the recipient, even when he or she is unconscious, deceived, or coerced. A transfusion would harm such a patient since the prospect of forgoing ever-lasting life is, for that patient, worse than death itself. Yet the informed-consent model allows for a blood transfusion to be administered without consent, if the physician can convince a court that the patient is incompetent. The problem with this approach is that, if the patient affirms or is known to affirm the doctrine of strict liability, a blood transfusion would harm him, whether or not he is conscious at the time, and whether or not he is considered competent. What further complicates the situation is that some Jehovah's Witnesses believe that what is prohibited is past, present, and future *consent* to blood transfusions. In this view, a court-ordered transfusion would not be the recipient's responsibility and would not deprive him of ever-lasting life. While many Witnesses secretly hope that physicians would order transfusions without their consent, the informed-consent model does not allow for this to happen. The only solution to this problem is for the physician to try, through communication with the patient or, where this is not possible, through discussion with the patient's relatives, to develop an understanding of the patient's values and beliefs, in order to treat the patient in a way that would be truly beneficial to that person.

A third shortcoming of the informed-consent model lies in its treatment of patients who choose not to exercise their autonomy. Henley *et al.* found that many doctors do not obtain informed consent for a variety of procedures and treatments on the basis that 'patients expect them to know best' (1995:1277). The USA studies similarly found that a number of doctors interpreted acquiescence as evidence of implied consent. A socio-biological explanation given by these authors is that acutely ill, hospitalised patients readily adopted a passive sick role in which they entrusted themselves to the care of the doctors whom they believed had the necessary technical expertise and were committed to delivering the best possible care.[7] Childress refers to such complacency as 'second-order autonomy', where the subject freely chooses to become the dependent or 'subordinate' of a health-care professional (1982:59, 62). The Kantian individualist would regard such submissiveness as a defect in autonomy, as a sign of weakness or moral inadequacy in persons who lack willpower and strength of determination to make their own decisions. They happily surrender themselves into the hands of a stranger, passively allowing themselves to be treated in any way the physician sees fit. By contrast, the compassionate physician recognises as a necessary fact that human beings depend upon each other for their welfare, and values the trust the patient places in her. She would still communicate with the patient and his relatives in an attempt to gain an empathic understanding of the unique circumstances of the individual and to help the patient to understand his suffering.

The legal requirement of informed consent, based as it is in a view of human beings as rational and self-sufficient, will often lead to preventable harms for individual patients by not paying heed to the vulnerability of human beings and the extent to which we depend upon each other for our welfare. It could also, ironically, lead to a failure to respect those patients who are judged to be incompetent or non-autonomous as well as those who willingly relinquish their right to make informed decisions.

## Conclusion

In the paternalistic version of the contractual relationship between physician and patient, the physician played the role of authoritarian decision-maker, while the good patient obeyed the regimen ordered by the superior. The informed-consent model has simply reversed the structure of the contractual relationship, so that the physician becomes a technician who obeys the orders of the patient as moral agent. This model neglects the fact that the moral agency of many patients is impeded. I hope that the model developed here points the way to consensus arising from dialogue and interaction, to a form of shared decision-making, as opposed to both paternalistic decision-making and the requirement of informed consent. The patient has to be respected as a self-realising individual, but this does not mean that the physician should abstain from any behaviour that would influence the patient's decision. Respecting the wishes of a person who refuses treatment due to fear or ignorance is not to further that person's growth as a self-realising person. As Shutte argues, 'it is only through a certain kind of dependence on other persons that personal freedom actually comes into being, grows and is perfected' (1993:77). Communication or dialogue thus has a twofold function: Firstly, it should be geared towards overcoming factors that may inhibit or prevent the patient's capacity for self-realisation. Secondly, communication should be geared towards gaining an understanding of what mode of treatment, if any, would be

---

7 Lidz *et al.* (1982) and Lidz *et al.* (1984).

most valuable in furthering a person's goals and ideals, without conflicting with his beliefs and values.

The advantage of this approach is that we need not distinguish and discriminate between 'competent' and 'incompetent' patients. The level of sophistication of the dialogue should be adapted to the patient's level of understanding. If the patient is totally unable to communicate, or not sufficiently so for the doctor to gain an understanding of his circumstances, other sources of understanding can be utilised, such as previous encounters with the patient, or communication with the family, close friends or religious leader. The focus should therefore not be on judging a patient as competent or incompetent and on obtaining the patient's signature on a consent form (if found to be competent), but to ascertain what course of treatment would promote the welfare and interests of the individual patient.

# Chapter Six

# Euthanasia and the Virtues

## Introduction

One of the most significant developments in ethical theory over the past few decades has been the revival of virtue ethics, which occurred mainly as a response to the perceived shortcomings of principle-based ethical systems. For the most part, virtue ethicists have focused on developing an account of morality that is theoretically sound, and have analysed the nature and significance of specific virtues. However, relatively few attempts have been made to apply virtue theory to specific moral issues. This, according to its critics, only serves to underline the fact that virtue ethicists are unable to shed light on the question of what ought and ought not to be done in specific situations. This shortcoming is seen as residing in the very structure of virtue ethics since it concerns itself primarily with character rather than action. In response to this charge Aristotelians usually emphasise that ethics is not a science that involves the application, in an impartial and consistent manner, of rules and principles to specific cases. To this end they often cite Aristotle's admonition that 'it is the mark of an educated man to look for precision in each class of things just so far as the nature of the subject admits' (*N. Ethics* I. iii). On a theoretical level we may well agree that the complexity of human needs, desires and interests, as well as the difficulty of balancing these when conflicts arise, rules out the sort of clear-cut formulae that may obtain in mathematics and science, so that it is to the credit of virtue ethics that it does not aim to codify morality. However, this does not eliminate the need for a clear set of moral guidelines that can be used as a basis for policy-making. We cannot discard all rules and policies and leave it to the discretion of individual physicians and other health-care workers to make morally-responsible decisions.

In this chapter I aim to outline a virtue-based approach to policy-making in the field of end-of-life decision-making. Although virtuous motives cannot be fully codified, this does not mean that the virtue-ethicist has to sit quietly in the corner during policy-making sessions. With this aim in mind I briefly discuss the most important features of the virtues of benevolence, compassion and respect, and relate them to the moral questions surrounding euthanasia, namely:

1. Under which conditions is compassion an appropriate motive for considering euthanasia?;

2. When is euthanasia an act of responsible benevolence; and
3. Does euthanasia ever allow a person to die with dignity?

This is followed by a discussion of a number of cases that typically arise in medical contexts, the aim of which is to clarify the conditions under which euthanasia is a morally-acceptable response to the problem of suffering. This makes it possible to formulate a set of rules or policies with regard to end-of-life decision-making. However, in many cases it will not be clear whether death is a desirable end. In such cases, I argue, involved family-members should make the decision based on a careful consideration of all morally-relevant aspects of the case, but without being required to produce conclusive evidence to the effect that the decision accords with the patient's previously-held wishes or serves to promote her interests. In these cases the decision-making process becomes more important than the actual decision made. First, however, a brief interlude follows in which I discuss the final feature of suffering that leads to a consideration of euthanasia as a means of ending a hopeless and desperate struggle.

## The Final Feature of Suffering: The Desperate Patient

Patients who suffer from terminal or chronic conditions may be faced with the same problems and dilemmas discussed in the previous chapters: a feeling of isolation, of helplessness and dependency, and a loss of self-respect. Yet their distress has a further dimension, which is brought about by the fact that their illness or disability is not a temporary phase which can be overcome through their own efforts or through the help of others. In *The Drowned and the Saved*, Primo Levi describes his suffering and despair as a survivor of Auschwitz. He contrasts the relentlessness of his own anguish to the popular image of suffering as follows:

> [A] certain fixed image has been proposed innumerable times, consecrated by literature and poetry, and picked up by the cinema: 'the quiet after the storm', when all hearts rejoice. 'To be freed from pain / is delightful for us'. The disease runs its course and health returns. To deliver us from imprisonment 'our boys', the liberators, arrive just in time, with waving flags; the soldier returns and again finds his family and peace (1993:181).

Overcoming hardship can be experienced as a temporary victory of the self and humanity over pain and death, as an opportunity for celebrating life. Yet neither modern medicine nor our personal efforts can eliminate the impending and unavoidable reality of death. Every triumph over pain serves as a reminder that destruction ultimately awaits us. Thus pain and suffering are intricate parts of the human condition, a bittersweet union of weakness and strength, of dependence and self-reliance, of isolation and community, and ultimately, of life and death. When pain or suffering becomes a permanent presence this union is upset. The person's efforts to rid himself of pain are frustrated, leaving him with a sense of helplessness and weakness. The cry for help is met by silence, by the inability of modern medicine to bring relief. The reliance upon others to restore health and to relieve suffering gives way to a permanent dependence. The purpose of pain in indicating disease seems no longer to preserve life but to destroy it. Thus pain gives rise to despair: a feeling of utter abandonment, of helplessness, and of frustration. The despair of Camus's absurd hero in 'The Myth of Sisyphus' is similarly met by the person who suffers from a terminal disease or a chronic condition:

> What, then, is that incalculable feeling that deprives the mind of the sleep necessary to life? A world that can be explained even with bad reasons is a familiar world. But, on the other hand, in a universe suddenly divested of illusions and lights, man feels an alien, a stranger. His exile is without remedy since he is deprived of the memory of a lost home or the hope of a promised land (Camus 1993:109-110).

For the sufferer of a terminal or incurable condition the question remains: 'What is to be done?' Feelings of isolation, degradation, weakness and despair often lead sufferers and bystanders to consider death as an answer to this question. Before committing suicide himself, Ambrose Bierce wrote that people are justified in 'removing themselves' when they find themselves in a desperate situation. This includes people who are afflicted with a painful and incurable disease, those who are a heavy burden to their friends with no prospect of their relief, those threatened with permanent insanity and those without friends, property, employment or hope (1993:235). In the same way, euthanasia is contemplated when we are faced with a situation where it is not a case of 'pleasure the son of misery' but of 'misery the son of misery' (Levi 1993:182), when the dying process is or can no longer be experienced as meaningful. Elizabeth Kübler-Ross has gained wide recognition for her work on death and dying, in particular her thesis that dying can be experienced as the final stage of growth.[1] She opposes euthanasia on the grounds that it deprives an individual of the possibility of finding meaning in the last days of his or her life. Yet without questioning the importance of her work, we are still able to ask: 'Is euthanasia really inconsistent with experiencing the dying process as a period of growth?'

Tolstoy's Ivan Ilyich dies after a long process of 'soul-searching', of attempting to discover the meaning of his life and of setting right the mistakes he has made and the lies he has deceived himself with. Euthanasia is never considered as an answer to his terrible suffering. Yet we should note that, when he finally does make peace with himself and others, when he reaches the final stage of

[1] Kübler-Ross (1975) outlines five stages of dying. The first is denial, where the patient reacts by refusing to believe that she is dying. The second stage is one of rage or anger, when the patient resents the fact that others remain healthy while she must die. Then follows the bargaining stage, when death is accepted but an attempt is made to strike bargains for more time. The fourth stage is one of depression, when the person mourns past losses, things not done and wrongs committed. From this time she enters the final stage of preparatory grief, getting ready for the arrival of death, of acceptance.

acceptance, it is only through the grace of the author that he dies a triumphant death. Reality does not always allow such happy endings. In real life, and especially with the aid of modern medicine, Ivan Ilyich might have continued to live long after he has lost the desire or ability to contemplate his life or to interact with others. In the film *The English Patient*, based on Michael Ondaatje's novel of the same title, we find a different ending to a similar story. After having suffered severe burn injuries, the English patient goes through a long process of reliving the loves, wrongs and mistakes of his past, making his peace with himself and others. He finally indicates to his nurse, Hana, to increase the dosage of morphine to what they both know is a lethal dosage. He dies peacefully while she reads to him. In Ondaatje's novel, the patient chooses a third way of dying. He refuses 'the tablet that brings painlessness' so that he can 'remain awake till the light dies out'. He dies alone (Ondaatje 1992:298). We are left to ask: 'Is there a difference, morally speaking, in the actions (and omissions) of caregivers in these three cases?'

## Virtues and Rules

One of the central objections to virtue-ethics is that is does not concern itself with formulating or discovering rules of right action. Against this I argued that the characterisation of Aristotle's virtue ethics, by both its proponents and its critics, as exclusively concerned with character rather than action is mistaken. To be virtuous is to act virtuously. It is true that virtue-ethicists cannot come up with a set of rules that will define the essential difference or the dividing line between right and wrong acts. Yet we should note that principle-based theories, though they put this forward as the ideal, have not had much success in discovering such a set of rules either. Instead of attempting to reduce the complexity of moral decision-making to evaluations about what is right and wrong we should accept that in many cases such answers will never be discovered since they do not exist. For instance, we cannot expect our moral deliberations about whether to withdraw life-support from a demented patient to always conclude with a simple 'yes' or 'no'.[2] There will usually be different judgements one can make concerning the moral acceptability of an act, depending upon whether one focused on (for example) the agent's motive, her intentions, or the consequences of the act for different parties involved. Instead of isolating one of these factors as constituting the essential difference between right and wrong, to make a morally-responsible decision we have to consider all of these factors as part of the complex web of moral decision-making. We should also accept that we will often be unable to

[2] A recently-published book, entitled *Euthanasia and Physician-Assisted Suicide: For and Against* (1998), is representative of the attempt to provide 'yes' or 'no' answers to questions concerning the morality of euthanasia. The two sides of the debate are dutifully put forward and defended by Gerald Dworkin and R.G. Frey (pro) and Sissela Bok (against).

make particular judgements about motives, intentions or consequences with any degree of certainty. For instance, it will often be difficult or impossible to come up with clear and convincing evidence that the burdens of life-sustaining treatment outweigh the benefits, or that cessation of treatment will be in accordance with the patient's wishes, beliefs and values.

Whereas principle-based theories seek to discover certain universal principles and more specific rules that can then be applied in every individual context, the Aristotelian views the moral enterprise as requiring the exercise of a certain amount of creativity. There is very little mention of moral rules in Aristotle's ethical writings. Yet he does emphasise the importance of adhering to laws, which are enacted by the city-state and absolutely prohibit (or prescribe) certain kinds of actions. The following passage illustrates Aristotle's attitude towards laws:

> With regard to the choice between abandoning an infant or rearing it, let there be a law that no cripple child be reared. But since the ordinance of custom forbids the exposure of infants on account of their numbers, there must be a limit to the production of children. If contrary to these arrangements copulation does take place and a child is conceived, abortion should be procured before the embryo has acquired life and sensation; the presence of life and sensation will be the mark of division between right and wrong here (*Politics* VII. xvi).

The fact that we find it unthinkable for our society to adopt a law requiring infanticide or abortion on the grounds specified by Aristotle should not be an embarrassment to contemporary Aristotelians. In contrast to Plato, who seeks to discover universal truths in an unchanging realm of ideas, Aristotle recommends that certain laws be adopted on the basis of a consideration of the particular circumstances and traditions in his society. He does not claim to have discovered moral rules upon which laws and policies may be based. The table of legal offences teaches its citizens what kinds of actions are intolerable *within that community*. These actions are the ones that, if they were permitted, would make it impossible for a community to create the kind of conditions that would allow its members to live good lives. Although he expected different communities to have different laws and penalties, Aristotle also thought that there would be some degree of resemblance in the kinds of activity they forbid. For instance, no community can thrive if acts such as assault, theft and perjury are tolerated.

However, for Aristotle obeying the laws enacted by a city-state accounts for a relatively small part of the moral enterprise. Apart from a table of legal offences, a community also had to teach its citizens what kinds of actions and qualities of mind would gain them merit and honour. The virtues ought to be encouraged in its citizens because they contribute to the realisation of the common good of the community. Yet they cannot be legislated for it belongs to the essence of virtue that it is exercised freely and willingly.

The challenge for contemporary virtue-ethicists, then, is to provide a set of guidelines for decision-making while also acknowledging the complexity and uncertainty that surrounds decision-making in most contexts. To meet this challenge we should begin by reformulating the moral questions in terms of the virtues. One of the reasons for the failure of virtue ethicists to come up with answers about the morality of euthanasia is that they have sought to answer the same questions posed by duty-ethicists, usually variations on the question, 'Is it always wrong to intentionally end the life of an innocent person?' But once we reject the idea that it is possible to discover a principle that captures the essence of morally right actions, we also have to rephrase the questions in terms of the virtues. In most cases such an inquiry would not conclude with the pronouncement that a certain kind of action, such as withdrawing life-sustaining treatment, is absolutely right or wrong, but would describe the treatment of, and attitude towards, the patient as more or less compassionate, benevolent and respectful.

In some cases it will be possible to provide conclusive reasons for why a certain action (or inaction) is not only less than virtuous, but intolerable both within the medical community and society at large. On the basis of the judgements in these specific cases we are able to clarify the conditions under which:

1. providing life-sustaining treatment is obligatory, since attempts to sustain life are clearly in the patient's best interest;
2. withdrawing life-sustaining treatment is obligatory, because the burdens of treatment would clearly outweigh the benefits;
3. hastening death is obligatory, since death is a desirable goal of treatment; or
4. shortening life is impermissible, since death is not a desirable goal of treatment.

What enables us to make these judgements is the extent to which human beings have similar needs and interests. Although people have different values and conceptions of the good life, certain things can be identified as necessary conditions for being able to live a good life. But in between the extremes of what would constitute obligatory and impermissible acts, we would be left with a fairly large grey area where it is unclear how the patient's interests could best be furthered. This is largely due to the differences between individuals with regard to what they experience as a meaningful life. In such cases, I shall argue, involved parties should be allowed the discretion to make the decision as they see fit, without being held to stringent standards of evidence requiring that their decision be uniquely correct.

## The Virtues in Dying

### *A Good Death: Benevolence*

The central moral questions we have to ask when deciding about the treatment of any patient concern the virtue of benevolence, namely (1) whether the proposed course of action or mode of treatment is intended to contribute to the patient's good, and (2) whether euthanasia is consistent with the goals of medical practice.

I have argued that Western medicine holds too-limited a view of the terms 'harm' and 'benefit'. This limitation is rooted in the Cabotean ethic of competence and supported by both the Kantian and rule-utilitarian approaches. The attempt to lay down universal rules commits one to the highly controversial view that death is a harm, and that continued life is always a benefit. The virtue of benevolence is much broader than the principle of beneficence as it operates within contemporary medical ethics. We cannot, as Beauchamp and Childress (1994) believe, specify a list of rules indicating which actions are beneficial towards patients in general. There are numerous ways, besides medical means, in which a patient's suffering can be alleviated. The patient's best interest does not only include the medical good, but also the good as interpreted by the patient in terms of his or her own values, lifestyle, aspirations, beliefs and so on. However, this does not mean that physicians should provide patients with religious or spiritual guidance, advice on relationships, tips on furniture arrangement, and whatever else the patient may need to flourish as a person, as the advocates of 'holistic medicine' sometimes suggest. Instead I have argued that the goal of medicine is to attempt to make it possible for people to live a good life or, in the context of terminal care, to die a good death, by removing the physical constraints such as pain, disability and discomfort. But since there is more than one conception of the good life, a physician can often only benefit patients if she is familiar with their values. For this reason responsible benevolence requires not only scientific knowledge and technical skill, but also practical wisdom. The most sincere desire and attempt to benefit others may, through ignorance of medical facts or lack of technical skills, lead to a failure to do so. However, nor will the physician be able to benefit her patient if her choice between alternative forms of medical treatment is not informed by an understanding of what a specific patient would experience as being beneficial, given his unique circumstances. In this way benevolence encompasses the virtue of respectfulness insofar as making a decision on which mode of treatment would best further the patient's good requires taking seriously the patient's life plan, values and beliefs.

Aristotle does not directly address the question of euthanasia, but to explore the implications of a teleological account of benevolence for the morality of euthanasia it is helpful to examine his discussion of the virtue of courage and the proper occasions for fear. He writes:

> With what sort of fearful things, then, is the brave man concerned? Surely with the greatest; for no one is more likely than he to stand his ground against what is awe-inspiring. Now death is the most fearful of all things; for it is considered the end, and nothing is thought to be any longer either good or bad for the dead. But the brave man would not seem to be concerned even with death in *all* circumstances, e.g., at sea or in disease.... Properly, then, he will be called brave who is fearless in face of a noble death, and of all emergencies that involve death; and the emergencies of war are in the highest degree of this kind. Yet at sea also, and in disease, the brave man is fearless, but not in the same ways as the seamen; for he has given up hope of safety, and is disliking the thought of death in this shape, while they are hopeful because of their experience. At the same time, we show courage in situations where there is the

> opportunity of showing prowess or where death is noble; but in these forms neither of these conditions is fulfilled (*N. Ethics* III. vi).

> [C]ourage is a mean with respect to things that inspire confidence or fear, in the circumstances that have been stated; and it chooses or endures things because it is noble to do so, or because it is base not to do so. But to die to escape from poverty or love or anything painful is not the mark of a brave man, but rather of a coward; for it is softness to fly from what is troublesome, and such a man endures death not because it is noble but to fly from evil (*N. Ethics* III. vii).

> Professional soldiers turn cowards, however, when the danger puts too great a strain on them and they are inferior in numbers and equipment; for they are the first to fly, while citizen-forces die at their posts, as in fact happened at the temple of Hermes. For to the latter flight is disgraceful and death is preferable to safety on those terms; while the former from the very beginning faced the danger on the assumption that they were stronger, and when they know the facts they fly, fearing death more than disgrace; but the brave man is not that sort of person (*N. Ethics* III. viii).

*Death and dignity* It is important to note that Aristotle does not consider death an evil because of any attributes it might have. Death is an evil and the proper object of fear because it deprives us of life. But life is not a good in itself. As a vehicle for consciousness life is a necessary (though not sufficient) condition for happiness or virtue. When life is such that it is no longer a sufficient condition for happiness, or when life can only be maintained at the cost of virtue or honour, death is not to be feared as the most dreadful of all things. Given that we will all die, it is not the fact of our death but the manner of our dying that is important. It is dishonour, rather than death itself, that is the appropriate object of fear. It is for this reason that Aristotle thinks that the man who commits suicide to escape life's misery and the soldier who tries to escape death are both cowards. A courageous person is afraid of a dishonourable death but is fearless in the face of an honourable death.

*The value of life* The implication of this for end-of-life decision-making is that life-sustaining treatment should only be employed if it contributes to the welfare or happiness of the specific person. We have seen that the Cabotean ethic of competence strives to produce certain clinical benefits, and the success of medical technology is measured on the basis of its effectiveness in producing certain results. If the ultimate goal and rationale of medicine is to procure health, death would always be seen as the worst possible clinical result. Combined with the Kantian view that the principle of beneficence is an imperfect duty, prolonging life is always morally praiseworthy, but never obligatory. Against this I have argued that decisions about treatment should not be made solely on the basis of a calculation of clinical harms and benefits, but on the basis of the contribution of medical treatment to a person's well-being. *The ultimate goal of medicine is not life as such, but life for something; not health as such, but health for something.* Of course, it is usually unnecessary or even pointless to distinguish between effective and beneficial treatment. If I could get a doctor to cure my migraine attacks, or at least to decrease their severity and duration, I would obviously consider the treatment both a clinical success and a contribution to my general welfare. But this is not always the case. For instance, the length of time a person spends in a comatose state before dying, or the success with which his bed-sores are treated while in this state, has no bearing on his welfare or happiness. Life-preserving and other measures should be employed only to the extent that they contribute to the patient's ability to lead a good life. The implication of this is that, *contra* Kant, prolonging life might sometimes be morally blameworthy.

*Death and mortality* Aristotle's approach to death also provides us with a method for determining when death is a desirable end. One of the arguments against euthanasia is that the opacity of death and its incommensurability with life has the implication that we can never safely say that a person is better off dead. Because we cannot compare the goods and evils experienced when alive with the goods and evils (if any) in death, the only safe choice is in favour of life. This argument fails to consider the obvious fact that human beings are mortal. Notions such as 'saving life' and 'choosing death' obscure the simple fact that, strictly speaking, decisions regarding euthanasia and suicide are never about a choice *between* life and death. Death is a given. What we do have some extent of control over is the time and manner of our death. The decision involved in suicide and euthanasia is therefore more accurately construed as a choice between 'death now' and 'death later'. It concerns the question whether to *advance* the date of a person's death, or, stated otherwise, to *shorten* her life. We should condemn most instances of killing because they deprive the other person of the life experience she would have had were it not for the killer's crude intervention. But is it true of all instances of killing that they deprive the person of something, or that they injure that person? Cannot killing sometimes be an act of benevolence or of non-injurious killing insofar as it saves, rather than deprives, a patient from certain life experiences?

*Ends and means* The virtue-based approach disposes us to think of the question of euthanasia primarily in terms of ends, rather than means or procedures. The rules and policies concerning the treatment of patients are all too often phrased in terms of the type of procedures that may or may not legitimately be forgone. As a consequence, many debates in bioethics focus on questions such as whether there is a moral difference between active and passive euthanasia, or between withholding and withdrawing life-sustaining treatment. This focus is the direct implication of an act- or principle-based ethic, which attempts to formulate a set of rules that are objective and universal. It is thought that a rule such as 'It is always wrong to withdraw nutrition and hydration' allows for more objectivity and impartiality than rules based on quality-of-life judgements.

As mentioned before, the changing connotations of the term 'euthanasia' reflects this shift of focus from the good of the individual patient to acts and procedures. Literally, it means 'a gentle and easy death', and in previous centuries was used to describe the dying process. A 'euthanasia' could refer to a heroic death, a quick and easy death, or a painless death, and was sometimes used metaphorically to refer to a peaceful political transition. Only in the twentieth century did the term come to be used to refer to the act of painlessly putting to death someone who suffers from a terminal condition.[3] The focus of moral assessment therefore shifted from the good of the dying person to the actions of the euthanist and the procedures employed by him. This shift constitutes one of the major shortcomings of advance directives, which generally provide a list of procedures to be forgone instead of focusing on the desirability of different possible outcomes. But as Joanne Lynn points out, for someone to be asked in advance whether he would want dialysis, ventilator, or feeding tubes, without knowing what using these procedures would yield, is incomprehensible. Good decision-making rests primarily on pursuing the best possible future from among those plans of care that can be achieved, with 'the best possible' being defined in terms of the patient's values. Nothing in this model needs to turn on the nature of the procedure involved, except as it shapes the desirability of various future courses to the patient. Sometimes ventilators are morally required, but sometimes even changing the sheets is contraindicated (1991:219).

A virtue-based approach draws the attention back to euthanasia in its original sense, with the central moral question no longer being 'Is a certain mode of action (or inaction) permissible?', but 'How can we make it possible for a person to live a good life?' Instead of drawing distinctions on the basis of the procedures or means used to shorten life, we need to develop a conceptual framework that focuses on the different kinds of situations patients may find themselves in. Our primary concern in deciding upon the means of death – whether it is by suicide, assisted suicide, active or passive euthanasia or from natural causes – should be the good of the patient. For example, whereas withdrawal of life-sustaining treatment and the provision of palliative care may allow some patients to die a relatively peaceful death, the same measures could have horrendous consequences for others.

*Death as personal responsibility* Some supporters of legalising euthanasia argue that patients have a *right* to euthanasia. The implication of acknowledging such a right is that assisted suicide would be included in the list of medical procedures that physicians are obliged to inform their patients of, and patients are entitled to demand if they are suitable candidates. For instance, the State of

---

[3] The *Oxford English Dictionary* gives the following uses of the term 'euthanasia':

**1646** BP. HALL *Balm Gil. 337* But let me prescribe and commend to thee, my sonne, this true spirituall meanes of thine happy Euthanasia. **1709** *Tatler No. 44 par. 3* Give me but gentle death: Euthanasia, Euthanasia, that is all I implore. **1768** BURKE *Corr. (1844) I.155* At her age, no friend could have hoped for your mother any thing but the Euthanasia. **1837** CARLYLEL *Fr. Rev. II. v.v*, Not a torture death, but a quiet euthanasia. **1875** H.C. WOOD *Therap. (1879) 239* It has been very largely employed to induce euthanasia in advanced stages of phthisis. *fig.* **1813** T. JEFFERSON *Writ. (1830) IV.224* We must leave.. to others.. to prepare this euthanasia for Platonic Christianity.

Oregon's Death With Dignity Act, known as Measure 16,[4] makes it legal for a physician to provide a terminally-ill patient who requests it a prescription for lethal drugs. Accordingly, physician-assisted suicide is included in the State's ranking system, which is used to ration health care on the basis of need. This obliges physicians to inform patients that they have a right to request medication for the purpose of ending their lives. Yet if we view euthanasia as *something the dying person does* rather than *something that is done to them,* it brings back the realisation that it is primarily the responsibility of each individual to live and die with dignity. Within a virtue-based approach, the most important question facing each person is, 'How can I live and die with honour and dignity?' Thus seen, the notion of a 'right to euthanasia' or a 'right to death with dignity' is nonsensical. There can be no right to a good death, just as there can be no right to beauty or intelligence. But because human beings depend upon each other, especially in times of sickness and hardship, to realise their goals, the central moral question for the caregiver is, 'How can I enable the patient to live a good life and die a good death?' Philoctetes's plight is tragic because circumstances beyond his control prevent him from making a choice that will enable him to live with dignity. His choice is between a dishonourable life and an honourable death, and it is only with the help of others that a third option, to live with dignity, becomes a possibility for him. In much the same way, medical professionals and other caregivers can never ensure that a patient actually reaches the desired goal of living and dying well. They can only attempt to remove certain impediments that make it difficult or impossible for the patient to die a good death, such as pain and discomfort, ignorance about the nature and seriousness of their medical condition, groundless fears and loneliness. These and other ways of bringing about or making possible a good or easy death need not directly concern us here. Our task in this chapter is a more modest one, namely to inquire when physicians should cease efforts to prolong life, and when, if ever, they are obliged to advance the hour of a patient's death. It is important, however, that we keep in mind that these decisions have to be made within the context of the complete narrative of the individual patient's life.

### *Mercy-Killing: Compassion and the Quality of Life*

This way of stating the question of euthanasia renders it essential to judge the quality of life remaining to the patient, not only considering the person's present capacities and experiences, but also his or her future possibilities and potential for happiness. As a criterion for decisions to forego life-sustaining treatment or to hasten the moment of death, quality of life has been severely criticised. A frequently-heard objection is that such judgements are equivalent to the 'social judgements' that involve discrimination on the grounds of morally-irrelevant criteria such as race and colour. Basing treatment decisions on quality-of-life judgements is seen as denying a view that has long formed the basis of Christian

---

[4] Measure 16 is reprinted as Appendix D in Battin *et al.* (1998:443-448).

ethics, namely that human life has infinite worth and thus cannot be measured in monetary terms. Human beings are equal and hence have an equal right to life.

Another objection to quality-of-life judgements takes the form of the slippery-slope argument. The fear is that such judgements form the first step on a slope that would ultimately lead to horrendous practices, like the execution of Jews in Nazi Germany. We might start off quite innocently by allowing euthanasia in cases where the patient is irreversibly comatose or where futile and unbearable suffering render life not worth living. Once we have accepted the notion that there is such a thing as a life not worth living, there would be nothing to stop us from killing defective infants whose lives would impose a financial burden upon their family and upon society in general. In this way, the sphere of those included in the category of those whose lives are not worth living will gradually be enlarged, eventually encompassing the socially unproductive, the ideologically unwanted and the 'racially impure'.[5]

This argument is certainly valid if quality-of-life judgements are based on utilitarian considerations such as a person's usefulness to society, whether she would impose a burden upon family members, her level of independent functioning, the financial cost of maintaining her life, and so forth. Because it is aggregative, the principle of utility requires a consideration not only of the present and future well-being of the specific patient, but also the pleasure and preferences of all those who will be affected by the decision or action. Peter Singer's position in favour of euthanasia for 'defective' infants offers a good example of this method of judging the value of life. Singer closely follows the basic tenets of classical utilitarianism with regard to the treatment of non-personal sentient beings, which includes human foetuses, infants and certain animals. He argues that the implication of the principle requiring that the sum-total of pleasure be maximised, is that the only moral objections relevant to killing infants are the indirect objection from side-effects (the bad effects it would have on others, most notably the parents) and the direct objection from decreasing the aggregate of happiness or pleasure in the world. If an infant's life is likely to include and bring about more pain than pleasure, and if the parents do not want the child to live and plan to replace it with another infant with a greater potential for happiness, it can be killed with full moral justification (1979:131-138). I argued in Chapter Two that Singer's position on infanticide entails a total utilitarian improvement policy in which those who will lead worthwhile, even happy lives, can justifiably be killed to make room for those who it is judged will lead happier or more valued lives.

[5] The Kantian version of the slippery-slope argument holds that allowing euthanasia would put us on a *logical* slippery slope, insofar as making exceptions to the rule that killing is wrong undermines the rule itself. In other words, it is claimed that once we allow euthanasia we are logically committed to accepting other forms of killing as well, whether in fact they happen or not. Utilitarians typically argue that allowing euthanasia in certain cases would put us on a *factual* slippery slope, in other words, that it will, as a matter of fact lead to morally-objectionable acts such as killing patients for trivial reasons, whether they are logically entailed or not.

Although Singer discusses the morality of infanticide under the heading of 'non-voluntary euthanasia', his is not an argument for euthanasia at all. He alternates between the characterisation of euthanasia as *mercy-killing*, where the reason for killing is to end the suffering of the patient herself, and the characterisation of euthanasia as *killing those whose lives are not considered to be worth living*. If quality-of-life judgements include consideration of the welfare of others and an increase in the aggregate happiness, killing an infant whose life is not considered worth living is not an instance of *euthanasia* at all, since the infant is not killed for its own sake. Most of us would be in trouble if the right to life depended on whether a person makes a positive contribution to the amount of happiness in the world.

However, the utilitarian method of judging the value of human life is not the only one available to us. Another way of making quality-of-life judgements – and one that is immune to the above objections – takes the patient's interests and experiences, rather than those of society or the family, as the primary consideration in decision-making. The most important consideration, according to this method, is whether euthanasia would benefit the actual recipient, and whether continued existence would be a harm to that individual. This requires us to understand or imagine the quality of a person's existence as it is lived or experienced by that person, rather than the value of his life as it is observed and judged from the outside. In this regard, the virtue of compassion is extremely important. Compassion involves an attempt to understand what the other person is going through, given her unique circumstances, and in this way it takes the range of experiences open to her as the primary consideration in judging quality of life. This does not involve a judgement to the effect that the person is worthless or that she has a lesser claim to be treated with respect than others. Choosing death because continued life is not worth experiencing does not necessarily amount to saying that the person's life is or has been without value. For instance, Socrates chooses death because he thinks that continued life would constitute a loss of virtue or integrity (on Plato's account), or that old age would deprive him of the joys of life (on Xenophon's account). His choice serves as an affirmation and protection of his values, and definitely not as a negation of his worth as a person.

Unfortunately, the dominant Cartesian-Newtonian scientific paradigm of medicine has rejected compassion and has focused instead on explaining pain and disease through the use of reason. The task of understanding and alleviating a patient's emotional and existential suffering is seen as a separate enterprise, best performed by psychologists and other human scientists. Although medical technology and scientific knowledge often tend to shift the focus from the person's suffering to her disease or medical condition, this shift is by no means a necessary one. I argued in Chapter Three that a compassionate understanding of a person's suffering involves holding certain beliefs and is therefore compatible with scientific knowledge and judgements. We cannot and need not reject reason in favour of compassion, or compassion in favour of reason. Medical science has developed precisely as a response to the need to reduce human suffering, so that scientific explanations form part of a compassionate understanding. An important part of a patient's suffering remains his illness or disease, which requires medical expertise, objective testing and scientific knowledge. Because of his medical knowledge the physician is able to help the patient and other concerned parties to understand the cause, nature and seriousness of her physical condition. We cannot appropriately identify with the suffering of patients if we remain isolated from, or choose to ignore, the latest scientific discoveries.

On the other hand, the distanced, rational attitude is insufficient for understanding suffering since quality-of-life judgements can only be subjective. Indeed, I find it entirely unclear what an 'objective' set of criteria for judging quality of life could possibly include. It is only because we possess certain capacities and share certain experiences that we are able to come to an understanding of the importance or value of these capacities and experiences. However, the subjectivity of these judgements does not mean that they are also arbitrary. The rational component of compassion allows us to determine whether and when compassion is an inappropriate motive for euthanasia. A compassionate identification does not solely involve imagining what we would feel like if something similar happened to us. As human beings, we are able to reconstruct someone else's condition, by imagining what she, given her circumstances, is undergoing, rather than what we ourselves would feel if faced with similar prospects. For instance, it is possible for me to imagine what the severity of the impact of the loss of a toe would be for an athlete, even though the same loss would not involve much more than a nuisance and embarrassment to me. I can understand the athlete's suffering because, as a human being, I know what it feels like to have one's ambitions, hopes and ideals irrevocably thwarted. We therefore have to distinguish between imaginatively projecting ourselves into the person's problem situation, and making the further adjustments required to imagine being *that person* in that person's situation. This difference, and the importance of noticing it, becomes clear when one examines Adam Smith's account of compassion:

> [O]f all the calamities to which the condition of mortality exposes mankind, the loss of reason appears, to those who have the least spark of humanity, by far the most dreadful and they behold that last stage of human wretchedness with deeper commiseration than any other. The anguish which humanity feels, therefore, at the sight of such an object, cannot be the reflection of any sentiment of the sufferer. The compassion of the spectator must arise altogether from the consideration of what he himself would feel if he was reduced to the same unhappy situation, and, what perhaps is impossible, was at the same time able to regard it with his present reason and judgment (Smith 1976:12).

Although there are certainly instances where a person may experience his deteriorating mental abilities as very distressing indeed (as, for example, is the case with Alzheimer's disease), what Smith has in mind here are cases where the loss of reason also deprives the person of the capacity for considering or experiencing it as a loss and of suffering as a result. Smith therefore misses the distinction between just imagining being in *x*'s situation, and making the further adjustments required to imagine being $x$ in $x$'s situation. Although people often do feel distress when watching the mental capacities of a loved-one deteriorate, this cannot be described as true compassion and cannot form the appropriate motive for euthanasia. If compassion is to be a rational response to a person's situation, that person has to possess the capacity to suffer (which requires at least a minimal level of consciousness) and also has to experience his or her suffering as serious indeed.

*Death with Dignity: Respect for Patients*

Within most religious contexts 'respect for persons' is understood as respect for the sanctity of human life, which has the implication that it is always wrong to intentionally end the life of a human being. In this view the wrongness of killing does not derive from the fact that it deprives the person of his or her life. It derives, instead, from the obligation to obey God's law. Killing is wrong because God, having created human beings in His image, has the sole right to give and take human life. In secular societies this view of the value of human life has gradually been eroded and replaced by the view that human beings are the agents and creators of their own destinies. Human dignity is no longer perceived as a gift from God. Instead, it derives from the ability to make rational decisions and to act upon those decisions free from interference or coercion. However, this shift in the dominant attitude towards human dignity does not mean that we can reject all appeals to the sanctity-of-life ethic as erroneous or out-dated. In liberal societies the rights to freedom and self-determination include the freedom to hold religious beliefs, so that respect for patient autonomy includes respecting whatever religious views a patient might have.

The autonomy model does not always ensure that a patient will be treated in accordance with her values, beliefs and ideals. There are two main reasons for this. Firstly, if a patient is found to be incompetent to participate in medical decision-making, the principle of beneficence regains priority over the principle of autonomy. This means that the physician may treat the patient according to his estimation of the patient's best interest, which will usually have the result that he will seek to maximise clinical benefits. For instance, an adult member of the Jehovah's Witness faith may be given a blood transfusion if she is unconscious, regardless of the fact that her beliefs may be well-known to the physician. Secondly, respect for patient autonomy, as it is understood in contemporary medical ethics, is a negative obligation. It requires the physician to refrain from intruding upon or interfering with the patient's privacy, and to obtain informed consent before subjecting the patient to treatment. However, in medical contexts various things, such as unconsciousness, fear, depression or lack of understanding, may impede the patient's ability to express her religious (and other) values or to clarify the implication of these for her treatment. Complying to the wishes of a patient who refuses treatment due to ignorance, trauma, shock, fear or the effects of premedication is not, I believe, to treat her with respect. Neither is respect conveyed by declaring a patient 'non-autonomous' or 'incompetent' and then proceeding to treat her according to the values of the physician or of 'the reasonable person'. In neither of these cases is the patient acknowledged as a person who has a history, who holds certain beliefs and values, and who lives in specific circumstances.

Respect in its more fundamental sense means to permit the other to be her own person, and to recognise her significance as a person. Although this would often require one to refrain from interfering with another's pursuit of his or her own ideals and interests, in medical contexts people are more likely to need the assistance of others to be able to assert their values and beliefs and to realise their goals. In a consensus-based model the task of the physician is not simply to inform the patient of the risks and benefits of alternative modes of intervention, but to assist her in elucidating and articulating her values and by determining which medical intervention, if any, would best realise these values. Instead of the one-way process in which the physician informs, while the patient consents (or refuses), the virtue of respect requires a conversation or dialogue between physician and patient in which the aim is to reach consensus on the desired goals of treatment. In this way the physician may help the patient to overcome obstacles that could prevent her from reaching a decision that truly expresses her religious beliefs and moral values. The conversation should also include involved family members and friends, who will be able to offer valuable insight into the patient's character, values and priorities. They should also be included in the decision-making process because they will often be directly affected by the decision, and because the success of a proposed mode of treatment may depend on their ability and willingness to assist in its implementation.

The compassionate physician conveys respect firstly by taking the patient's suffering seriously, that is, by acknowledging that she has good reason to suffer as she does; secondly, through his belief that her suffering is the result of our shared vulnerability to misfortune, and that she does not deserve to suffer as she does; and finally, by his attempt to form an empathetic understanding of and promote her values, beliefs and ideals.

## Moral Decision-Making at the End of Life

In what follows I discuss a number of cases involving life-and-death decision-making in which we are able to reach a conclusion about whether to withdraw life-sustaining treatment or to advance the hour of a patient's death. In each case I will consider whether compassion is an appropriate motive for euthanasia, whether the choice of treatment is an instance of responsible benevolence, and whether it conveys respect for the patient.

### *Comatose or Unconscious Patients*

A necessary condition for being able to suffer, and hence to be the appropriate object of compassion, is that the person is conscious and able to interpret his own condition or situation as one of loss or deprivation. In 'The Myth of Sisyphus' Albert Camus writes:

> If this myth is tragic, that is because the hero is conscious. Where would his torture be, indeed, if at every step the hope of succeeding upheld him? The workman of today works every day in his life at the same tasks, and his fate is no less absurd. But it is tragic only at the rare moments when it becomes conscious. Sisyphus, proletarian of the gods, powerless and rebellious, knows the whole extent of his wretched condition: it is what he thinks of during his descent (1993:115).

In the case of patients who are comatose, brain dead or have suffered severe brain damage, compassion cannot be an appropriate motivation for shortening their lives. It is not uncommon for onlookers to have deep feelings of sympathy towards such patients, evoked by their attempt to imagine what such patients are experiencing, and to hope that they themselves never end up in such a miserable state. However, advances in medical science and technology have shown such feelings of sympathy to rest on erroneous beliefs about the extent to which patients in an irreversible coma are aware of their surroundings. For instance, the reaction by comatose patients to painful physical stimuli is often the cause of much distress in onlookers. Yet these reactions are merely reflex activities controlled by the brain-stem but, in the absence of upper-brain functioning, are not and cannot be *experienced* by the individual as a painful sensation. Those who consider it appropriate for onlookers to have compassion for these patients fall prone to the objection that compassion precludes rational judgement. Our inability to imaginatively reconstruct their situation does not simply stem from the fact that their experiences are wholly different from our own, but from the fact that they do not have experiences at all.

It follows that benevolence is not a sufficient motive for ending their lives, since the question, 'How can we relieve their suffering?' does not even arise. The central moral question then becomes whether the virtue of respect for patients requires us to prolong the lives of these patients. The sanctity-of-life ethic seems to require that we do so, since people have a right to life regardless of their quality of life. In recent decades adherents of the autonomy model have argued that incompetent patients have a right to refuse life-sustaining treatment. They can exercise this right by drawing up an advance directive while still competent to do so. Alternatively, a surrogate decision-maker can exercise an incompetent patient's rights on his or her behalf. The rationale behind both these alternatives is to ensure that decisions are made in accordance with the wishes of the patient, thus rendering the decision to withdraw life-sustaining treatment somehow 'voluntary' and hence morally permissible. One of the problems with this model is that there is usually a lack of clear and reliable evidence regarding whether the patient would want treatment to be withdrawn. It is my view that a more responsible decision about their treatment can be made on the basis of their capacity to benefit. To determine the relative weight that a patient's previously stated wishes should carry vis-à-vis his or her potential to benefit from continued treatment, we can examine the following cases:

> Dr. Clarke was an active member of the Voluntary Euthanasia Society and had previously signed an advance directive to the effect that his life should not be maintained artificially if there is no reasonable expectation of him recovering from extreme mental or physical disability. In 1991 he suffered cardiac arrest and lapsed into an irreversible coma. His wife requested that life-sustaining treatment be withdrawn, since this is clearly what he had wanted. The court eventually granted permission to discontinue naso-gastric feeding, but did not do so on the basis of the patient's previously expressed wishes. Instead, they considered the quality of his life and reasoned that 'maintenance of biological life such as heartbeat and respiration unaccompanied by any function of the brain cannot be equated with living in the human context'.[6]

> Nancy Cruzan had been in a state of irreversible coma for eight years. Her guardians sought court permission to withdraw artificial feeding. The court refused. It held that since Cruzan was not competent to refuse treatment, and since the state had an interest in preserving life, it could only give permission for life-sustaining treatment to be withdrawn if there were clear and convincing evidence that this was what Cruzan would have wanted. She remained in this state until former friends recalled that she had said things to them indicating that she would wish to die if she were ever in such a situation. The court subsequently accepted that there was now clear and convincing evidence of her desire not to have her life sustained artificially and gave permission to discontinue treatment.[7]

The court's reasoning in the Clarke case was based on a quality-of-life judgement, which disregarded the patient's previously-stated wishes. In contrast, the judges in the Cruzan case considered patient autonomy to be a more important value, and disregarded her quality of life. The latter approach is problematical for a number of reasons. Quite apart from the fact that I have strong suspicions as to the authenticity of her friends' sudden recollections, the court's approach to the question simply contains too many 'ifs' to be tenable. Giving absolute priority to the principle of patient autonomy requires one to attempt to decide *what the patient would have wished if she were capable of wishing and if she were at the same time capable of experiencing her current situation*. This, to my mind, is a thoroughly nonsensical question. The fact is simply that these patients, lacking intellectual or cognitive awareness of their present condition, do not and never will have or be able to express any preferences, desires or needs, and this is exactly why termination of life-support is considered. The court seems to have allowed for the possibility that Cruzan might actually have thought it in her best interest to continue living in her present state. Yet convincing medical evidence exists which shows that continued life can be of no benefit to patients in an irreversible coma, and that treatment would be futile in attempting to restore their health or improve

---

6 *Clarke v. Hurst NO and Others 1992 (4) SA 630.*

7 *Cruzan v. Director, Missouri Department of Health, 110 S.Ct. 2841 (1990).*

their quality of life. While it is true that contemporary societies are characterised by a vast plurality of views concerning the content of the good life, our views on what constitutes the level of functioning necessary for being able to live a good life are certainly not *that* diverse. I am yet to meet the person who would prefer to live in a comatose state for an indefinite period rather than die immediately. And even if we were to find a person who made such a request, perhaps this is the kind of wish that should not be respected. We cannot always get what we want, especially when what we want comes at a significant cost to others yet with no benefit to ourselves. Whether or not permanently comatose patients previously stated any wishes should have no bearing on the outcome of the decision.

Where there is a good chance of restoring an unconscious or comatose patient to health, yet where he or she has previously signed an advance directive or stated a clear wish to die, I would similarly argue that we should not abide by such wishes. The hypothetical case of Gary Austin can be used as an illustration:

> Gary informs Rob, his physician and good friend, of his intention to commit suicide. He complains that he lost his job after being made redundant a few weeks ago, and then his wife left him for a younger man, taking the car and the dog. He is clear in his mind that he wishes to die, and adamant for his desire not to be thwarted. Rob tries to support his friend, but Gary remains convinced that life will never again be worth living. Two weeks later Rob finds Gary unconscious in the casualty department, having swallowed an overdose of sleeping pills. Gary left a suicide note in his pocket, in which he threatens to take legal action if anyone were to interfere in his suicide attempt.

In their discussion of voluntary euthanasia, Beauchamp and Childress (1994:236) argue that if a person desires death rather than life's more typical goods and projects, then causing that person's death at his autonomous request neither harms nor wrongs him. It is for this reason that they think voluntary euthanasia (which for them includes cases where the patient signed an advance directive) is morally justifiable. The implication for this case would be that failing to interfere in Gary's suicide attempt at his autonomous request would not constitute a failure to benefit him. Indeed, by providing the treatment necessary to save his life physicians will be guilty of harming and wronging Gary, who has clearly stated that he thinks it in his best interest not to continue living.

Most people would agree that the physician should resuscitate his friend, despite Gary's clearly expressed wishes. To justify such interference some would argue that we need not respect Gary's wishes since his very desire to commit suicide demonstrates Gary's incompetence or lack of autonomy. However, in my view we need not take such detours in trying to justify our interference. I argued before that the Aristotelian recognises that there may be a discrepancy between what a person thinks to be in his own good, and what is really in his best interest. The reason we feel entitled or, indeed, obliged to intervene in such circumstances is that we cannot agree with the terms on which Gary is not prepared to accept life. Overriding his wishes would only be disrespectful if we interpret respect in the negative sense of 'not intruding upon or not interfering with another person's privacy'. In its more fundamental sense, however, respect means to recognise the significance of others, to permit them to be their own person. As we have seen, respect for persons usually requires one to keep a certain distance, but in some circumstances it may require positive interference. Not to interfere with Gary's suicide attempt would be to allow him to die a cowardly death, which is certainly not the most benevolent or the respectful thing to do in these circumstances. Underlying Beauchamp and Childress's view is the assumption that the value of a person's life depends on the degree to which he or she values it. But that this is not always the case can be seen from the simple fact that most people who seriously attempt suicide and are saved do not persist in their wish to die. The wish to die is reversible, and it is often reversed in response to the compassion and care of others.

### *Medical Hopelessness and the Desperate Patient*

It is often argued that euthanasia is unnecessary since modern palliative measures provide effective means of pain management. But pain is by far not the only or even the main cause of suffering. Certain conditions do not involve physical pain at all. Some diseases lead to death by suffocation, while strokes leave previously intelligent people mentally crippled and often hugely distressed at their condition. If someone is suffering from a fatal progressive paralysis, the mere tragic contrast in that person's mind between what she once was and what she has become may be sufficient to make her life intolerable to her. In a study of the practice of euthanasia in the Netherlands, the most important reasons for the request of euthanasia were found to be futile suffering (29 percent), avoidance of humiliation (24 percent), and unbearable suffering (18 percent). Although pain was among the reasons in 40 percent of cases, only in 5 percent of cases was pain mentioned as the most important reason (Van der Wal and Dillmann 1994:1374). These findings suggest that the different forms of emotional, psychological and existential suffering, such as despair, a feeling of helplessness and isolation or a loss of self-respect, constitute the most important features of suffering at the end of life. Even when the primary source of suffering is pain, the methods of pain management available are not without side effects. For instance, the medication used to alleviate pain in cancer patients is extremely addictive, so that they may experience withdrawal symptoms if they do not receive their medication on time. It often happens that the dosage has to be increased, not because pain has increased in severity, but to prevent the unpleasant symptoms of withdrawal. Many individuals who discover themselves to be addicted to a substance in the final years of their lives experience this as a further attack on their dignity and self-respect. What determines that a state is intolerable for a particular individual is therefore extremely complex and subtle, involving significantly more than physical pain or discomfort.

One of the implications of the subjectivity of suffering is that the quality of the life that remains for the person has no fixed nature or content before it has been lived. The Netherlands studies found that there were three times as many requests for euthanasia or assisted suicide as there were deaths from these causes. Among the reasons given for this discrepancy is that in many cases, alternative ways have been found of relieving suffering and of providing an acceptable level of comfort. The discrepancy between the frequency of the occurrence of euthanasia in hospitals (one out of 75 deaths) and in nursing homes (one out of 800 deaths) further supports the claim that suffering can often be relieved through adequate emotional and psychological support (Van der Wal and Dillmann 1994:1346-1347). Caregivers can usually help to improve a person's seemingly desperate situation. In this regard it is important to draw attention to the difference between being in a *medically hopeless* condition and being in a state of *despair*. While the latter is an internal or existential state of being, the first entails an objective judgement to the effect that there is no statistically significant chance of recovery or remission from disease.

Medical hopelessness is cited in a surprising number of cases as a justification for euthanasia. Another major study conducted in the Netherlands found that, of the 2,300 yearly deaths from active euthanasia, 1,000 occurred without explicit request. Another thousand died as the result of treatment for pain, and in 5,000 other cases medical decisions were taken with the intention to end life (passive euthanasia) but without consulting competent patients. The Commission lumped all of these together by claiming that in the overwhelming majority of instances where patients were killed or allowed to die without explicit request, they were already in the dying phase, and that ending their lives was normal medical practice (Van der Maas *et al.* 1992).

By itself, medical hopelessness is not a sufficient reason for considering euthanasia. Although there may be little or nothing that can be done to improve the patient's medical condition, this does not necessarily mean that there is no cure for his despair. The compassionate support of family and friends can play an important role in restoring hope and meaning in a patient's life, even if there may be only days or weeks left. I would therefore strongly object to euthanasia if it is considered solely on the basis that there is no hope of recovery or of continuing to live life with the same degree of independence and self-sufficiency as before. Dependency is an intricate part of human existence, and the Western liberal ideal of total individual freedom and autonomy too often generates intolerance towards dependency in both the patient and his family. Strictly speaking, the excuse 'she is going to die anyway' applies to every human being. Citing the victim's mortality does not justify ending her life.

For the same reason despair is not a sufficient justification for euthanasia. No doubt a patient may consider her desperate situation to be a sufficient motive for committing suicide. However, as soon as she requests others to assist in her suicide, they too become morally responsible for the outcome chosen. The question is no longer simply whether the patient has an authentic and autonomous desire to die. Those who are called upon to assist in her suicide have to determine whether rendering such assistance would be an act of responsible benevolence. For euthanasia to be an act of responsible benevolence, it has to be considered as the last resort, when nothing else can be done to provide sufficient relief from suffering. Death does not only release a person from suffering, it also deprives her of all that is good in life. The 'Assen Case' (named after the Dutch city in which the case was heard) can be used to illustrate this point. The details of the case are as follows:

> On September 27, 1991, 'Netty Boomsma' (a pseudonym) committed suicide by taking medication provided by Dr Boudewijn Chabot. According to the official report Chabot filed after Boomsma's death (the report was required under the Dutch legislation permitting euthanasia), Boomsma was neither physically nor psychiatrically ill, but was suffering from a deep bereavement brought on by a combination of factors. Netty had had an unpleasant relationship with her domineering mother and father, and married an abusive husband at 22 in order to escape her parents. The first of their two sons committed suicide when he was 20. At the end of 1988 Netty's father died, and two weeks later she left her husband, who had blamed her for their son's death. Her remaining son became her only solace, and her only reason for continuing to live. But in November 1990 doctors discovered he had a teratoma of the lung, which had become malignant and inoperable. He died in May 1991 as a consequence of chemotherapy. The same day Netty attempted to commit suicide. Netty met Dr Chabot for the first time in July of 1991, and Chabot spent the next few weeks counselling her. On August 25 Netty told Chabot that they had gone into all of the details of her life and that she had not come for bereavement therapy, nor for medication. She wanted him to assist in her suicide. Netty told Chabot that she was not coming back unless he agreed to help her. If he did not agree to help, she added, she might have to take her life herself. Chabot made a complete written summary of the case as he knew it, and asked a number of experts for their opinion. Two of them recommended that Chabot not go forward with the assisted suicide. The others experts agreed that Netty's suffering was unbearable, with little prospect that bereavement therapy would help, especially if Netty did not enter into it willingly. Chabot compared Netty to a patient who can refuse chemotherapy for cancer and request euthanasia if the chances for treatment to succeed are small. On September 24 Chabot went to Netty's house, accompanied by another physician (to witness the death), and assisted in her suicide by providing her with rapidly lethal compounds. He followed the approved procedure for officially reporting an unnatural death. In December 1992 Chabot was called to court to prove that Netty's case met the Dutch criterion for *force majeure*, meaning he was compelled by an overpowering force to put the welfare of his patient above the law. The case was heard in Assen in April 1993, and the judges decided that the *force majeure* criterion was satisfied. The decision was upheld in the appeals court in September of 1993, and affirmed by the Dutch Supreme Court in June 1994. The Assen Case was seen as a triumph by euthanasia advocates, since it established a legal basis for assisting in the suicide of Dutch patients who were in psychological distress but had no physical illness.[8]

One possible objection to Chabot's actions is that it is unclear why he thought Netty had a right to demand assistance in her suicide. Arguably, she has a right to take her own life, and can demand that others not interfere in her attempts to do so,

---

8 See Hendin (1998:76-91) for further detail and a discussion of this case.

but this is very different from claiming that it is her right that others provide her with the assistance necessary to carry out her own goals. I argued earlier that neither the right to autonomy nor the right to self-determination support the contention that patients have a right to receive assistance in their suicide. Patients can only be said to have such a right within a system that already accepts physician-assisted suicide as among the legitimate medical procedures on offer. A separate argument, one that is not derived from autonomy rights, is needed to show that euthanasia is among the appropriate tools at the disposal of medicine. However, this argument is not applicable to the Assen Case since, at the time that Chabot assisted in Netty's suicide, *de facto* legalisation of euthanasia and physician-assisted suicide already existed in the Netherlands. Patients knew that they had a right to request euthanasia if they were chronically or terminally ill.[9] It only remained for Chabot to convince judges that, to be consistent with already established medical practice, they had to allow euthanasia in cases where patients suffer from psychological distress but have no physical illness. Although many felt uncomfortable with Chabot's decision, they could not deny the soundness of his reasoning. If patients who suffer from somatic diseases are granted a right to euthanasia, it would be unfair discrimination to deny assisted death to people who endure psychological pain when it is not associated with physical illness.

Within a rights-based approach the only avenue left for objecting to euthanasia for people like Netty Boomsma is to argue that they are not competent to make such a decision. Yet this avenue holds little promise. Chabot insisted that Netty was not depressed and had no psychiatric illness, and all the experts consulted agreed that she was competent. We might find it highly questionable whether this was indeed the case. If someone suffers such extreme psychological distress that they become obsessed with death, we have to wonder whether they are indeed thinking clearly and rationally. Another indication that Netty was deceiving herself about the nature of her choice is that, although she was not religious, she believed that death would reunite her with her sons. Despite these reservations we should note that Netty was, in all likelihood, no less competent or autonomous than most patients who suffer from chronic or terminal conditions. To demand a stricter criterion of competence or to judge competence on the basis of the outcome chosen would border on paternalism, which is exactly what the rights-based approach seeks to avoid. It is also to discriminate between patients on irrelevant grounds. If patients have a right to demand euthanasia on the basis of intolerable suffering, it is irrelevant whether the source of that suffering is somatic or psychological.

---

9 Although Dutch criminal law provides punishment for euthanasia and a lesser punishment for assisted suicide, the same code stipulates circumstances for exceptions to the law. In a series of cases over the last twenty years the Dutch courts have ruled that *force majeure* is such a special circumstance; euthanasia is thus permitted when a doctor faces an unresolvable conflict between the law, which makes euthanasia illegal, and his responsibility to help a patient whose irremediable suffering makes euthanasia necessary (Hendin 1998:64).

The virtue-based approach developed here provides us with another way of substantiating the counter-intuitive implications of the ruling in the Assen Case. It does so by altogether rejecting the rights-based approach to euthanasia. Assisted suicide is not the kind of thing one can have a right to but has to be seen and assessed as a last and courageous gesture of compassion, benevolence and respect. Chabot's compassion for Netty Boomsma was clearly warranted, and it is understandable that it would motivate him to end her life. But when we ask the question, 'Is euthanasia the kindest or most benevolent thing to do in this situation?', the answer is 'No'. Assisting in Netty's suicide was clearly not an act of responsible benevolence. It is simply not true to suggest that there was nothing more that could have been done to alleviate her suffering or to help her find meaning in life. I am in no position to judge the opinion of the experts who studied the case and concluded that bereavement therapy is unlikely to succeed. However, we should note that the main reason experts reached this conclusion is that Netty made it clear that she did not want bereavement therapy or medication. Her declining the offer of help does not detract from the fact that the kindest thing that Chabot (as well as her family and friends) could do was to persist in their efforts to help her. I argued previously that the role of medicine should be to remove certain impediments that make it difficult or impossible for a patient to live and die virtuously. Although we cannot underestimate the intensity of her suffering, it is important to note that the only impediment to her happiness could not be removed by physicians since it consisted of Netty's own refusal to accept help. In the final instance, individuals should take some responsibility for living and dying with dignity.

### *Deciding for Infants*

In the previous section I argued that neither medical hopelessness nor despair is a sufficient reason for considering euthanasia, for in both types of cases something can be done to alleviate the person's suffering. The overwhelming majority of terminally- or chronically-ill patients fall in this category, but there are certainly exceptions. Aristotle remarks that 'what is fearful is not the same for all men; but we say there are things fearful even beyond human strength' (*N. Ethics* III.vii). When a patient's medical condition prohibits or prevents the possibility of him or her finding continued life at all meaningful or even bearable, it becomes appropriate to consider euthanasia as a final act of benevolence. Some patients experience relentless pain or extreme discomfort, but lack the cognitive ability or potential to find that suffering meaningful. Cases of this kind include infants suffering from Tay-Sachs disease, which involves increasing spasticity and dementia and usually results in death by age three or four, and Lesch-Nyhan disease, which involves uncontrollable spasms, compulsive self-mutilation, mental retardation and early death. These infants are unable to live without severe pain, and because they are unable to survive infancy or will never develop sufficient mental abilities, they will never reach a stage where they will be able to perceive their struggle to be meaningful. There are also cases when attempts to sustain life, while not altogether futile, would sustain a harm that would clearly be out of proportion to any benefit it could secure, for instance where a short prolongation of conscious life can only be secured at the cost of a massively distressing and burdensome resuscitation or surgical operation. In such cases life-sustaining treatment should be withheld or discontinued as a matter of policy. Consider the following case:

> J, an infant, had suffered severe brain damage at the time of his birth. He had a limited life expectancy, was unlikely to develop even limited intellectual abilities or be able to sit up or hold his head upright. Yet he was able to feel pain to the same extent as other infants. He suffered respiratory failure on several occasions, but was successfully resuscitated every time. Given his bleak prognosis, some members of the health-care staff thought that the infant should be allowed to die. However, the parents insisted that everything possible be done to save the infant's life. Finally the court was faced with the decision whether J should be ventilated again in the event of respiratory failure. The official solicitor thought that the court could not give an order to the effect that life-saving treatment be withheld because 'the Court is unable to evaluate the consequences of death, i.e., non-existence'. He reasoned that, however severe the infant's current sufferings and however bleak his prospects for the future, we cannot be sure that death would not be an even greater harm. He further argued that respect for the sanctity of human life and the requirements of public policy preclude attempts by the court to evaluate the quality of a disabled person's life.[10]

In recent decades much emphasis has been placed on the right of parents to make decisions on behalf of minor children, subject only to the condition that they do not neglect or abuse their children. This right, together with the assumption that continued life is a benefit, has made it difficult to object when parents want everything possible to be done to save the life of an infant or child whose life can only be one of suffering. Under certain circumstances, a utilitarian approach also lends support to the conclusion that doctors should respect the parents' decision in such cases. The implication of the aggregative nature of the principle of utility is that the parents' preferences and the satisfaction or happiness they might derive from raising such a child could outweigh the suffering experienced by the infant. Hence Singer argues that it would be wrong to end the life of the most gravely defective infant if its parents want it to live as long as possible (1979:132).

From a virtue-based perspective it is clear that prolonging the life of an infant whose life would be one of gross, irremediable and uncompensated pain and suffering, would certainly not be an act of kindness or respect. Saving its life would impose upon it a life sentence of suffering. We should note that there is a significant difference between infants and adults in this regard. An adult who suffers from a terminal condition may experience the last months or days of her life as a stage of growth, despite severe pain or discomfort. However, an infant suffering from a similar condition lacks the ability to interpret its situation, whatever its level of consciousness, so that its suffering can only be devoid of

---

[10] *Re J (a minor), 1990, 3 All England Rights 930.*

meaning. In such cases it would be the utmost gesture of kindness to end life as quickly and painlessly as possible, thus not condemning the infant to death, but sparing him or her from the agony of a prolonged dying process. To conclude on the basis of a quality-of-life judgement that the infant should be allowed to die does not amount to a judgement about the infant's inherent value or 'social worth'. In an ethic guided by the virtue of compassion, taking account of quality of life means being concerned on behalf of the patient about his or her capacity for future happiness, development and well-being. Such assessments exclude consideration of the likely financial cost of long-term care to the family, hospital and society.[11]

No doubt those who favour continuing treatment in such cases mean well (i.e., have benevolent intentions). However, being truly virtuous does not only involve having certain inclinations and sentiments; it also requires the possession of certain skills necessary for accomplishing one's goals. We can describe someone as having the virtue of benevolence if he tries to be beneficent, whether or not he has much success at accomplishing his goals. But to be benevolent in its full or ideal form one must also possess the other skills or virtues needed for doing what, as a benevolent person, one wishes to do. Responsible benevolence requires the intellectual virtues of *phronesis* (practical wisdom), which allows one to judge whether a certain end is worth striving for; as well as technical skills (*techne*) and medical knowledge (*episteme*) necessary to diagnose accurately, predict the likely outcome and assess the patient's current level of functioning.

If the morality of euthanasia depends on the agent's motivation and intention, there is no significant moral difference between active and passive euthanasia. Once it has been decided that death is a desirable end, the means by which death is brought about should be dictated by the specific circumstances. In most cases these infants will die soon after life-sustaining treatment is withdrawn, and can be kept free of pain or discomfort. However, in some cases withdrawal of life-sustaining treatment will leave the infant to suffer for days or weeks, so that it might be necessary to actively hasten death.

The above kinds of cases have to be distinguished from cases where the infant's medical condition, although properly described as an abnormality, does not necessarily involve an extraordinary amount of suffering, such as haemophilia, Down's syndrome, blindness, less severe forms of spina bifida and some forms of infantile paralysis. Infants born with such abnormalities are sometimes allowed to die because it is felt that as their abilities and potential for development are limited, their lives are not worth living. Parents are often less than willing to raise such infants since they will lack some or all of the qualities that are highly valued in contemporary societies, such as physical beauty, intelligence, athletic prowess and independence. Although these considerations are clearly not sufficient to justify euthanasia, what allows for the justification of letting such infants die is the

---

[11] Of course, lack of resources might make it impossible to provide each and every patient with the necessary care. It is important to notice that allowing an infant to die because of a shortage of resources does not amount to euthanasia at all. Instead, it is a decision about the distribution of resources based on considerations of justice.

view that the obligation of beneficence is not as stringent as the obligation of non-maleficence, with the implication that failing to prevent death from natural causes is acceptable while direct killing is wrong.

A virtue-based approach shows the error of this kind of reasoning. It is clear that we cannot cite compassion as an appropriate motive for euthanasia, since strictly speaking, these people do not (or need not) 'suffer from' these abnormalities. Of course, their medical condition does create special needs, and these needs can be the cause of much suffering if they are not met. Yet it is true of all human beings that they will suffer if their needs are not met. The mere fact that certain groups of individuals are more dependent than others or have needs that differ from the needs of the majority, is not sufficient reason for making them the objects of one's compassion. For instance, infants with Down's syndrome are capable of living very contented and happy lives, of forming affectionate relationships, of playing simple games, and so forth. The abilities of people with spina bifida may be limited, but their capacity for living worth-while lives are not.

Allowing such an infant to die usually does not stem from compassion or a consideration of the infant's good, but from the judgement that it would be a burden on its parents or on society. Those who do feel compassion for such infants do so on the basis of an erroneous belief that they will lead impoverished lives. It is true, for instance, that most of us would not be happy spending our days playing simple games, but people with Down's syndrome simply do not feel deprived because they are unable to participate in all kinds of 'higher intellectual activities'. The erroneously compassionate imagine being in *x*'s situation, but fail to make the further adjustments required to imagine being *x* in *x*'s situation. People without disabilities often imagine that the experience of disability is one of hopelessness, limitation and loss. A good illustration of how the unwarranted presumption of dysfunction is based on inappropriate feelings of compassion is the State of Oregon's 1992 attempt to ration health care. The aim was to ration health care by disallowing or diminishing medical treatment with reference to whether the patient would be left with a disability. Oregon's policies grew out of a telephone survey of able-bodied individuals who surmised, for example, that if they were confined to a wheelchair, they would rather be dead. Because people without disabilities believe that impairment must be experienced as irrevocable loss, it seems plausible to them that individuals with disabilities are likely to be depressed and despondent. Yet there is no evidence to support the conclusion that individuals with disabilities are at special risk of depression or suicide (Silvers 1998:139-141).

### *Involuntary Euthanasia*

In my discussion of the Assen case I argued that neither Netty's desire to die, nor her own perception of her situation as one of despair, justify euthanasia since bringing about an earlier death was not the only way to end her suffering. In this section I discuss a case where the patient does not wish to die, but suffers such extreme agony that we might think it in her best interest to be euthanised. If consideration of a patient's best interest and her capacity to benefit overrides her wishes, it would seem to follow that involuntary euthanasia is sometimes morally acceptable.

The following case is reconstructed from one mentioned by Hendin (1998:95) in his study of the practice of euthanasia in the Netherlands:

> Maria is a Catholic nun and dying of ovarian cancer in a nursing home in Rotterdam. She has long accepted death and has spent many hours praying to God for mercy. Pain medication has brought some relief, and although she never complains about pain or discomfort, Dr. van Riet can see that for long periods of the day she is in excruciating pain. He also knows that she only has a few days, perhaps weeks, to live. Knowing that her religious convictions do not permit her to ask for death, Van Riet decides it would be better to terminate her life quickly and painlessly. He later justifies his decision by explaining that the severity of her suffering rendered Maria incompetent to make a rational decision. Any reasonable person would want their lives to be ended in similar circumstances, and her wish to struggle to the end demonstrates her lack of autonomy.

It was certainly appropriate for the physician to feel compassion for the dying nun, and it is understandable that he thought someone who suffers such excruciating pain would be better off dead. But had Van Riet taken her religious beliefs seriously, had he respected her as a person, he would have realised that it was not in her best interest to avoid suffering. Her religious conviction not only prevented her from requesting death, it also provided her with a means of rendering that suffering meaningful. It is irrelevant whether the nun was competent to make a decision, whatever the criterion of competence one uses. For devoted members of the Catholic Church avoiding hardship is not of central importance, since they believe suffering has a divine purpose.

Involuntary euthanasia is morally unacceptable because patients who choose to struggle to the end clearly find life meaningful, despite (or even because of) what might appear to others to be intolerable suffering. As we have seen in previous chapters, human beings have devised various ways of coping with pain or suffering by interpreting it as a meaningful experience in life. For instance, John Hick (1966) argues that suffering forms part of the process of 'soul-making' by providing both the sufferer and the compassionate onlooker with an opportunity for moral growth. But it is not only religious people who think it very important to struggle to the end. For instance, Nietzsche criticises those who 'have no thought of the personal necessity of distress' (1974:269). He thinks that suffering serves to strengthen one's character by providing an opportunity for courage: '[A] loss is a loss for barely one hour; somehow it brings us some gift from heaven – new strength, for example, or at least a new opportunity for strength' (1974:256).

Although we might be of a different opinion, there is no need to enter into a debate with the Christian martyrs or the Nietzschean heroes about whether suffering is indeed meaningful. Here we have to agree with post-modernists that there can only be different interpretations of suffering, and that there is no Truth to be discovered regarding its meaning or significance. However, although these opinions may be characterised by a certain arbitrariness or relativity, this does not mean that we need not take them seriously. It is important for physicians and other caregivers to respect these deeply held beliefs and opinions, not because they are rational or expressed by autonomous individuals, but for the simple reason that a patient's view on the meaning of suffering will, to a significant extent, determine what it means for him or her to die with dignity. Only in this way we can combine the Aristotelian pursuit of the single goal of a virtuous life with the reality of cultural and religious pluralism that has come to characterise contemporary Western societies.

That involuntary euthanasia is morally wrong does not imply voluntary euthanasia is always acceptable. Whereas the desire or wish to continue living indicates that the person finds his life meaningful – despite what others might consider to be unbearable suffering – the wish to die does not necessarily show that the person's life is or should remain devoid of meaningful experiences. The attempt by many supporters of the autonomy movement to specify a set of absolute rules and regulations based on the competent patient's right to self-determination ignores the fallibility not only of patients, but of human beings in general. The shortcomings of the autonomy model are most apparent in the context of end-of-life decision-making. While causing significant pain or suffering, terminal or chronic diseases often rob patients of the ability to make decisions based on a rational calculation of the harms and benefits of alternative modes of treatment. The following case, related by a doctor at a nursing home in Amsterdam, illustrates the moral dilemma that arises as a result:

> Dolf is 43 and has been ill with AIDS for a few years. About ten months ago he asked first his GP, then his consultant, then his neurologist and finally his psychiatrist for an end to his life. They all said 'No, you're doing far too well at the moment'.
>
> He now repeats his request to Dr. Bert Keizer, whose answer to Dolf's sister is, 'No, he's too far gone now'.
>
> Dolf's sister replies: 'First he's not ill enough, now he's too ill. What kind of game is this? How in God's name should that boy time his downfall so he can call you at precisely the right moment? Who knows that point in time where his misery and his intellect, the one going up, the other going down, intersect? Is there a consensus about this? And you were the one who gave us the impression that we could always talk about the possibility of euthanasia. But now when it comes down to it, you run away'.
>
> Keizer muses to himself, 'It really can't be done, for Dolf is rather empty inside. It doesn't matter what you ask him, his strangely emphatic answer is always, "Right, that's exactly what I mean"' (Keizer 1997:300).

Keizer continues his discussion of this case by explaining in quite some detail why he thinks Dolf is incompetent. Yet there is no discussion of the nature or seriousness of Dolf's suffering. Dolf's sister might be wrong in thinking that his suffering has become worse – gradual loss of mental awareness tends to decrease, not increase, a patient's mental anguish. One is also left to wonder why Dolf, when he was considered to be 'doing far too well' to be a suitable candidate for euthanasia, repeatedly asked to be killed. Dolf was either depressed by the thought of a premature and undignified death, or the team of doctors underestimated the extent of his physical pain and discomfort.

Even if we accept Keizer's judgement of incompetence, the lack of information about the nature and seriousness of Dolf's suffering renders us unable to make a conclusive judgement about the acceptability of euthanasia in his case. To be able to determine whether euthanasia will be an act of compassion and benevolence, we need the kind of knowledge and skills that only physicians can offer. For the sake of argument, we can assume that Dolf, like the typical AIDS-patient, suffered from a series of opportunistic infections, such as *Pneumocystis carinii* pneumonia (PCP), meningitis, ear infections and sinusitis. These infections, together with the cocktail of drugs taken to combat them, are usually the cause of extreme pain and discomfort to patients, who also know that the chances of recovering from AIDS are very low indeed, perhaps even non-existent. Apart from the assault of bacterial infections on the body, AIDS-patients often develop a brain infection, such as toxoplasmosis or brain lymphoma. Initially, these infections cause memory loss, light-headedness, dizziness and loss of balance, and finally result in loss of consciousness.

If his sister is correct in thinking that Dolf's suffering has become more severe, despite his fading mental abilities, it seems arbitrary to refuse euthanasia solely on the basis of an assessment of his present level of competence. The fact that he has recently repeated his wish to die to Keizer need not be seen as the fully voluntary and rational decision of an autonomous person, but does indicate that Dolf is still suffering unbearably. And given his repeated requests to be killed over the past few months, before the onset of the brain infection, it is clear that hastening death will not conflict with Dolf's values and beliefs. It will also put an end to the suffering he is no longer able to find meaningful yet from which there is no respite other than loss of consciousness.

If, on the other hand, the brain infection has robbed him of awareness of pain and discomfort, euthanasia is no longer necessary. The significance of Dolf's mental condition is not, as Keizer would have it, the fact that it renders him incompetent to make a decision. The reason that euthanasia is morally inappropriate is not that Dolf cannot give his free and fully informed consent to life-shortening treatment, but that he is no longer suffering. The most important thing Keizer can do under these circumstances is to alleviate the sister's fears and concerns by assuring her that her brother has already been released from suffering, for she has now become the appropriate object of compassion.

## The Role of Family in Death and Dying: The Area of Uncertainty

Having identified the kinds of cases in which euthanasia is or is not morally acceptable, we are still left with a fairly large grey area in which the moral status of euthanasia is uncertain. In some cases it is unclear whether to provide or to continue providing life-sustaining treatment. Examples include cases in which the chances of treatment achieving something worthwhile are, while not hopeless, very low indeed, or where the harm-benefit ratio of a particular treatment would be regarded by some as tolerable while others would consider it disproportionate. In other cases, for example where there is uncertainty as to whether or to what extent a patient is experiencing significant pain or discomfort, it is unclear whether the moment of death should be advanced. There might also be uncertainty with regard to the patient's wishes or beliefs regarding euthanasia. When the morality of a proposed course of action falls into this grey area, the only way in which a responsible choice can be reached is through a discussion, involving all interested parties, of the patient's best interest, his values and beliefs, as well as the way in which the decision will affect family members. In what follows, I discuss each of these factors in more detail.

### *The Patient's Interests*

When attempting to determine whether continued life would be in a patient's best interest, it is important to understand the nature or quality of the patient's experiences. Compassion plays a central part in such decision-making since, as we have seen, it involves an attempt to understand a person's situation by imagining what she, given her beliefs, values and circumstances, is undergoing. Compassion is a mean between sympathy, which involves a complete emotional identification with the sufferer and failure to take a critical or objective distance, and the scientific attitude that regards the patient as an object or an instance of disease. To reach a responsible decision it is necessary that family members and health-care professionals engage in a discussion of the patient's interests. Family members will usually be in the best position to form a compassionate understanding of the patient's situation because they are familiar with her values and beliefs. But they cannot be left to make the decision on their own. Health-care professionals should make sure that the family understands the relevant medical facts, including, for instance, the extent to which the patient is aware of her surroundings, her capacity for experiencing pleasure and pain, her life expectancy and the quality of life she is likely to have if she survives.

It is important that those charged with the responsibility to make the decision understand that there is no single right answer to moral questions such as these. Too often people feel haunted by the thought that they might have made the wrong decision, as if the 'right decision' already exists and will one day be revealed to them. In a virtue-based approach the way in which the decision is made will be just as, if not more significant than the content of the decision. The best that can be done in such cases is to come to a decision based on a careful consideration of the patient's medical condition, her future possibilities, and the way in which her values and beliefs might impact on her ability to appreciate life despite pain and discomfort.

*The Patient's Wishes, Values and Beliefs*

Perhaps the most difficult kind of case is where patients with limited mental capacities refuse to consent to treatment thought to be in their best interest. In such cases the autonomy model allows forcible intervention on the grounds that the patient is incompetent to refuse or consent to treatment. I have argued that respect for patients should not simply be interpreted as requiring respect for the wishes of a competent patient. Autonomy should not be a requirement or condition for being treated with respect. Autonomists often overlook the fact that forcing medical treatment on an incompetent patient can be a source of great pain and humiliation. A patient can have strong preferences against treatment, even if he is considered to be incompetent or non-autonomous, and even if these preferences are not well grounded in reality or in the patient's previously authentic value system. When deciding whether to provide such treatment it should be considered whether the benefits do outweigh the pain and suffering brought about by forcing it on an unwilling patient.

If the patient is unconscious or semiconscious the goal of medical decision-making should be to further the patient's interests and to treat the patient in ways that do not conflict with her values and beliefs. In my discussion of the cases of Nancy Cruzan, Dr. Clarke and 'Gary Austin' I argued that the wishes of comatose or unconscious patients, whether they were verbally expressed or stated in the form of an advance directive, should not be the decisive factor in determining whether to provide life-sustaining treatment. Since these patients are unable to experience such treatment as invasive or burdensome, the most important consideration is their capacity to benefit from it. However, when it is unclear whether treatment will be beneficial, advance directives can give those who have to make the decision an indication of whether the patient is likely to find continued life worth living.

*The Family's Interests*

In modern medical contexts patients are often expected to make autonomous decisions about their own health without consulting family members and without considering their wishes and interests. A patient who chooses to die because she thinks it will relieve the burden on her family is often seen as less than autonomous. In the same way, surrogate decision-makers are expected to make a decision about an individual patient's medical treatment without considering the way in which they themselves will be affected by the decision. However, such individualistic decision-making conflicts with the way in which family members reach important decisions. Within families it is usually understood that the interests of all members have to be considered when deciding about the treatment of one member. It is therefore to be expected that the family's decision will be influenced by the impact on their own lives of continued treatment. This should not be a cause of concern so long as the case originally falls within the area of uncertainty. As I have argued in Chapter Four, being moral does not require self-sacrifice. We cannot expect or demand of people that they sacrifice their own interests – whether these be occupational, educational, financial, or otherwise – to care for a chronically-ill patient at home for indefinite periods, or to keep him alive for a few more weeks.

We also need to keep in mind that the patient's potential or ability to live a tolerable life may well turn on the family's willingness to spend a considerable amount of their time and resources in order to care for the sick person. If an infant with major physical and mental disabilities is kept alive against the parents' wishes it is extremely unlikely that it will ever be able to live a decent or tolerable life. When reaching a decision in difficult cases it is also necessary to consider the socio-economic circumstances of the family or those who would be responsible for taking care of the patient, since these circumstances will have a significant bearing on the patient's quality of life. It needs to be considered, for instance, whether they have sufficient financial resources to take care of the patient, whether the family can afford the loss of income brought about by having to provide this care, how it will affect their ability to meet responsibilities towards dependent children or elderly people, whether an adequate support network is available, and so forth.

A possible objection to this line of argument is that it can be used to justify euthanasia whenever parents or family-members are unwilling or unable to take care of the patient. After all, no one is able to live a tolerable life if their basic needs are not met, and all infants and old or fragile persons place a significant burden on caregivers. I argued before that it is morally unacceptable to allow infants with conditions such as Down's syndrome to die, since it would stem from self-interest rather than a consideration of the infant's interests. The question is therefore whether there is any difference between an infant with Down's syndrome, and an infant who has more severe abnormalities yet who is capable, with a considerable amount of care, of enjoying an acceptable quality of life. If the burden on the parents of raising the infant does not count as a justification for euthanasia in the first case, why should it be accepted as justification in the second?

In response I must admit that the difference is one of degree, rather than kind. The acceptability of euthanasia in these cases will to a large degree depend on the available resources within the family and the community to care for children with disabilities. In developing countries it may be impossible for a child with Down's syndrome to live a happy life or even to survive. In most developed countries it is not plausible to argue that it is in the best interest of such infants to die, since it is possible to provide in their needs and to ensure that they continue to live happy lives. It is for this reason that we cannot make a universal judgement about the morality of treating such infants. We can only formulate a policy, or create a law based on a consideration of the circumstances of the specific society. Yet there will remain cases where significant doubt exists as to whether an infant will ever be able to live a fulfilling life. In such cases the parents' decision should be respected since their willingness to sacrifice almost all of their time and resources to provide it with the best care possible could make the decisive difference as to whether the infant is able to live a good life. We cannot expect any person to sacrifice his or her life for another human being whose potential for living a good life, even with constant care and attention, is highly questionable.

## Conclusion

Michael Ondaatje's film, *The English Patient,* contains many images of healing and nurturing, set against the background of an arid and hostile landscape and the cruelties of war. The patient survives an aeroplane crash and is found in the desert by a group of Bedouin men, who dress his wounds and take care of him. Given the severity of his injuries one wonders whether it would have been kinder to let him die, but the journey that ensues shows that life can be meaningful despite pain and disability. The patient finally ends up in the care of a nurse who leaves the travelling group of patients and nurses so that he can be made more comfortable. The various roles played by morphine represent some of the faces of medicine. The traditional or 'proper' function of morphine is to relieve physical pain, which the nurse Hana does routinely. Caravaggio uses it to relieve his mental suffering brought about by the horrors of war. Hana appears to know that he steals morphine from her but turns a blind eye. Finally, morphine becomes the instrument of euthanasia. Apart from the different functions or uses of medicine, we see different sides of Hana's character. We meet her as a nurse in uniform, who is motivated by a sense of duty to relieve the patient's pain and to offer comfort and companionship. For instance, when he asks her why she has taken it upon herself to care for him, she answers, 'Because I am a nurse'. As she sheds the uniform we become acquainted with her as a lover and friend so that, when the English patient finally indicates that he is ready to die, it is as a friend that she complies. We are left to wonder which of these uses or roles of medicine constitute its true or legitimate role.

If 'euthanasia' is understood in the traditional sense of 'a good death', the central moral question we must ask is 'How can we make it possible for the suffering person to live and die with honour and dignity?' Although this question is far too broad to be dealt with in a single book, I have made an attempt to go some way towards addressing it in the previous chapters. The virtues of compassion, benevolence, and respect are a response to the various features of suffering: loneliness, helplessness and loss of self-respect. My focus in the present chapter was with the morality of euthanasia, understood in the narrower sense of intentionally ending a person's life or allowing a person to die. The first question that can be asked in this regard is whether and when euthanasia can be justified as a compassionate, benevolent and respectful response to the patient's plight. The second is whether euthanasia is consistent with the goals of medicine, in other words, whether physicians and other health-care professionals should become involved in euthanasia and assisted-suicide. One might agree that euthanasia or assisted suicide is sometimes a virtuous act motivated by compassion and intended to be for the benefit of the patient, but for precisely this reason think it more appropriate for a close relative or friend to perform it.

With regard to the first question, I have argued that a virtue-ethical approach to the questions surrounding euthanasia does allow us to formulate a set of rules that can be used to decide about the moral acceptability of intentionally terminating or shortening a person's life. Such rules may include:

1. Patients in an irreversible coma should be allowed to die, regardless of their previously stated wishes or the wishes of the family.
2. Patients who are currently unconscious but who have a good chance of being returned to reasonable health should receive life-sustaining treatment, regardless of their previously stated wishes or the wishes of the family.
3. Infants should be allowed to die if their medical condition causes them to suffer unmitigated and incessant pain and/or discomfort, regardless of the parents' wishes.
4. Euthanasia should not be considered solely on the basis of either medical hopelessness (terminal or incurable disease or illness) or psychological suffering.
5. Where a patient is able to communicate his views but has not requested euthanasia, it is impermissible to end his life (or allow him to die) as a means of relieving suffering (involuntary 'euthanasia').
6. Euthanasia is acceptable if a patient's physical condition brings about extreme suffering, and if it is known with reasonable certainty that that patient has no religious or other objections to euthanasia.

These rules do not express the essential difference between right and wrong and are not based on a single moral principle. Instead, they are summaries of decisions made on the basis of three considerations in particular, namely whether compassion is an appropriate motive for euthanasia, whether death is a desirable end, and whether euthanasia conveys respect for the patient. The consensus reached in specific kinds of cases can be translated into policies that outline the conditions in which withdrawing or withholding life-sustaining treatment is morally required. A set of rules can also be formulated that would state the conditions in which intentionally ending a patient's life is not only immoral, but intolerable within the medical community as well as society in general. These policies, if adequately formulated, should provide us with some protection against abuse by individual health-care professionals. They should also help to safeguard us against the threat of the slippery slope. Yet it is important to note that no set of rules and no policy will ever provide a guarantee that physicians and other health-care professionals will not abuse their power. No matter how carefully formulated, a rule or policy will always leave room for interpretation. We can only rely on the relevant authorities to enforce these rules and to see to it that the correct procedures are followed, and trust, as we already do, that medical professionals are able to make morally-responsible decisions.

With regard to the second question mentioned above, I hope to have shown that physicians are in the best position to practise euthanasia or assisted suicide as an act of *responsible* benevolence, since they are able more accurately to assess the patient's condition, including such factors as whether and how much the patient is suffering, whether there is significant hope of recovery, and the quality of life they can expect to have if they survive the illness. Their special knowledge and skills also enable physicians to bring about death while minimising pain and discomfort. For instance, they will be able to predict more accurately whether withdrawing life-sustaining treatment will result in the patient dying a slow and painful death, which could make active euthanasia a morally-desirable alternative.

Yet we cannot expect to completely substitute rule-following for careful and arduous moral decision-making. It is not only impossible, but also undesirable to attempt to specify universal rules and regulations that are supposed to provide an answer to every ethical dilemma we may encounter. In many cases it will be impossible to determine with any degree of certainty whether compassion is an appropriate motive for euthanasia, whether death is a desirable end, and whether euthanasia will be an act of respect. Once it has been decided that a case falls into the grey area of uncertainty, a decision can only be reached after a careful discussion involving all interested parties. In these cases family and friends have a central role to play in the decision-making procedure. They should be informed by physicians of the relevant medical facts and assisted, if possible, by an independent third party, such as a member of an ethical committee or a social worker. While time-consuming and emotionally demanding, this discussion has the value of providing some comfort and reassurance to everyone involved that the decision taken was in the patient's best interest and did not conflict with her values and beliefs.

Advancing the hour of a patient's death should only be considered as a last resort, for it is only then that we are able to say that euthanasia is the kindest or most benevolent act among the available alternatives. The Hospice movement has argued that euthanasia is unnecessary because all suffering can be relieved if caregivers are sufficiently skilful and compassionate, and to a certain extent I agree. Caregivers can have a significant influence on whether a person is able to find the dying process meaningful and to bear the pain and discomfort that often precede death. Yet I have attempted to show that euthanasia and compassionate care are not mutually exclusive. We should not and cannot *demand* of someone to endure suffering with heroic courage. Gay-Williams writes that every human being has a natural inclination to continue living, and that the organisation of the human body and our patterns of behavioural responses make the continuation of life a natural goal. Euthanasia therefore does violence to our dignity, which comes from seeking our ends (1992:222-223). He fails to note that the organisation of the human body also makes death inevitable, and a persistent and obsessive denial of this reality by those who hope for a miraculous recovery or a spontaneous remission amounts to demanding of medicine a power it does not possess. If our dignity comes from seeking our ends, there are certainly circumstances in which death is a desirable end.

# Bibliography


Abernethy, V. 1984. 'Compassion, control, and decisions about competency', *American Journal of Psychiatry*, 141(1):53-58.

Acton, H.B. 1970. *Kant's Moral Philosophy*. London: Macmillan.

Anscombe, G.E.M. 1997. 'Modern moral philosophy', in R. Crisp and M. Slote (eds.) *Virtue Ethics*. New York: Oxford University Press.

Aristotle. 1990. *Nicomachean Ethics*. D. Ross (trans.) Oxford and New York: Oxford University Press.

Aristotle. 1991. *On Rhetoric. A theory of civic discourse*. G.A. Kennedy (trans.) New York and Oxford: Oxford University Press.

Aristotle. 1992. *Politics*. T.A. Sinclair (trans.) London: Penguin Books.

Aristotle. 1999. *Poetics*. K. McLeish (trans.) London: Nick Hern Books.

Battin, M.P. 1998. 'Physician-assisted suicide: Safe, legal, rare?', in M.P. Battin, R. Rhodes and A. Silvers (eds.) *Physician Assisted Suicide: Expanding the debate*. New York and London: Routledge.

Battin, M.P., Rhodes, R. and Silvers, A. 1998. *Physician Assisted Suicide: Expanding the debate*. New York and London: Routledge.

Baumrin, B. 1998. 'Physician, stay thy hand!', in M.P. Battin, R. Rhodes and A. Silvers (eds.) *Physician Assisted Suicide: Expanding the debate*. New York and London: Routledge.

Beauchamp, T.L. and Childress, J.F. 1994. *Principles of Biomedical Ethics* (4th edition). New York and Oxford: Oxford University Press.

Beiner, R. 1992. 'The moral vocabulary of liberalism', in J.W. Chapman and W.A. Galston (eds.) *Virtue*. New York and London: New York University Press.

Bernstein, R.J. 1986. *Philosophical Profiles: Essays in a pragmatic mode*. Philadelphia: University of Pennsylvania Press.

Bierce, A. 1993. 'Taking oneself off', in J. Miller (ed.) *On Suicide: Great writers on the ultimate question*. San Francisco: Chronicle Books.

Blum, L. 1980. 'Compassion', in A.O. Rorty (ed.) *Explaining Emotions*. London: University of California Press.

Bodemer, C.W. 1979. 'Physicians and the dying: A historical sketch', *The Journal of Family Practice*, 9(5):827-832.

Boeyink, D.E. 1974. 'Pain and suffering', *Journal of Religious Ethics*, 2:85-98.

Bok, S. 1998. 'Euthanasia', in G. Dworkin, R.G. Frey, and S. Bok (eds.) *Euthanasia and Physician-Assisted Suicide: For and against*. Cambridge: Cambridge University Press.

Borchert, D.M. and Stewart, D. 1986. *Exploring Ethics*. New York: Macmillan.

Brazier, M. 1991. 'Competence, consent and proxy consents', in M. Brazier and M. Lobjoit (eds.) *Protecting the Vulnerable: Autonomy and consent in health care.* London and New York: Routledge.

Buytendijk, F.J.J. 1961. *Pain.* E. O'Shiel (trans.) Westport, Connecticut: Greenwood Press.

Campbell, A.G.M. and McHaffie, H.E. 1995. 'Prolonging life and allowing death: infants', *Journal of Medical Ethics*, 21:339-344.

Campbell, A.V. 1984. *Moderated Love: A theology of professional care.* London: S.P.C.K.

Campbell, A.V. 1991. 'Dependency revisited: The limits of autonomy in medical ethics', in M. Brazier and M. Lobjoit (eds.) *Protecting the Vulnerable: Autonomy and consent in health care.* London and New York: Routledge.

Campbell, C. 1993, 'Dying well: Hospice confronts physician-assisted suicide', *Biolaw* 11(4):29-36.

Camus, A. 1993. 'The myth of Sisyphus', in J. Miller (ed.) *On Suicide: Great writers on the ultimate question.* San Francisco: Chronicle Books.

Childress, J.F. 1982. *Who Should Decide? Paternalism in health care.* Oxford and New York: Oxford University Press.

Choron, J. 1963. *Death and Western Thought.* New York: Macmillan.

Collins, D.B. 1992. *Medical Law in New Zealand.* Wellington: Booker and Friend.

Conrad, L.I., Neve, M., Nutton V., Porter, R. and Wear, A. 1995. *The Western Medical Tradition: 800 BC to AD 1800.* Cambridge: Cambridge University Press.

Deigh, J. 1995. 'Ethics and universalizability', *Ethics*, 105(July):743-763.

Dworkin, G. 1998. 'The nature of medicine', in G. Dworkin, R.G. Frey, and S. Bok (eds.) *Euthanasia and Physician-Assisted Suicide: For and against.* Cambridge: Cambridge University Press.

Dworkin, G., Frey, R.G. and Bok, S. 1998. *Euthanasia and Physician-Assisted Suicide: For and against.* Cambridge: Cambridge University Press.

Dyck, A. 1975. 'Beneficent euthanasia and benemortasia: Alternative views on mercy', in M. Kohl (ed.) *Beneficent Euthanasia.* Buffalo, NY: Prometheus Books.

Feinberg, J. 1978. 'Voluntary euthanasia and the inalienable right to life', *Philosophy and Public Affairs*, 7(2):93-123.

Feldman, F. 1988. 'Kantian Ethics', in L.P. Pojman (ed.) *Ethical Theory: Classical and contemporary readings.* Belmont, CA: Wadsworth.

Fletcher, J. 1960. *Morals and Medicine.* Boston: Beacon Press.

Fletcher, J. 1975. 'The "right" to live and the "right" to die', in M. Kohl (ed.) *Beneficent Euthanasia.* Buffalo, NY: Prometheus Books.

Flyvbjerg, B. 1993. 'Aristotle, Foucault and Progressive *Phronesis*: Outline of an applied ethics for sustainable development', in E.R. Winkler and J.R. Coombs (eds.) *Applied Ethics: A reader.* Cambridge, MA: Basil Blackwell.

Foot, P. 1977. 'Euthanasia', *Philosophy and Public Affairs*, 6(2):85-112.

Foot, P. 1994. 'Nietzsche's immoralism', in R. Schacht (ed.) *Nietzsche, Genealogy, Morality: Essays on Nietzsche's 'Genealogy of Morals'*. Berkeley and Los Angeles: University of California Press.

Frankena, W.K. 1987. 'Beneficence/benevolence', *Social Philosophy and Policy*, 4(2):20.

Frankena, W.K. 1988. 'A critique of virtue-based ethical systems', in L.P. Pojman (ed.) *Ethical Theory: Classical and contemporary readings*. Belmont, CA: Wadsworth.

Freeman, J.M. 1972. 'Is there a right to die – quickly?', *The Journal of Pediatrics*, 80(5):904-905.

Furlow, T.W. 1975. 'Euthanasia and the tyranny of technology', in M. Kohl (ed.) *Beneficent Euthanasia*. Buffalo, NY: Prometheus Books.

Gay-Williams, J. 1979. 'The Wrongfulness of Euthanasia', in R. Munson (ed.) *Intervention and Reflection: Basic issues in medical ethics*. Belmont, CA: Wadsworth.

Gennaro, R.J. 1996. 'The relevance of intentions in morality and euthanasia', *International Philosophical Quarterly*, 36(2):217-227.

Gillon, R. 1969. 'Suicide and voluntary euthanasia: Historical perspectives', in A.B. Downing (ed.) *Euthanasia and the Right to Death: The case for voluntary euthanasia*. London: Peter Owen.

Gillon, R. 1991. 'Research on the vulnerable: An ethical overview', in M. Brazier and M. Lobjoit (eds.) *Protecting the Vulnerable: Autonomy and consent in health care*. London and New York: Routledge.

Gillon, R. (ed.) 1994. *Principles of Health Care Ethics*. Chichester: John Wiley and Sons.

Gillon, R. 1995. *Philosophical Medical Ethics*. London: John Wiley and Sons.

Glaser, B.G. and Strauss, A.L. 1968. *Time For Dying*. Chicago: Aldine.

Gordon, R.M. 1995. 'Sympathy, simulation, and the impartial spectator', *Ethics*, 105(July):727-742.

Hamlyn, D.W. 1988. *A History of Western Philosophy*. Middlesex: Penguin Books.

Hare, R.M. 1977. 'Medical ethics: Can the moral philosopher help?', in S.F. Spicker and H. Engelhardt (eds.) *Philosophical Medical Ethics: Its nature and significance*. Boston and Dordrecht: Reidel.

Hauerwas, S. 1986. *Suffering Presence*. Indiana: Notre Dame Press.

Hendin, H. 1998. *Seduced by Death: Doctors, patients, and assisted suicide*. New York and London: W.W. Norton and Company.

Henley, L., Benatar, S.R., Robertson, B.A. and Ensink, K. 1995. 'Informed consent – a survey of doctors' practices in South Africa', *South African Medical Journal*, 85(12):1273-1278.

Hick, J. 1966. *Evil and the God of Love*. London: Macmillan.

Hilberg, R. 1985. *The Destruction of the European Jews*. New York: Holmes and Meier.

*Holy Bible.* 1983. (Good News edition) Bible Society of South Africa: Cape Town.

Hume, D. 1960. *A Treatise of Human Nature.* L.A. Selby-Bigge (ed.) Oxford: Clarendon Press.

Hume, D. 1961. *An Enquiry Concerning the Principles of Morals.* L.A. Selby-Bigge (ed.) Oxford: Clarendon Press.

Hursthouse, R. 1987. *Beginning Lives.* Oxford: Basil Blackwell.

Hursthouse, R. 1991. 'Virtue theory and abortion', *Philosophy and Public Affairs*, 20:223-246.

Hursthouse, R. 1995. 'Applying virtue ethics', in R. Hursthouse, G. Lawrence and W. Quinn (eds.) *Virtues and Reasons: Philippa Foot and Moral Theory.* Oxford: Clarendon Press.

Illich, I. 1975. *Medical Nemesis: The expropriation of health.* London: Calder and Boyars.

Jeske, D. 1997. 'Friendship, virtue, and impartiality', *Philosophy and Phenomenological Research*, 57(1):51-72.

Jones, W.H.S. 1923. *Hippocrates (vols. I and II).* London: William Heinemann.

Jonsen, A.R. 1977. 'Do no harm: Axiom of medical ethics', in S.F. Spicker and H. Engelhardt (eds.) *Philosophical Medical Ethics: Its nature and significance.* Boston and Dordrecht: Reidel.

Jonsen, A.R. 1990. *The New Medicine and the Old Ethics.* Cambridge, MA: Harvard University Press.

Kant, I. 1964. *The Metaphysical Principles of Virtue: Part II of the Metaphysics of Morals.* J. Ellington (trans.) New York: The Bobbs-Merill Company.

Kant, I. 1988. *Fundamental Principles of the Metaphysics of Morals.* T.K. Abbott (trans.) Buffalo, NY: Prometheus Books.

Kass, L.R. 1989. 'Neither for love nor money: Why doctors must not kill', *The Public Interest*, 94:25-46.

Kass, L.R. 1990. 'Death with dignity and the sanctity of life', *Commentary*, 89(3):33-43.

Keizer, B. 1997. *Dancing with Mister D: Notes on life and death.* London: Black Swan Books.

Kekes, J. 1987. 'Benevolence: A minor virtue', *Social Philosophy and Policy*, 4(2):21-36.

Keown, J. 1997. *Euthanasia Examined.* Cambridge: Cambridge University Press.

Kohl, M. 1974. *The Morality of Killing: Sanctity of life, abortion and euthanasia.* New York: Humanities Press.

Kohl, M. 1975. 'Voluntary beneficent euthanasia', in M. Kohl (ed.) *Beneficent Euthanasia.* Buffalo, NY: Prometheus Books.

Kohl, M. 1977. 'Euthanasia and the right to life', in S.F. Spicker and H. Engelhardt (eds.) *Philosophical Medical Ethics: Its nature and significance.* Boston and Dordrecht: Reidel.

Kübler-Ross, E. 1975. *Death: The final stage of growth.* New Jersey: Englewood Cliffs.

Landman, W.A. 1990. 'The morality of killing and causing suffering: Reasons for rejecting Peter Singer's pluralistic consequentialism', *South African Journal of Philosophy*, 9(4):159-171.

Lasagna, L. 1977. 'Discussion of "do no harm"', in S.F. Spicker and H. Engelhardt (eds.) *Philosophical Medical Ethics: Its nature and significance*. Boston and Dordrecht: Reidel.

Leary, P.M. 1997. 'History taking – a disappearing art?', *Pedmed*, 10(1):2.

Levi, P. 1993. 'Shame' (Excerpt from *The drowned and the saved*), in J. Miller (ed.) *On Suicide: Great writers on the ultimate question*. San Francisco: Chronicle Books.

Lidz, C.W., Meisel, A., Holden, J.L., Marx, J.H. and Munetz, M.R. 1982. 'Informed consent and the structure of medical care', in *President's Commission for the Study of Ethical Problems in Medicine and Behavioral Research. Making health care decisions: The ethical and legal implications of informed consent in the patient-practitioner relationship.* Vol. 2. Appendix C: *Empirical Studies of informed consent.*

Lidz, C.W., Meisel, A., Zerubavel, E., Carter, M., Sestak, R.M. and Roth, L.H. 1984. *Informed Consent. A study of decision making in psychiatry*. New York: Guilford Press.

Longrigg, J. 1993. *Greek Rational Medicine: Philosophy and medicine from Alcmaeon to the Alexandrians*. London and New York: Routledge.

Louden, R.B. 1997. 'On some vices of virtue ethics', in R. Crisp and M. Slote (eds.) *Virtue Ethics*. New York: Oxford University Press.

Lynn, J. 1995. 'Why I don't have a living will', in J.D. Arras and B. Steinbock (eds.) *Ethical Issues in Modern Medicine* (4th edition). Mountain View, CA: Mayfield.

MacIntyre, A. 1977. 'Patients as agents', in S.F. Spicker and H. Engelhardt (eds.) *Philosophical Medical Ethics: Its nature and significance*. Boston and Dordrecht: Reidel.

MacIntyre, A. 1990. *After Virtue: A study in moral theory* (2nd edition). London: Duckworth.

Martin, M.W. 1994. *Everyday Morality: An introduction to applied ethics* (2nd edition). Belmont, CA: Wadsworth.

McGee, R.R. 1976. 'To hell with those laws – Let's be good doctors', *Medical Economics*, 53:92-100.

Menard, B. and Perrone, C. 1994. *Hospice Care: An introduction and review of the evidence*. Arlington, VA: National Hospice Organization.

Menkiti, I.A. 1979. 'Person and community in African traditional thought', in R.A. Wright (ed.) *African Philosophy*. New York: University Press of America.

Mill, J.S. 1924. *Autobiography*. J.J. Coss (ed.) New York: Columbia University Press.

Mill, J.S. 1985. *On Liberty*. G. Himmelfarb (ed.) Middlesex: Penguin Books.

Mill, J.S. 1987. 'Utilitarianism', in A. Ryan (ed.) *Utilitarianism and Other Essays: J.S. Mill and Jeremy Bentham*. Middlesex: Penguin Books.

Morrison, K.F. 1988. *I am You: The hermeneutics of empathy in Western literature, theology and art*. Princeton: Princeton University Press.

Nesbitt, W. 1993. 'Euthanasia and the distinction between acts and omissions', *Journal of Applied Philosophy*, 10(2):253-256.

Nietzsche, F. 1967a. *On the Genealogy of Morals.* W. Kaufmann and R.J. Hollingdale (trans.) New York: Vintage Books.

Nietzsche, F. 1967b. *The Will to Power.* W. Kaufmann and R.J. Hollingdale (trans.) New York: Vintage Books.

Nietzsche, F. 1969. *Thus Spoke Zarathustra: A book for everyone and no one*. R.J. Hollingdale (trans.) Middlesex: Penguin Books.

Nietzsche, F. 1974. *The Gay Science With a Prelude in Rhymes and an Appendix of Songs.* W. Kaufmann (trans.) New York: Vintage Books.

Nietzsche, F. 1982. *Daybreak: Thoughts on the prejudices of morality.* R.J. Hollingdale (trans.) Cambridge and New York: Cambridge University Press.

Nietzsche, F. 1986. *Human, All Too Human: A book for free spirits.* R.J. Hollingdale (trans.) Cambridge: Cambridge University Press.

Nietzsche, F. 1989. *Beyond Good and Evil: Prelude to a philosophy of the future.* W. Kaufmann (trans.) New York: Vintage Books.

Nietzsche, F. 1990. *Twilight of the Idols* and *The Anti-Christ.* R.J. Hollingdale (trans.) London: Penguin Books.

Norman, R. 1986. *The Moral Philosophers*. Oxford: Clarendon Press.

Nozick, R. 1974. *Anarchy, State, and Utopia*. Oxford: Basil Blackwell.

Nuland, S.B. 1994. *How We Die.* London: Chatto and Windus.

Nussbaum, M.C. 1992. 'Tragedy and self-sufficiency: Plato and Aristotle on fear and pity', in A.O. Rorty (ed.) *Essays on Aristotle's Poetics*. Princeton: Princeton University Press.

Nussbaum, M.C. 1994. 'Pity and mercy: Nietzsche's stoicism', in R. Schacht (ed.) *Nietzsche, Genealogy, Morality: Essays on Nietzsche's 'Genealogy of Morals'*. Berkeley and Los Angeles: University of California Press.

Nussbaum, M.C. 1996. 'Compassion: The basic social emotion', *Social Philosophy and Policy*, 13(1):27-58.

Ondaatje, M. 1992. *The English Patient.* London: Picador Books.

Ortony, A., Clore, G.L. and Collins, A. 1988. *The Cognitive Structure of the Emotions*. Cambridge: Cambridge University Press.

Owens, J. 1977. 'Aristotelian ethics, medicine, and the changing nature of man', in S.F. Spicker and H. Engelhardt (eds.) *Philosophical Medical Ethics: Its nature and significance.* Boston and Dordrecht: Reidel.

*The Oxford English Dictionary* (OED). 1989. (2nd edition) Prepared by J.A. Simpson and E.S.C. Weiner. Oxford: Clarendon Press.

Paris, J.J. and Moreland, M.P. 1998. 'A Catholic perspective on physician-assisted suicide', in M.P. Battin, R. Rhodes and A. Silvers (eds.) *Physician Assisted Suicide: Expanding the debate*. New York and London: Routledge.

Pellegrino, E.D. and Thomasma, D.C. 1988. *For the Patient's Good: The restoration of beneficence in health care.* New York and Oxford: Oxford University Press.

Pellegrino, E.D. and Thomasma, D.C. 1993. *The Virtues in Medical Practice.* New York and Oxford: Oxford University Press.

Peschel, R.E. and Peschel, E.R. 1993. 'Selective empathy', in H.M. Spiro, M.G. McCrea Curnen, E.R. Peschel and D. St. James (eds.) *Empathy and the Practice of Medicine: Beyond pills and the scalpel.* New Haven and London: Yale University Press.

Plato. 1959. *The Last Days of Socrates: Euthyhro, The Apology, Crito, Phaedo.* H. Tredennick (trans.) Middlesex: Penguin Books.

Plato. 1994. *Republic.* R. Waterfield (trans.) Oxford and New York: Oxford University Press.

Pojman, L.P. (ed.) 1988. *Ethical Theory: Classical and contemporary readings.* Belmont, CA: Wadsworth.

Potts, S.G. 1988. 'Looking for the exit door: Killing and caring in modern medicine', *Houston Law Review*, 25:498-515.

Prejean, H. 1996. *Dead Man Walking: An eyewitness account of the death penalty in the United States.* London: Fount Paperbacks.

Rachels, J. 1975. 'Active and passive euthanasia', *New England Journal of Medicine*, 292(2):78-80.

Rachels, J. 1986. *The End of Life: Euthanasia and morality.* Oxford: Oxford University Press.

Rachels, J. 1989. 'More impertinent distinctions', in R.M. Baird and S.E. Rosenbaum (eds.) *Euthanasia.* Buffalo, NY: Prometheus.

Rawls, J. 1971. *A Theory of Justice.* Cambridge, MA: Harvard University Press.

Reiser, S.J. 1993. 'Science, pedagogy, and the transformation of empathy in medicine', in H.M. Spiro, M.G. McCrea Curnen, E.R. Peschel and D. St. James (eds.) *Empathy and the Practice of Medicine: Beyond pills and the scalpel.* New Haven and London: Yale University Press.

Robinson, V. 1943. *The Story of Medicine.* New York: The New Home Library.

Rosenberg, J.F. 1983. *Thinking Clearly About Death.* New Jersey: Prentice-Hall.

Ross, W.B. 1930. *The Right and the Good.* Oxford: Clarendon Press.

Rousseau, J.-J. 1909. *Rousseau's Emile or Treatise on Education.* W.H. Payne (trans.) New York: D. Appleton and Company.

Sacks, O. 1991. *A leg to stand on* (2nd edition). London: Picador Books.

Sartre J.-P. 1993. *Being and Nothingness: An essay on phenomenological ontology.* H.E. Barnes (trans.) London: Routledge.

Sauerbruch, F. and Wenke, H. 1963. *Pain: Its meaning and significance.* E. Fitzgerald (trans.) London: George Allen and Unwin.

Scarry, E. 1985. *The body in pain: The making and unmaking of the world.* Oxford and New York: Oxford University Press.

Schacht, R. 1992. *Nietzsche.* London and New York: Routledge.

Shelp, E.E. (ed.) 1985. *Virtue and Medicine: Explorations in the character of medicine.* Dordrecht, Boston and Lancaster: Reidel.

Shutte, A. 1993. *Philosophy for Africa.* Cape Town: University of Cape Town Press.

Sigerist, H.E. 1933. *Great Doctors: A biographical history of medicine.* London: George Allen and Unwin.

Silvers, A. 1998. 'Protecting the innocents from physician-assisted suicide: Disability discrimination and the duty to protect otherwise vulnerable groups', in M.P. Battin, R. Rhodes and A. Silvers (eds.) *Physician Assisted Suicide: Expanding the debate*. New York and London: Routledge.

Singer, P. 1979. *Practical Ethics*. Cambridge: Cambridge University Press.

Singer, P. 1995. *Rethinking Life and Death: The collapse of our traditional ethics.* Oxford: Oxford University Press.

Singer, P. and Kuhse, H. 1993. 'More on euthanasia: A response to Pauer-Studer', *Monist*, 76(2):158-173.

Skevington, S.M. 1995. *Psychology of Pain.* Chichester and New York: John Wiley and Sons.

Smith, A. 1976. *The Theory of Moral Sentiments.* D.D. Raphael and A.L. Macfie (eds.) Oxford: Clarendon Press.

Sophocles. 1906. *The Seven Plays in English Verse.* L. Campbell (trans.) London: Oxford University Press.

Sophocles. 1986. *Electra and Other Plays: Ajax, Electra, Women of Trachis, Philoctetes.* E.F. Watling (trans. and introduction). Middlesex: Penguin Books.

South African Law Commission (SALC). 1997. *Euthanasia and the Artificial Preservation of Life*. Discussion paper 71.

Spicker, S.F. 1977. 'Medicine's influence on ethics: Reflections on the putative role of medicine', in S.F. Spicker and H. Engelhardt (eds.) *Philosophical Medical Ethics: Its nature and significance.* Boston and Dordrecht: Reidel.

Spiro, H.M. 1993. 'What is empathy and can it be taught?', in H.M. Spiro, M.G. McCrea Curnen, E.R. Peschel and D. St. James (eds.) *Empathy and the Practice of Medicine: Beyond pills and the scalpel.* New Haven and London: Yale University Press.

Spiro, H.M., McCrea Curnen, M.G., Peschel, E.R. and St. James, D. (eds.) 1993. *Empathy and the Practice of Medicine: Beyond pills and the scalpel.* New Haven and London: Yale University Press.

Steinbock, B. 1979. *Ethics in Science and Medicine.* Pergamon Press.

Sternbach, R.A. 1974. *Pain Patients: Traits and treatment*. New York: Academic Press.

Stewart, D. 1980. *Exploring the Philosophy of Religion* (2nd edition). New Jersey: Prentice-Hall.

Strauss, S.A. 1991. *Doctor, Patient and the Law: A selection of practical issues* (3rd edition). Pretoria: JL van Schaik.

Tauber, A.I. 1999. *Confessions of a Medicine Man: An essay in popular philosophy.* Cambridge, MA: MIT Press.

Taylor, J.V. 1963. *The Primal Vision*. London: S.C.M.

Taylor, R. 1970. *Good and Evil.* Buffalo, NY: Prometheus Books.

Temkin, O. 1991. *Hippocrates in a World of Pagans and Christians.* Baltimore and London: Johns Hopkins University Press.

Tolstoy, L. 1960. *The Cossacks, The Death of Ivan Ilyich, Happy Ever After*. R. Edmonds (trans. and introduction). Middlesex: Penguin Books.

Trubo, R. 1973. *An Act of Mercy: Euthanasia today*. Los Angeles: Nash Publishing.

Van der Maas, P.J., van Delden, J.J.M. and Pijnenborg, L. 1992. *Euthanasia and Other Medical Decisions Concerning the End of Life.* New York: Elsevier.

Van der Wal, G. and Dillmann, R.J.M. 1994. 'Euthanasia in the Netherlands', *British Medical Journal*, 308:1346-1349.

Wallace, J.D. 1978. *Virtues and Vices*. Ithaca and London: Cornell University Press.

Young, R. 1976. 'Voluntary and nonvoluntary euthanasia', *Monist*, 59(2):264-283.

Zola, I. 1972. 'Medicine as an institution of social control', *Sociological Review*, 20:487-503.

# Index

References from footnotes indicated by 'n' after page reference